PERSPECTIVES IN CROSS-CULTURAL PSYCHIATRY

PERSPECTIVES IN CROSS-CULTURAL PSYCHIATRY

Edited by

ANNA M. GEORGIOPOULOS, MD
Department of Psychiatry
Massachusetts General Hospital
Boston, Massachusetts

JERROLD F. ROSENBAUM, MD
Chair of Psychiatry
Massachusetts General Hospital
Boston, Massachusetts

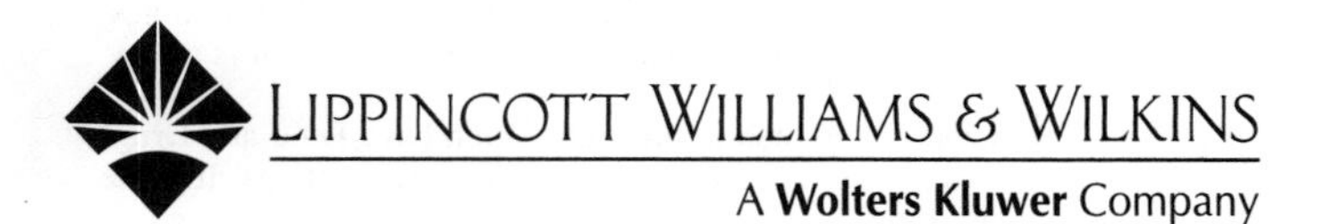

Philadelphia • Baltimore • New York • London
Buenos Aires • Hong Kong • Sydney • Tokyo

Acquisitions Editor: Charley Mitchell
Project Manager: Jennifer Jett
Cover Designer: Lou Moriconi
Compositor: Maryland Composition
Printer: R.R. Donnelley-Crawfordsville

530 Walnut Street
Philadelphia, PA 19106 USA
LWW.com

Printed in USA

Library of Congress Cataloging-in-Publication Data

Perspectives in cross-cultural psychiatry / edited by Anna M. Georgiopoulos, Jerrold F. Rosenbaum.
p. ;cm.
Includes bibliographical references and index.
ISBN 0-7817-5794-0
1. Psychiatry, Transcultural. 2. Psychotherapy—Cross-cultural studies. 3. Mental health policy. I. Georgiopoulos, Anna M. II. Rosenbaum, J. F. (Jerrold F.)
[DNLM: 1. Mental Disorders—ethnology. 2. Mental Disorders—therapy. 3. Cross-Cultural Comparison. 4. Ethnic Groups—psychology. 5. Psychiatry—methods. WM 400 P467 2005]
RC455.4.E8P476 2005
616.89—dc22

2004021744

---

10 9 8 7 6 5 4 3 2 1

Dedication

To my family, without whose support this book would not have been possible.
—AMG

To the promise of the International Division, MGH Department of Psychiatry.
—JFR

Contents

Foreword

This modestly titled volume, *Perspectives in Cross-Cultural Psychiatry*, represents a significant effort to chart cross-cultural studies as a critical domain of research, knowledge, and practice for contemporary psychiatry. Although the book provides relatively little explicit theorizing aimed at reframing what constitutes knowledge in this field, the volume as a whole stands as a challenge both to outmoded forms of cross-cultural research and to everyday assumptions of much clinical and basic science research in psychiatry today. On the one hand, there is no neat distinction in this volume between disorders common to all cultures (depression, schizophrenia, etc.) and the culture-bound disorders, forms of psychopathology assumed to be highly specific to particular societies of subcultures, viewed as exotic characteristics of distant 'Others' (even if they are occasionally found in 'our' midst) or even earlier stages of human development, as in an older cross-cultural psychiatry. The book makes universalistic assumptions. But what emerges as universal in the chapters of this volume is a deep and fundamental diversity. Individuals and groups are shown to be genetically and biologically diverse in ways that have great practical importance for mental illness and for psychiatric practice and research. But this biological diversity is shown to be interwoven with social and cultural diversity in ways that challenge any simplified assumptions about universal disease entities or culture as strange 'beliefs' that influence (or disguise) 'expression' of the underlying entities. Diversity is assumed to be much more fundamental in this volume than in standard psychiatric epistemology, thus offering a challenge to build a less parochial human science than what presently exists.

The book is organized in three sections. The first provides specific studies of the implications for psychiatric diagnosis and treatment of biological and cultural diversity. This section includes chapters that begin to show how fundamental a concept of diversity may be for psychiatry, and how wide the implications are if diversity is taken seriously. For example, human populations are biologically diverse in very specific ways, with significant implications for pharmaceutical practice. Research is beginning to show that biological differences are differentially distributed across populations. However, genetic diversity is ultimately individual, and great differences are found within ethnic and national groups and between groups; no stereotypes or simple rules of thumb about drug doses will do. Implications for research and routine practice are thus significant. But populations and individuals are also diverse in terms of trauma histories, cognitive structures, and networks of meaning, so that panic symptoms may result from quite different patterns of traumatic cognitions, triggering quite different physiological processes. Culture makes illness heterogeneous, interacting with biology to constitute different conditions. Cultural forms and local categories and nosologies also map in complex ways onto diagnostic categories, as nearly two decades of research on *ataques de nervios* now shows. Nonetheless, tendencies to stereotype, which are always present as shorthand forms of knowledge, combine with persistent forms of racism and sexism to produce systematic and routine biases in judgment. The continued tendency in the United States to overdiagnose schizophrenia among African Americans, particularly young men, is testimony to the pernicious effects of a misguided formulation of diversity. This section thus begins to sketch out where a fundamental understanding of diversity would take us.

The second section of the book focuses on the cultural and political context of psychotherapy. It is perhaps less surprising that cultural diversity is significant in this domain. However, rather than characterizing culture in terms of beliefs or cultural traits, this section begins to show how a variety of language practices, modes of self-revelation and reflection, attempts to make meaning, and understandings of hierarchy provide the very stuff of everyday clinical practice. When clinicians and patients are culturally different, practices that often seem invisible and work seamlessly suddenly break down. Misunderstandings become the source for recognition and knowledge. At the same time, as Hickling demonstrates, diversity is not politically neutral or easily overcome by cultural sensitivity or even professional translators. Diversity is rooted in colonial history, longstanding theories of race and racial difference, and violence, and postcolonial encounters, whether they take place in the psychiatric clinic or elsewhere, are heirs to that history. Neutrality, conflict, and advocacy stand in uneasy relationship in such encounters, shaping the work of psychiatry in everyday clinical practice.

The third section of the book looks explicitly to the global. Mental health has finally begun to be recognized as one of the major burdens of international public health (1), on par with infectious diseases and chronic medical conditions. This section points in two directions. On the one hand, medical care is woefully and desperately inadequate in many parts of the world for conditions for which there are now good—and inexpensive—treatments. Schizophrenia and depression are, in this way, like tuberculosis. But there are few examples of mental health programs akin to the best national tuberculosis control programs, and there is no consensus model for a 'DOTS' program for depression. Given a tremendous shortage of resources—imagine creating a mental health system for Boston with five psychiatrists, I challenge my students—the need to develop and evaluate treatment programs and implement them among low and middle income populations is an enormous challenge. On the other hand, this section points to even greater challenges. The chapters in this section demonstrate that psychopathology, whether in men, women, or children, is inseparable from large-scale, transnational social forces, producing violence and warfare, trauma and dislocation, astonishing inequalities of basic human resources and access to health care, and unprecedented movements of populations within nations and globally. Cross-culture psychiatry today can hardly be framed purely in relation to local, cultural forms, and global and national policy work may be as relevant for mental health as the development of services. Building a knowledge base and training a new generation of global mental health specialists is thus a major project for our times.

This book is as much a sketch of an agenda as a statement for where the field is. But it provides a major challenge to the field, suggesting just how parochial is much psychiatric research and publication. In this text, Becker quotes a finding that only 6% of the studies published in six major psychiatric journals derive from regions that comprise 90% of the global population. The assumption that 'universal' knowledge can result from studies of a tiny minority of the world's population—because 'basic processes' are being studied—is simply untenable. A fundamental conception of diversity in psychiatry requires a new science. This book is a contribution to that new science.

REFERENCES

1. Desjarlais R, Eisenberg L, Good B, et al. *World mental health. Problems and priorities in low-income countries.* New York: Oxford University Press, 1995.

Byron Good, PhD
Department of Social Science
Harvard Medical School
Cambridge, Massachusetts

Introduction

The importance of understanding cultural issues to the task of understanding psychiatric disorders and caring for psychiatric patients has been increasingly recognized in recent years. Appreciation for the complexity of diagnosis and treatment across cultural contexts internationally is accelerating, and growing ethnic diversity has lent special urgency to these efforts within the United States (1,2). Heeding the wisdom of these observations, the Massachusetts General Hospital (MGH) Department of Psychiatry has recently launched its first International Division to pursue work in cross-cultural psychiatry. The *Diagnostic and Statistical Manual of Mental Disorders* (DSM) now includes an appendix outlining cultural formulation and "culture-bound syndromes" that emphasizes taking into account a patient's cultural identity, cultural meanings of illness, cultural influences on the psychosocial environment and functioning of the patient as well as on the relationship between patient and clinician, and anticipated cultural effects on diagnosis and treatment (3).

As Kirmayer notes, however, our understanding of culture itself is increasingly complex: "Older notions of cultures as self-contained systems (implicit in the concept of culture-bound syndromes) have given way to a view of cultural worlds as temporary, ever-changing constructions that emerge from interactions between individuals, communities, and larger ideologies and institutional practices"(4). It is not only patients, then, but also clinicians, researchers, and larger institutions (including the field of psychiatry) that function within and take part in constituting specific cultures (4). This knowledge complicates and enriches our understanding of the processes of diagnosing and treating individual patients, of systematically studying psychiatric illness, and of working within—and in some cases to reform—existing systems of care for mental illness (5,6).

The traditions of Western psychiatry have advanced knowledge and technique through work in subfields that often remain largely distinct: biologically-oriented, symptom-focused, evidence-based research; psychotherapeutic methods; and attention to the larger psychosocial environment affecting patients. However, it is clear that a full understanding and effective treatment of the individual patient is best promoted using a combination of quantitative and qualitative methods in a biopsychosocial approach (7). Systematic research in psychiatry also will become more valid, reliable, and useful as its conceptualization and execution increasingly incorporate multiple approaches, including methods from psychiatry, anthropology, epidemiology, and related disciplines (8,9). Further, it has become evident that optimally addressing health-care disparities and promoting "cultural competence" will likely require not only skill development for clinical care providers, but also structural and organizational responses within health-care systems (2).

This book grew out of a recent lecture series on cross-cultural psychiatry held in Boston at MGH. Like the lecture series, the book seeks to highlight cutting-edge work in the field of cross-cultural psychiatry by clinicians, researchers, and leaders in mental health policy at MGH, Harvard Medical School, and beyond. This volume does not attempt the impossible task of representing work from all areas of the world. Even so, a multitude of cross-cultural settings are studied here, including people of Asian, African, and Hispanic origin living in the United States, as well as populations in Europe and developing countries. The chapters in this collection also recognize the need for psychiatrists to attend not only to identified psychiatric patients from a variety of cultural backgrounds, but also to the wider human landscape: primary care patients, postpartum women, medical interpreters, individuals and families traumatized in the course of conflict, mental health systems, government agencies, and nongovernmental/international organizations.

The methodologies drawn upon in this volume to study these groups and institutions are equally diverse, including evidence-based psychiatric approaches, psychodynamic psychiatry, biological and genetic techniques, qualitative and ethnographic methods, and public policy. Many chapters feature an integrated approach to these methods. Nonetheless, and perhaps somewhat artificially, we have divided the book into three sections to highlight the contributions of each of these perspectives to cross-cultural psychiatry. The first section includes chapters focusing on the intersection of biological and cultural diversity and the implications for psychiatric diagnosis and treatment. The second section concentrates on psychotherapeutically-oriented work. Chapters in the third section elucidate important topics in international mental health policy. Following is an overview of the chapters included in this volume.

Ng et al. begin the first section by showing that even the most seemingly "universal" aspect of psychiatric care—that of biologically-based therapies—can be sharply affected by ethnicity and culture. They describe the impact of genetic polymorphisms distributed unevenly across world populations on the dosing and side effects of psychopharmacologic agents and on therapeutic response. They also note that significant environmental effects on gene expression, including diet and tobacco exposure, often vary by ethnic group and that nonbiological cultural factors can play a critical role in the effectiveness of psychopharmacologic treatment. Given the real risk of clinicians misattributing genetically-based variability in drug response to personal or cultural factors (assuming, for example, that a Somali CYP-2D6 ultrarapid metabolizer is noncompliant with medications) and of researchers neglecting to take ethnic differences into account in psychopharmacology studies, this burgeoning area of study is of critical importance.

Yeung and Kam examine the explanatory models of illness in Chinese-speaking patients attending a primary care clinic in Boston who meet criteria for major depression. Their data provides a suggestive response to the controversial question of "somatization" frequently cited in Asian populations. They note that although their presenting complaints are rarely psychologically framed, Chinese American patients readily endorse depressive symptoms on standardized instruments and are often amenable to treatment for depression. Understanding the cultural context can help increase recognition of symptoms, but can also force clinicians to skillfully confront the clash of explanatory models, recognize the potential for stigma, and consider treatment models, such as integration of mental health into primary care settings, that are likely to improve outcomes.

Hinton et al. describe a model of panic among Southeast Asian refugees to the United States, focusing on Cambodians. Their model is informed by both cognitive-behavioral and fear network theory, but also by a subtle understanding of Southeast Asian cultures and history, and the experiences of conflict, trauma, and displacement. Their careful exegesis of the application of this model in work with Cambodian refugees fosters recognition of culturally-specific panic variants that appear amenable to medications and to a culturally-adapted cognitive-behavioral therapy. In addition, this work advances our theoretical understanding of how symptoms of panic and PTSD may interact in traumatized populations more generally, providing a testable template with potential for fruitful application to other groups.

Similarly, Lewis-Fernández et al. combine an ethnographic understanding of Caribbean Latino communities with strong evidence-based research to elucidate the phenomenon of *ataque de nervios.* They note that this syndrome can serve as an idiom of distress ranging from a normative response to crisis to a marker of psychopathology sometimes overlapping with DSM-IV diagnostic categories, including panic attacks, dissociative disorders, and PTSD. They describe evaluation of *ataques* using the DSM-IV cultural formulation model and suggest a treatment approach that integrates psychotherapy, social activism, and where indicated, psychopharmacology. Their nuanced presentation of *ataque de nervios* will be invaluable to clinicians working with these populations, but also serves as a model for cross-cultural research that forces us to carefully reevaluate psychiatric nosology.

The growth of cross-cultural psychiatry has been accompanied by a backlash against the overgeneralization, stereotyping, and false sense of knowing about individual patients that can result from descriptions of cultures as homogeneous entities (8). Although addressing each patient as an individual is critical (10), there is also some risk in not examining broader cultural themes when training psychiatrists in cultural competence (2). This can leave clinicians with a lack of hypotheses to explore in their interactions with patients from an unfamiliar culture; the ensuing mutual discomfort may damage the treatment alliance. Mischoulon reminds us that it is possible to fruitfully discuss an ethnic group that is large and heterogeneous in order to broaden clinicians' conceptual frameworks of diagnosis and treatment. His overview of working with Hispanic psychiatric patients includes information about culture bound syndromes, ethnopsychopharmacology and key alternative medications, and cultural issues that may affect the relationship with a psychiatrist.

Combining a biologically well-defined event with highly culturally variable manifestations of social role change, childbirth provides a unique opportunity for cross-cultural study. Georgiopoulos et al. review cross-cultural data on postpartum mood disturbance to learn what cross-cultural epidemiology, varying patterns of distress, and the ameliorative effects of social support can teach us about the nature of this disorder. Although postpartum distress may not be universally experienced or recognized as a mental disorder, postpartum illness consistent with the biomedical nosologic category of postpartum depression appears to be globally widespread. Research to date has been limited by methodologic inconsistencies, and the importance of integrated ethnographic and quantitative approaches to future research efforts in prevention and treatment is critical in this arena.

Bipolar disorder is often underrecognized in African Americans and access to effective care can be limited. Lawson reviews current information about bipolar disorder in this population, noting that African Americans are often misdiagnosed with unipolar depression or schizophrenia; consequences include inappropriate treatments, such as overreliance on conventional antipsychotics, depot medications, and tricyclic antidepressants. Lawson explores contributing factors, including stereotyping or failure to elicit symptoms by clinicians, differences in symptom expression and approaches to treatment by patients, and selection bias in research. The research and educational efforts he suggests could decrease the burden of illness for African Americans with bipolar illness, while serving as a model for investigation of health disparities more generally.

The second section of the book is devoted to psychotherapeutic approaches to cross-cultural psychiatry. Roland demonstrates how the Western psychoanalytic model can be productively applied to treatment with Asian and Asian American patients, noting how culture and social change affect the psyche, and conceptualizing psychoanalysis in this context as a form of depth ethnography. He discusses the adaptations that can help this work proceed more smoothly, noting that psychopathology, transference, and countertransference often emerge in ways unaccustomed to Western-raised and trained therapists, in part due to differences in self-conceptualization. Noting how the self is constituted in these societies also helps us understand what is societally constructed about Western concepts of psychic health.

In their moving study of the transgenerational transmission of trauma in Cambodian families living in the United States, Rubin and Rhodes use the qualitative method of focused ethnography with participant observation to examine the importance of family cultures in the perpetuation of distress. Using a narrative approach, Rubin and Rhodes explore the meaning of trauma experience in the context of parenting and the consequences for children; their parents' experiences can remain powerfully unspeakable or can emerge in a way that may secondarily traumatize them. This chapter, set alongside the work of Hinton et al., Lopes Cardozo and Fricchione, and McDonald et al. in this volume, constitutes a powerful argument for the importance of outreach and culturally-appropriate treatment for individual Cambodian refugees, but also for the need and complexity of creating a plan for recovery for the broader community.

Language is central to cultural and personal identity. Drawing on her experience running debriefing and process groups for interpreters at MGH, O'Neill explores issues that arise when treating patients in psychotherapeutic and medical settings who are not native English speakers. While emphasizing the importance of skilled medical interpretation, she addresses the group dynamics and other challenges that may arise in the encounter among patient, clinician, and interpreter. Clinicians have much to learn from interpreters who can act as culture brokers, while a familiarity with group process can help clinicians and interpreters handle difficult situations more effectively. Understanding the psychodynamic and cross-cultural phenomena that can develop when patient and clinician do not share a mother tongue is key to optimizing patient care.

Drawing on psychoanalysis, social anthropology, and social and cultural psychiatry and psychology, Stylianidis et al. examine attempts to dismantle the asylum culture in a children's psychiatric hospital in Greece. Using participant observation and discourse analysis, the authors decipher psychodynamic and social processes arising during the process of deinstitutionalization. Placed within the broader context of systems of care and politics, their work demonstrates how particular cultural influences become manifest through such phenomena as prejudice, bureaucracy, and the institution. The chapter also reveals how ethnographic principles can be usefully applied to the culture of psychiatry itself, creating movement toward reform.

Promoting the mental health of people of African descent worldwide requires addressing the psychology of centuries of racism and colonialism. Originally presented at MGH as part of an international conference on psychiatric issues in the African diaspora, Hickling's chapter confronts this legacy using the method of psychohistoriography. Originally developed in a Jamaican mental hospital, the technique was designed to elicit reality-based insight in a group setting to promote productivity and change. His psychohistoriographic analysis, set in a postcolonial frame, argues the existence of a collective delusion incorporating beliefs in the subhumanity of people of color and the right to European ownership of the world. Hickling identifies key historical periods—emancipation, national independence, the end of apartheid—in which this "European psychosis" has been modified by the struggles of African people for self-determination. His provocative, multidisciplinary approach suggests that improving mental health in the African diaspora will require developing not only better mental health services, but also developing the psychological processes necessary to counter racism and colonialism, navigate capitalism, and promote African unity.

The final section of the book focuses on international mental health policy. Mental illness has become increasingly recognized in the public health community as a costly problem with severe impacts on populations around the world. Fricchione delineates challenges in settings of poor resource availability and political instability, focusing particular attention on the case of Ethiopia, with only nine psychiatrists for a population of 70 million. Describing models for providing mental health services in primary care settings in the developing world, he emphasizes the need for targeted intervention studies. The innovative strategies he highlights, including the WHO Mental Health Global Action Program and the newly-created Division of International Psychiatry at MGH, represent important steps toward reducing the global burden of disease due to mental illness.

Despite the special vulnerabilities of young people, minimal resources are dedicated to them in many countries. Belfer reviews the mental health status of children worldwide, addressing the developmental effects of malnutrition, violence, exploitation, and HIV/AIDS. He explores our limited knowledge of the global epidemiology of psychiatric disorders in children and how cultural factors complicate the assessment of psychopathology. Recognizing the need for effective mental health policy for children, he discusses challenges in developing prevention and treatment services. Calling for accelerated research in such areas as epidemiology, child-rearing, and service delivery, Belfer argues for careful attention to the needs of children worldwide who cannot advocate for themselves.

A wide range of mental health effects is associated with violence worldwide, from exhaustion, hopelessness, or a drive for revenge, to severe psychiatric illness. Lopes Cardozo and Fricchione review how our understanding of the effects of mental trauma among combatants and civilians has evolved, including important data about psychiatric morbidity and disability emerging from recent studies of refugee populations in Asia, Africa, and Europe. They address the role of psychological factors in the perpetuation of cycles of violence and suggest approaches to the challenging task of planning psychosocial interventions to address the intersecting burdens of violence and mental illness.

Noting the critical lack of adequate research-generated data on mental illness in the developing world, Becker provides perceptive recommendations for fostering the development of both local and global research cultures. The cross-cultural applicability of research approaches encouraged by major psychiatric journals and sources of research funding within the Western model of evidence-based medicine has not been demonstrated. Becker notes the need for community-based research in the developing world, addressing local agendas and producing findings with contextual relevance. She describes innovative approaches for attracting and training researchers, inviting the participation of local populations, and promoting the development of sustained, bidirectional collaborations between researchers in developing and Western countries.

Project 1 Billion represents a landmark collaborative effort among scientists, international agencies, and national health authorities in countries affected by violence. Drawing on the experience of the Harvard Program in Refugee Trauma, McDonald et al. describe the limitations of current models of providing care in postconflict societies and propose a comprehensive action plan for mental health recovery. The Project 1 Billion action plan addresses the interrelated domains of policymaking, financing, evidence-based care, multidisciplinary mental health education, coordination of international agencies, economic development, and human rights. This interdisciplinary approach integrates scientific knowledge with political, financial, and field realities, raising the field to a new level of sophistication. Project 1 Billion's mental health action plan should result in wiser use of limited human and capital resources as well as recognition of mental health as a linchpin of recovery for devastated societies.

Lewis-Fernandez and Kleinman emphasize that culture is "located not in the minds of individuals, but between people"(8). The chapters in this volume make clear that our field can no longer afford a parochial approach to clinical care or research, neither in the subjects and goals of study, nor in the methods used. Despite the abundance of perspectives presented, each of these chapters in its own way transgresses traditional boundaries that delineate psychiatric dogma, that separate subfields within psychiatry, and that prevent interaction between psychiatry and other disciplines such as anthropology, epidemiology, and sociology, and between academia and institutions with other forms of political and economic power. The great synergy that can be created by using integrative approaches in diverse populations is evident here. It is our hope that this book will help to foster a new culture of collaboration to promote global mental health.

REFERENCES

1. *Mental Health: Culture, Race, Ethnicity—A Supplement to Mental Health: A Report of the Surgeon General*. Rockville, MD: US Department of Health and Human Services, Substance Abuse and Mental Health Services Administration, Center for Mental Health Services, 2001.
2. Betancourt JR, Green AR, Carrillo JE, et al. Defining cultural competence: a practical framework for addressing racial/ethnic disparities in health and health care. *Public Health Rep* 2003;118:293–302.
3. American Psychiatric Association. *Diagnostic and statistical manual of mental disorders. 4th edition, text revision.* Washington, DC: American Psychiatric Association, 2000.
4. Kirmayer LJ. Cultural variations in the clinical presentation of depression and anxiety: implications for diagnosis and treatment. *J Clin Psychiatry* 2001;62 [Suppl 13]:22–28.
5. Kleinman A. *The illness narratives: suffering, healing, and the human condition.* New York: Basic Books, 1988.
6. Kleinman A. *Rethinking psychiatry: from cultural category to personal experience.* New York: Free Press, 1988.
7. Jellinek MS, McDermott JF. Formulation: putting the diagnosis into a therapeutic context and treatment plan. *J Am Acad Child Adolesc Psychiatry* 2004;43: 913–916.
8. Lewis-Fernandez R, Kleinman A. Cultural psychiatry: theoretical, clinical, and research issues. *Psychiatr Clin North Am* 1995;18:433–449.
9. Oates MR, Cox JL, Neema S, et al. Postnatal depression across countries and cultures: a qualitative study. *Br J Psychiatry* 2004;184[Suppl 13]:10–16.
10. Tseng W. Culture and psychotherapy: an overview. In: Tseng W, Streltzer J, eds. *Culture and psychotherapy: a guide to clinical practice.* Washington, DC: American Psychiatric Press, 2001:3–12.

Anna M. Georgiopoulos
Jerrold F. Rosenbaum

Contributing Authors

Anne E. Becker, MD, PhD *Associate Professor of Medical Anthropology, Assistant Professor of Psychiatry, Department of Social Medicine, Harvard Medical School, Department of Psychiatry, Massachusetts General Hospital, 15 Parkman Street, WAC 816, Boston, Massachusetts 02114*

Myron L. Belfer, MD, MPA *Professor of Psychiatry, Department of Social Medicine, Harvard Medical School, Senior Associate in Psychiatry, Boston Children's Hospital, 641 Huntington Avenue, Boston, Massachusetts 02115, Senior Adviser, Child and Adolescent Mental Health, World Health Organization, Geneva, Switzerland*

Robina Bhasin *Research Assistant, Harvard Program in Refugee Trauma, 22 Putnam Avenue, Cambridge, Massachusetts 02139*

Panayiotis Chondros, MS *Scientific Association for Regional Development and Mental Health (EPAPSY), Grammou 61–63, 15124 Maroussi, Athens, Greece*

Naelys Díaz, MSW *PhD Candidate, Fordham University, Graduate School of Social Service, 1780 Broadway, Suite 900, New York, New York 10019*

Gregory L. Fricchione, MD *Associate Chief of Psychiatry, Director, Division of International Psychiatry, Massachusetts General Hospital, 55 Fruit Street, Warren 6, Boston, Massachusetts 02114*

Anna M. Georgiopoulos, MD *Department of Psychiatry, Massachusetts General Hospital, 15 Parkman Street, WAC 725, Boston, MA 02114*

Peter J. Guarnaccia, PhD *Professor and Medical Anthropologist, Institute for Health, Health Care Policy and Aging Research, Rutgers, The State University of New Jersey, 30 College Avenue, New Brunswick, New Jersey 08901*

Frederick W. Hickling, DM, MRCPsych (UK) *Professor of Psychiatry, Department of Community Health and Psychiatry, University of the West Indies, Mona, Kingston 7, Jamaica, West Indies*

Devon E. Hinton, MD, PhD *Department of Psychiatry, Massachusetts General Hospital, 15 Parkman Street, WAC 815, Boston, Massachusetts 02114*

Raymond Kam, MD, MPH *Children's Hospital, 300 Longwood Avenue, Fegan 8, Boston, Massachusetts 02115*

William B. Lawson, MD, PhD, FAPA *Chairman, Department of Psychiatry, Howard University Hospital 5B03, 2041 Georgia Avenue NW, Washington DC 20060*

Roberto Lewis-Fernández, MD *Director, Hispanic Treatment Program, New York State Psychiatric Institute, Lecturer, Department of Social Medicine, Harvard Medical School, Associate Professor, Department of Psychiatry, Columbia College of Physicians & Surgeons, 1051 Riverside Drive, Room 3200, Unit 69, New York, NY 10032*

Keh-Ming Lin, MD, MPH *National Health Research Institutes, Division of Mental Health and Drug Abuse Research, 3F, 109, Ming-Chuan E. Rd., Sec. 6, Taipei 114, Taiwan, R.O.C.*

Dana Lizardi, PhD *Fordham University, Graduate School of Social Service, 1780 Broadway, Suite 900, New York, New York 10019*

Barbara Lopes Cardozo, MD, MPH *National Center for Environmental Health, International Emergency and Refugee Health Branch, Centers for Disease Control and Prevention, 1825 Century Center Boulevard, Room 3005, Atlanta, Georgia 30345*

Laura S. McDonald, MALD *Research Associate, Harvard Program in Refugee Trauma, 22 Putnam Avenue, Cambridge, Massachusetts 02139*

David Mischoulon, MD, PhD *Assistant Professor of Psychiatry, Harvard Medical School, Staff Psychiatrist, Depression Clinical and Research Program, Massachusetts General Hospital, 15 Parkman Street, WAC 812, Boston, Massachusetts 02114*

Richard F. Mollica, MD, MAR *Professor of Psychiatry, Harvard Medical School, Director, Harvard Program in Refugee Trauma, 22 Putnam Avenue, Cambridge, Massachusetts 02139*

Joann Ng, MD *Department of Psychiatry, Research Center on the Psychobiology of Ethnicity, Harbor-UCLA Medical Center, 1124 West Carson Street, B-4 South, Torrance, California 90502*

Siobhan M. O'Neill, MD *Department of Psychiatry, Massachusetts General Hospital, 15 Parkman Street, WAC 812, Boston, Massachusetts 02114*

Sapana Patel, PhD *Research Fellow, New York State Psychiatric Institute and Department of Psychiatry, Columbia College of Physicians & Surgeons, 1051 Riverside Drive, Unit 69, New York, New York 10032*

Vuth Pich *Social Worker, Southeast Asian Clinic, Arbour Counseling Services, 10 Bridge Street, The Simpson Block, Lowell, Massachusetts 01852*

Mark H. Pollack, MD *Associate Professor of Psychiatry, Harvard Medical School, Director Anxiety and Traumatic Stress Disorders Program, Department of Psychiatry, Massachusetts General Hospital, 15 Parkman Street, WAC 815, Boston, Massachusetts 02114*

Lorna Rhodes, PhD *Professor, Department of Anthropology, University of Washington, Seattle, Washington 98195*

Alan Roland, PhD *National Psychological Association for Psychoanalysis, 274 West 11 Street, New York, New York 10014*

Jerrold F. Rosenbaum, MD *Chair of Psychiatry, Massachusetts General Hospital, 15 Parkman Street, WAC 812, Boston, Massachusetts 02114*

Audrey Rubin, MD *Clinical Assistant Professor, Department of Child and Adolescent Psychiatry, Boston University School of Medicine, 715 Albany Street, Boston, Massachusetts 02118*

Amy B. Saltzman *Department of Anthropology, Princeton University, Princeton, NJ 08544*

Michael Smith, MD *Associate Professor of Psychiatry, Research Center on the Psychobiology of Ethnicity, Harbor-UCLA Medical Center, 1124 West Carson Street, B-4 South, Torrance, California 90502*

Stelios Stylianidis, MD, PhD *Director, Children's Psychiatric Hospital of Attica, Scientific Association for Regional Development and Mental Health (EPAPSY), Grammou 61–63, 15124 Maroussi, Athens, Greece*

M-G Lily Stylianoudi, JD, PhD *Social and Legal Anthropologist, Research Professor, Director of the Research Center for Greek Society, Academy of Athens, Solonos 84, 10680 Athens, Greece*

Albert Yeung, MD, ScD *Depression Clinical and Research Program, Massachusetts General Hospital, 50 Staniford Street, Suite 401, Boston, Massachusetts 02114*

Acknowledgments

We would like to thank all those who have helped to bring this project to fruition. We are grateful to the many colleagues from MGH and beyond who have generously shared their work in this volume and the lecture series that preceded it. Along with many others, Devon Hinton, Ruta Nonacs, Maurizio Fava, Roy Perlis, David Mischoulon, Albert Yeung, Greg Fricchione, Peter Guarnaccia, Lawrence Kirmayer, and Chester Pierce each provided useful suggestions and encouragement at critical steps along the way. Special thanks are due to Anne Becker for her guidance throughout the process. We would also like to express appreciation for the expert efforts of Charlie Mitchell, Jennifer Jett, and others at Lippincott Williams & Wilkins to facilitate publication of this volume.

SECTION I

Biological and Cultural Diversity: Implications for Psychiatric Diagnosis and Treatment

1

Psychopharmacotherapy in the Age of Accelerating Diversity

[*]Joann Ng, [†]Keh-Ming Lin, and [*]Michael Smith

[*]Department of Psychiatry, Harbor-UCLA Medical Center, Torrance, California 90502 and [†]National Health Research Institutes, Division of Mental Health and Drug Abuse Research, Taiwan ROC

I. INTRODUCTION

The use of psychiatric medication has transcended geographic, cultural, and ethnic boundaries during the past several decades. Within a few years of their discovery, modern psychotropics have achieved worldwide acceptance as the mainstay for the treatment of the mentally ill (1). This notwithstanding, until most recently, clinicians and researchers have paid little attention to potential influences of ethnic and cultural factors on pharmacotherapeutic responses. With a few prominent exceptions, practically all psychiatric medications have been developed and tested in North America and Western Europe, and often on "young, white males." In addition, because these research efforts usually aim at defining what is "typical," variations in responses are often regarded as "noise" and consequently ignored. Therefore, although substantial differences in psychotropic responses have been repeatedly observed and documented in the literature, such information has not been widely disseminated, and our knowledge in this regard is still sparse and unsystematic. Treatment decisions are not individualized; choice of medication and dosing routines are largely based on "trial and error" practices rather than on rational principles.

For a number of reasons, such a "one dose fits all" approach is increasingly problematic. All over the world, communities have become increasingly multiethnic and multicultural, and clinicians no longer have the luxury of neglecting these issues. This is clearly reflected in the demographic trends in this country as well as worldwide. The United States 2000 census shows that approximately 30% of the country's population comes from "ethnic minority" backgrounds; 13% are Hispanics, 12% African Americans, 4% Asians, and 1% American Indians. By 2050, there will no

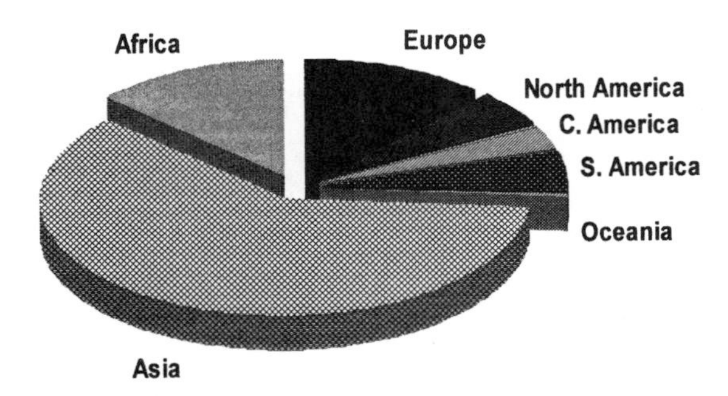

FIG. 1-1. The population of the world.

longer be a majority group in this country, with a projected 49% white population, 25% Hispanic, 13% African American, 11% Asian, and 2% American Indian. In California, this is already the case: the population is 43% white, 35% Hispanic, 11% Asian, 10% African American, and 1% American Indian. Indeed, as shown in Figure 1-1, what we are used to labeling as the "majority"—those classified as whites—represents a relatively small fraction (roughly 25%) of the human race populating the world. Yet what we believe to be true in psychiatry and human behavior has been largely based on experience, observations, and research focusing only on this relatively small segment of the world's population. Too often, we tend to implicitly assume that information thus derived should apply to all peoples. That such an assumption could lead to salutary outcomes attests to the profound universality in human behavior and psychobiological processes. Nevertheless, the prudent and responsible clinician should be mindful of the knowledge gaps, and be cognizant of patients' ethnic and cultural backgrounds as potentially potent factors in determining their responses to psychiatric interventions, including psychopharmacological treatments.

II. RACE, ETHNICITY, AND CULTURE

Similar to most concepts of fundamental importance (e.g., *self, society, life, consciousness*), the meaning of terms such as *culture, ethnicity,* and *race* are seemingly self-evident yet difficult to define. Traditionally, culture represents attributes that are learned and passed down from generation to generation, whereas race and ethnicity are regarded as more biologically and genetically based (1). Among the three, race may be the most difficult and most controversial. Based on skin color and presumed ancestral origin, the concept of race has long been entwined with biological determinism, and tainted with a long history of discrimination, slavery, and even genocide (2). In contrast, the concept of ethnicity is not primarily tied to any specific physical characteristics, but according to McGoldrick (3) "refers to a common ancestry through which individuals have evolved shared values and customs. It is deeply tied to the family, through which it is transmitted." Finally, as noted by Brislin (4), culture is most commonly defined as "patterns, explicit and implicit, of and for behavior acquired and transmitted by symbols, constituting the distinctive achievements of human groups...; culture systems may, on the one hand, be considered as products of action, on the other as conditioning elements of further action."

It is important to keep in mind the fluidity of these concepts. Racial/ethnic classifications are inherently arbitrary at some level (e.g., How similar or different are Southern and Northern Chinese? Are Somalians and Nigerians both African blacks? Should Americans of Mexican and Puerto Rican backgrounds be grouped together, or treated as separate groups?). The ambiguity inherent in these boundaries is further complicated by the intermixing of people over generations. Similarly, the concept of culture cannot be easily defined. Cultural traditions are not static, even though there is an implicit sense of continuity when one speaks of culture. Cultural traditions change constantly, not only due to the evolving nature of people's thoughts and aspirations, as well as their relationship with the environment, but also to extensive cultural exchanges that have occurred throughout the millennia, and have been taking place at an accelerating pace in recent decades. It is thus of utmost importance to avoid an overly rigid interpretation of findings in relation to these categories, in order to minimize stereotyping and stigmatization.

III. INDIVIDUAL AND ETHNIC VARIATIONS IN DRUG RESPONSE

Keeping the previously stated caveats in mind, it is nevertheless important to point out at the outset that, no matter how these concepts are defined, ethnicity and culture powerfully determine individuals' pharmacological responses. As shown in Figure 1-2, these responses are shaped simultaneously by genetic and environmental factors.

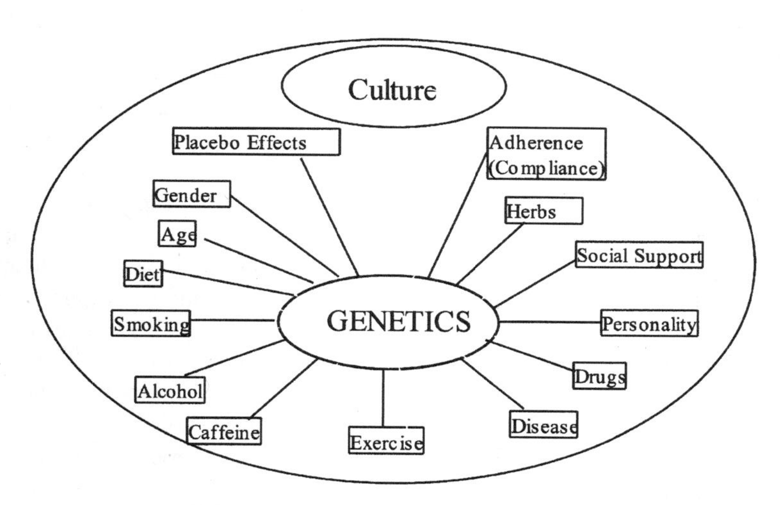

FIG. 1-2. Factors affecting drug response.

On the genetic side, genetic polymorphisms with functional significance have been identified in most genes encoding drug-metabolizing enzymes as well as in those encoding the putative targets of pharmaceutical agents, such as neurotransmitter receptors and transporters. Patterns of these genetic polymorphisms often vary substantially across ethnic groups, resulting in variations in the activities of proteins controlling both the fate and the effects of pharmacotherapeutic agents. In addition, the expression of these genes is often significantly modified by a large number of environmental factors, including diet and exposure to various substances like tobacco and herbal preparations.

Of even greater importance, the success of any therapy, including pharmacotherapy, depends on the relationship between patient and therapist. The nature and quality of the interaction between the clinician and the patient, flavored by both of their cultural backgrounds, values, attitudes, and expectations, serve as the backdrop against which drugs work, or fail to work. Attention to and successful management of transference and counter-transference are key to the success of not only psychotherapy, but also pharmacotherapy. The importance of culture in this regard cannot be disregarded.

The literature documenting cultural and ethnic influence on pharmacological responses has been reviewed and commented on by various authors in recent years (1,5), and will not be discussed in great detail here. However, it is important to point out that these data came from reports derived from sources and studies using divergent designs, including surveys of drug utilization and dosing patterns, case reports, chart reviews, pharmacokinetics/pharmacodynamics, and prospective treatment studies. Findings from these studies convincingly demonstrate that significant cross-ethnic drug-response variations exist in practically all classes of medications, especially with regard to psychotropic, cardiovascular, and antineoplastic medications. For example, a series of studies demonstrated that, in comparison with their white counterparts, Asians are often successfully treated with lower dosages of haloperidol and other neuroleptics in the inpatient hospital setting (6). When given comparable doses of medication, Asian schizophrenic patients (7) and Asian normal volunteers (8) exhibited plasma haloperidol concentrations that were approximately 50% greater than those of their white counterparts.

At the same time, the study also showed a greater prolactin response to haloperidol in Asians than in whites. When receiving comparable doses of intramuscular haloperidol, Asian patients had higher plasma prolactin concentrations than their white counterparts (8). This difference remained statistically significant after controlling for ethnic variations in plasma haloperidol concentrations. In a subsequent clinical treatment study (9), Asian schizophrenic patients responded optimally to significantly lower plasma haloperidol concentrations when compared with their white counterparts. This finding was replicated by Jibiki et al. (10), who demonstrated that their Japanese schizophrenic patients responded to haloperidol with a therapeutic range between 0.8 and 2.3 ng/mL. Together, these data suggest that both pharmacokinetic and pharmacodynamic mechanisms are responsible for previous observations

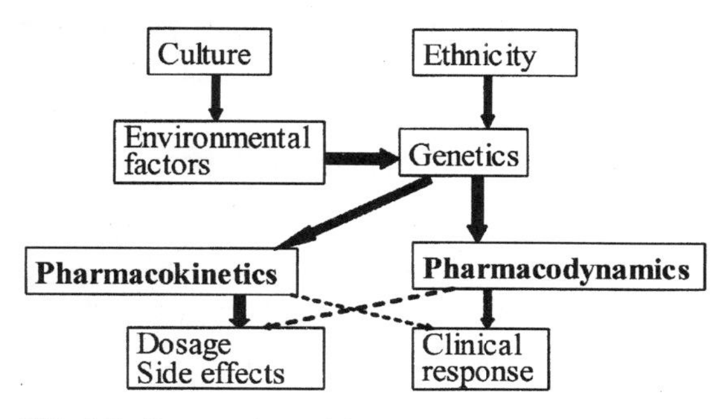

FIG. 1-3. Factors determining pharmacological response.

of Asians requiring lower doses of neuroleptics for similar therapeutic responses (Fig. 1-3).

The importance of pharmacodynamics in determining ethnic variation in drug responses is further demonstrated in the following two examples. First, studies in Asia show that the optimum range of lithium dosing is two thirds of that used in most Western countries. For example, Yang (11) studied 101 Taiwanese bipolar patients who were treated over a 2-year period with clinically determined doses of lithium. He found that the plasma lithium level of the majority of good responders ranged between 0.5 and 0.79 mEq/L, compared to the 0.8–1.2 mEq/L therapeutic range that is commonly reported in literature from Europe and North America. Second, the dose of propranolol prescribed in the United States has long been known to be three to four times higher than that prescribed in Asia. In a cross-ethnic pharmacokinetic/pharmacodynamic study, Zhou et al. (12) showed no significant pharmacokinetic differences between Chinese and white normal volunteers treated with a test dose of propranolol. However, Chinese subjects required between one fifth and one tenth of the dose and plasma concentration of propranolol to achieve a 10% decrease in heart rate and blood pressure as compared to those needed by their white counterparts.

IV. DRUG-METABOLIZING ENZYMES

A limited number of enzymes are involved in the biotransformation of all drugs, including psychotropics. Among the four factors (absorption, distribution, metabolism, and excretion) that together determine the fate and disposition of most drugs, variability in the process of metabolism is most substantial and usually is the reason for interindividual and cross-ethnic variation in drug responses (13). As the human genome project rapidly advances, the role of genetic polymorphism in drug metabolism is becoming an important adjunct for rational drug therapy, and for the explanation of drug toxicity and interactions.

Most drugs are metabolized via two phases: Phase I, commonly mediated by one or more of the cytochrome P-450 enzymes (CYPs), leads to the oxidation of the

	CYP1A2	CYP2D6	CYP3A4
Haloperidol	++	++	--
Phenothiazines	+	++	--
Clozapine	++	+	++
Olanzapine	+++	++	--
Risperidone	--	+++	+
Quetiapine	--	--	+++
Ziprasidone	--	--	+++
Aripiprazole	-	++	++

FIG. 1-4. Cytochrome P450 enzymes and neuroleptics.

substrate; Phase II involves conjugation, and is usually mediated by one of the transferases. There is clear evidence of interindividual and interethnic variation in the activity of the enzymes in both phases (5,14). Because far more information is currently available in regard to the CYPs than the Phase II enzymes, and because the CYPs appear to control the rate-limiting steps in the metabolism of most psychotropics, the following discussion will focus mainly on the CYP 450 enzymes.

With very few exceptions (e.g., lithium does not require biotransformation; lorazepam and oxazepam are directly conjugated without first going through oxidation), the pharmacokinetics of practically all psychotropics are dependent on one or more of the CYPs. The activities of these cytochrome enzymes significantly influence the tissue concentrations, dose requirement, and side-effect profiles of their substrates.

Figure 1-4 includes a list of major CYPs that are responsible for the Phase I metabolism of commonly used antipsychotics. Figure 1-5 lists the cytochrome enzymes primarily involved in metabolizing the common antidepressants. Most psychotropics are metabolized by one or more of the following four cytochrome enzymes: CYP2D6, CYP3A4, CYP1A2, and CYP2C19. CYP2D6 is not easily induced, but rather is easily inhibited. CYP3A4 and CYP1A2 are highly inducible.

V. GENETIC POLYMORPHISMS IN THE CYP450 METABOLIZING ENZYMES

Functionally significant genetic polymorphisms exist in most of the cytochrome enzymes (14), leading to extremely large variations in the activity of these enzymes in any given population. CYP2D6 represents the most dramatic example, with more than 50 mutations that inactivate, impair or accelerate its function (15). Most of these mutant alleles are to a large extent ethnically specific. For example, *CYP2D6*-4(CYP2D6)*, which leads to the production of defective proteins, is found in approxi-

	CYP1A2	CYP2C19	CYP2D6	CYP3A4
TCA's (tertiary)	++	+	++	++
TCA's (secondary	-	-	++	+
Fluoxetine	+	++	+++	++
Paroxetine	+	-	+++	+
Sertraline	+	++	+	++
Mirtazapine	+	-	+	+
Nefazodone	+	-	+	+++
Venlafaxine	+	+	+	+
Bupropion	+	+	+	-
Fluvoxamine	+++	++	+	-
Citalopram	=	++	-	++

FIG. 1-5. Cytochrome P450 enzymes and antidepressants.

mately 25% of whites, but is rarely identified in other ethnic groups. This mutation is mainly responsible for the high rate of poor metabolizers (PM) in whites (5–9%), who are expected to be inefficient in metabolizing CYP2D6 substrates, such as risperidone and paroxetine (Fig. 1-5). Instead of *CYP2D6*4,* high frequencies of *CYP2D6*17* (16–18) and *CYP2D6*10* (19–21) were found among those of African and Asian origins, respectively. Both of these alleles are associated with lower enzyme activities and slower metabolism of CYP2D6 substrates (Fig. 1-5). "Slow" metabolizers are likely to develop higher plasma concentrations and require lower therapeutic doses. The higher frequency of alleles that encode less effective CYP2D6 in Africans and Asians may explain the lower therapeutic dose ranges of neuroleptics and antidepressants observed in Asians and lower doses of tricyclic antidepressants needed in African Americans (14). Interestingly, our recent study showed that Mexican Americans had very low rates of any of these "impairing" mutations (22), leading to significantly faster overall CYP2D6 activity in subjects with this ethnic background.

CYP2D6 also is unique in that the gene often is duplicated or multiplied (up to 13 copies). Those possessing these duplicated or multiple genes have proportionally more enzymes and faster enzyme activity, and are termed "ultra-rapid" metabolizers (UM). This is found in 1% of Swedish, 5% of Spaniards (white Americans are in between these two figures), 19% of Arabs, and 29% of Ethiopians. UM patients are likely to fail to respond to usual doses of medications metabolized by CYP2D6, since they typically will fail to achieve therapeutic levels unless treated with extremely high doses of the same drugs. There have been reports of UM patients being regarded as noncompliant because they did not show any evidence of drug effect while given standard doses of medications (23). This may be a particularly important issue for Ethiopians because one third of Ethiopians genotyped were UMs, and therefore possibly needed higher doses of medicines whose biotransformation is mediated by CYP2D6, such as risperidone and paroxetine, in order to achieve therapeutic response.

The measurement of CYP2D6 activity, as well as the determination of CYP2D6, may be of particular relevance for the care of geriatric patients, for whom it is more crucial to accurately gauge therapeutic dose range and to avoid drug toxicity. CYP2D6 genotyping will serve to identify patients with heightened likelihood for developing side effects when treated with medication dependent on CYP2D6 for metabolism. In addition, the measurement of CYP2D6 activity may also be indicated in this population, because they often are treated with multiple drugs, some of which (e.g., paroxetine and fluoxetine) are likely to inhibit the enzyme to the extent that a "phenocopy" is created, converting an ''extensive metabolizer'' (EM), with previously ''normal'' ability to metabolize the drug, into a PM). When compounded by other factors, such as impairment in hepatic and renal clearance (24), the consequence of such drug–drug and drug–gene interactions could be disastrous.

CYP2C19 represents another dramatic example of the existence of both cross-ethnic and interindividual variations in drug metabolism. This enzyme is involved in the metabolism of commonly used psychotropics such as diazepam and tertiary tricyclic antidepressants, as well as one of the new antidepressants, citalopram. Using S-mephenytoin as the probe, earlier studies demonstrated that up to 20% of East Asians (Chinese, Japanese, and Koreans) are PMs, which is true only in 3% to 5% of whites. After the gene for the enzyme had been identified and sequenced, it became clear that such enzyme deficiency is mostly caused by two unique mutations, *CYP2C19*2* and *CYP2C19*3*. Whereas the *2 mutation can be found in all ethnic groups, the *3 mutation appears to be specific to those with Eastern Asian origins. The presence of *3, together with a higher rate of *2, are responsible for the higher rate of PMs among Asians. This explains why Asians often have increased sensitivity to drugs such as diazepam and other substrates of CYP2C19 (25,26).

VI. DIET AND ITS EFFECT ON P450 ENZYMES

Dietary habits affect pharmacokinetics because they change the body's ability to absorb, distribute, and metabolize medications. A high-protein diet, for example, has been shown to enhance drug metabolism through increased oxidation and conjugation. A high-protein diet accelerates the metabolism of drugs such as antipyrine and theophyllines, whereas a high-carbohydrate diet appears to have the opposite effect (27–29). In addition to the "macronutrients" (i.e., proportion of carbohydrates, proteins, and fat in the diet), numerous "micronutrients" also exert major effects on the expression of many drug-metabolizing enzymes. For example, CYP1A2 is inducible by charbroiled beef and cruciferous vegetables, and certain citrus fruits and plant products, such as grapefruits and corn, potently inhibit CYP3A4 (30,31).

A series of studies conducted in the 1970s clearly highlights the importance of culture and cultural change in determining drug metabolism. Conducted among Sudanese and South Asians before and after their migration to England, these studies showed a substantially slower rate of metabolism of some of the CYP1A2 substrates, such as antipyrine and clomipramine, among these "non-Westerners" as compared to their white British counterparts. Once they immigrated to London and took on new dietary habits, these immigrants' metabolic profiles for CYP1A2 substrates became indistinguishable from those of the "native" Westerners' (27,32). Figure 1-6 compares the clearance rate of antipyrine between the Sudanese in Sudan (far left), the Sudanese immigrants in London (center), and the British natives in London (far right).

The central importance of CYP3A4 in the metabolism of the majority of psychotropics is clearly demonstrated in Figures 1-4 and 1-5. This enzyme is highly inducible by a large variety of commonly prescribed and used synthetic drugs (e.g., carbamazepine) and plant products (e.g., St. John's wort), and at the same time also is potently inhibited by various other medications (e.g., terfenadine and ketoconazole) as well as common foodstuffs (e.g., grapefruit juice). Since individuals and ethnic/cultural groups vary dramatically in their exposure to these inducers and inhibitors, it stands to reason that there should be significant variations in the expression of this enzyme, which then should be translated into differences in the metabolism and effects of psychotropics and other medications.

A recent example further illustrates the importance of taking such interactions into consideration in clinical decisions. Although drugs used for the control of hypercholesterolemia such as simvastatin, atorvastatin, and lovastatin are safe at the usual dose range, they carry a risk for serious side effects when the tissue drug concentrations become excessive due to drug–drug or drug–nutrient interactions. Since the metabolism of these antihypercholesterolemic drugs is dependent on CYP3A4, coadministration of these drugs with inhibitors of the enzyme (e.g., nefazodone and grapefruit juice) may render them toxic. This may be the reason for cases of rhabdomyolysis or myositis that developed in several patients treated with both simvastatin

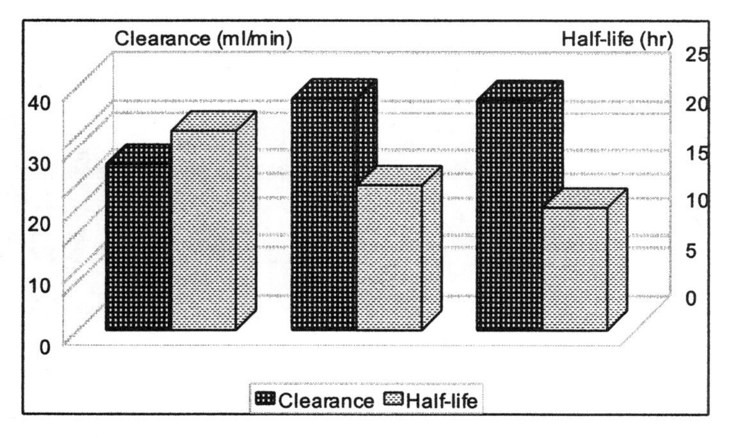

FIG. 1-6. Pharmacokinetics of antipyrine: Sudanese and British.

and nefazodone (33–35). Such a thesis was further supported by a study in healthy adults, where coadministration of simvastatin and nefazodone resulted in an approximately 20-fold increase in simvastatin and simvastatin acid (35).

VII. SMOKING AND ITS EFFECT ON P450 ENZYMES

Compared to those without psychiatric disorders, psychiatric patients are significantly more likely to be addicted to nicotine, and also are more likely to become heavier smokers. The heavier exposure to tobacco carries with it significant health risks for this vulnerable population that have not been adequately addressed. In addition, even less known is the fact that exposure to tobacco often significantly alters the pharmacokinetics of psychotropics (and other medications), resulting in changes in dosing requirements, side-effect profiles, and ultimately patients' response to pharmacotherapy (36). Polycyclic aromatic hydrocarbons present in cigarette smoke induce several hepatic cytochrome P450 isozymes, including CYP1A2 and CYP2E1. Whereas the induction of CYP2E1 has been implicated in cancer risks associated with smoking, CYP1A2 induction has been identified as the main reason for the reduction of the plasma concentrations of antidepressants (e.g., imipramine, clomipramine, fluvoxamine, and trazodone, but not bupropion), antipsychotics (e.g., chlorpromazine, clozapine, thiothixene, fluphenazine, haloperidol, and olanzapine), and anxiolytics (e.g., alprazolam, lorazepam, oxazepam, diazepam, and demethyldiazepam, but probably not chlordiazepoxide). Surprisingly, carbamazepine appears to be minimally affected by cigarette smoking, although it has been shown to be a substrate of as well as a potent inducer for CYP1A2. Perhaps this is because hepatic enzymes are already maximally stimulated by the autoinductive properties of this unique medication. Taken together, it is clear that cigarette smoking affects the pharmacokinetics of a large number of psychotropic drugs. Separately, it could also alter drug response via pharmacodynamic mechanisms. It is thus crucial that clinicians consider smoking as an important factor in prescribing these medications. Figure 1-7 shows the percentage of depressed and schizophrenic patients that smoke

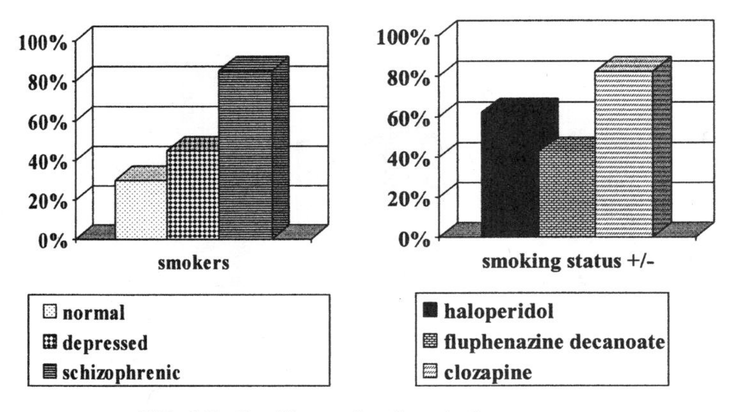

FIG. 1-7. Smoking and antipsychotic responses.

as compared to the general population, demonstrated on the left panel. The right panel shows the decrease in plasma drug concentration from baseline after initiation of smoking. For example, subjects taking haloperidol who began smoking had drug levels that were only 60% of their levels measured before they started smoking.

VIII. GENETIC POLYMORPHISMS IN GENE ENCODING RECEPTORS, TRANSPORTERS OR OTHER THERAPEUTIC TARGETS

Although most await further clarification, a large number of genes have already been identified as exerting major influences on therapeutic targets' response to psychotropics. These include genes encoding transporters and receptors of key neurotransmitters believed to be involved in mediating the clinical effects (therapeutic as well as toxic) of most commonly used psychotherapeutic agents. Genes controlling the biosynthesis and catabolism of these neurotransmitters also have been extensively studied. Most of these genes have been found to be polymorphic, and the patterns of these polymorphisms also typically vary significantly across ethnicity (37–41). Because of space limitations, in the following we will focus our discussion on the two most extensively studied genes, namely the serotonin transporter (5-HTT) and the catecholamine-*O*-methyl transferase (COMT).

A. Genetic Polymorphism of 5-HTT

Responsible for the reuptake of serotonin back to the presynaptic neuron, 5-HTT is the target of most of the newer antidepressants, whose demonstrated efficacy supports the thesis that 5-HTT indeed plays a crucial role in the pathogenesis of depression, as well as in mediating the effect of antidepressants. A functional insertion/deletion polymorphism in the promoter region of the 5-HTT gene (*HTTLPR*) has been shown to modulate its transcription, resulting in differential 5-HTT expression and serotonin cellular uptake (42). Hariri et al. (43) reported that subjects who are homozygotic for the *l* allele for *HTTLPR* showed less fear and anxiety-related behaviors and exhibited less amygdala neuronal activity, as assessed by functional magnetic resonance imaging, in response to fearful stimuli. Of note, the prevalence of the *l* allele varies substantially across ethnic groups, ranging from approximately 70% among populations with Sub-Saharan African origin to 30% among East Asians (see Fig. 1-8).

The relationship between *HTTLPR* polymorphisms and antidepressant response has been intriguing. Since 1998, at least five studies conducted in Italy and North America (with predominantly white patient populations), as well as one from Taiwan (44), showed that the 5-HTTLPR *l* allele is associated with better or more rapid selective serotonin reuptake inhibitor (SSRI) response (45–49). Two recent studies also implicate the 5-HTTLPR *s* allele in SSRI-emergent adverse effects (50,51). In contrast, two of three studies conducted in Asia (52,53) found that the *s* allele was predictive of better SSRI response. Although the mechanism(s) responsible for such

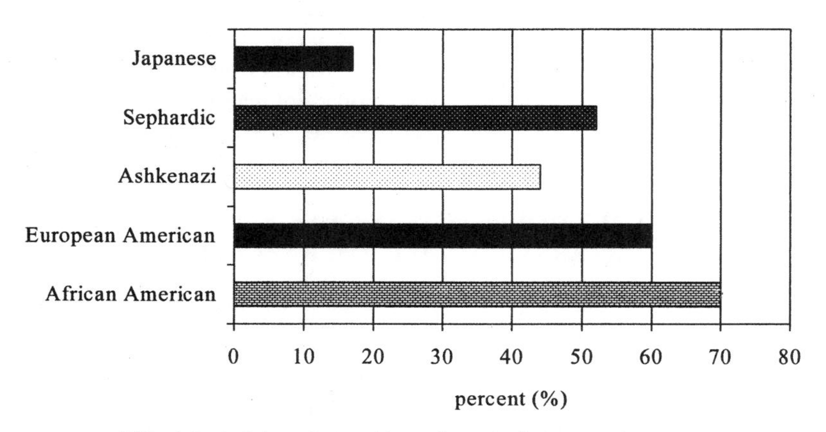

FIG. 1-8. *l* allele polymorphism of serotonin transporter gene.

cross-ethnic discrepancies in the effect of the *HTTLPR* polymorphisms remain unclear, they do serve to highlight the importance of taking ethnicity into consideration in designing pharmacogenetic and other genetic studies.

B. Genetic Polymorphism of COMT

COMT mediates one of the most important pathways for the metabolism of catecholamines, including dopamine and norepinephrine. COMT activity has long been known to have a trimodal distribution (54,55). Recent studies demonstrate that the reduction of its activity is caused by a single nucleotide mutation whose *L* allele frequency is approximately 26% in African Americans, 18% in Asians, and 50% in whites. Higher COMT activity is correlated with the ratio between 3-*O*-methyldopa and levodopa, which in turn predicts the occurrence of side effects of levodopa in treating Parkinsonism. Reflecting this, a higher percentage of Asians have been found to be poor responders to levodopa (56).

The COMT gene has long been implicated in playing a role in the pathogenesis of schizophrenia, as well as in the risk and treatment response of panic disorders. In terms of schizophrenia, a series of studies conducted by Weinberger and associates (57) demonstrated that COMT polymorphism is responsible for approximately 4% of the risk for schizophrenia, and it also is associated with the severity of neurocognitive deficits. Similarly, in a study of 103 Korean inpatient schizophrenics, Park et al. (58) found that cases with COMT *L* allele–containing genotypes (*L/L* and *L/H*) as well as a positive family history had an almost fourfold higher risk of schizophrenia compared to controls. The COMT *L/L* genotype has also been associated with more severe clinical signs in a group of Turkish schizophrenics (59).

A recent study suggests that a COMT genetic polymorphism may be an important factor in the development and treatment response of panic disorder. COMT activity might be related to susceptibility to panic disorder in that significantly higher proportions of the COMT *L* allele and *L/L* genotype were observed in patients with panic disorder than in healthy comparison subjects (60). In addition, patients with the *L/L* genotype also showed poorer treatment response to pharmacotherapy than did patients with other genotypes (60). If the *L/L* genotype indeed represents a significant factor in the development of panic disorder, it would be tempting to speculate that the low frequency of this genotype in Asian populations may be partially responsible for the relatively lower rate of panic in Asia, which ranges from 0.4% to 1.7% (61–63), substantially lower than the US rate of 3.5%, according to estimates from the National Comorbidity Study (64).

IX. NONBIOLOGICAL FACTORS THAT AFFECT DRUG RESPONSE

We have thus far focused on the biological factors that affect drug response, but healing often takes place in the context of interactions among individuals. In these interactions, both patient and clinician bring their own knowledge, predispositions, values, priorities, modes of thinking, and belief systems into play. Within this transaction, issues such as patient compliance, "expectation effect" (including the placebo effect), clinician ideology, and past experiences impact drug responses. These "nonbiological" factors, which are in a large part shaped by culture, powerfully determine the success or failure of any pharmacological treatment, regardless of drug receptor specificity or drug potency. Figure 1-9 shows the various determinants of the sociocultural milieu in which the patient and clinician are both enmeshed.

Because of space limitations, these issues will not be discussed in detail here, but can be found in some of our review articles published elsewhere (14,65,66). However, the following example is included to highlight the enormity of these cultural influences on "pharmacological" responses (67). Buckalew and Coffield (68) reported findings from a well-controlled study showing significant ethnic differences in response to placebo pills with different colors. In this study, white capsules were seen as analgesics by white subjects but as stimulants by their African American counterparts. In contrast, black capsules were seen as stimulants by whites and as analgesics by African Americans. The color of the pill impacted the subject's expectations and response differently, depending on each subject's belief of the purpose of the drug. This and other studies indicate that it is important to take the patient's cultural norms and expectations into consideration in pharmacotherapy.

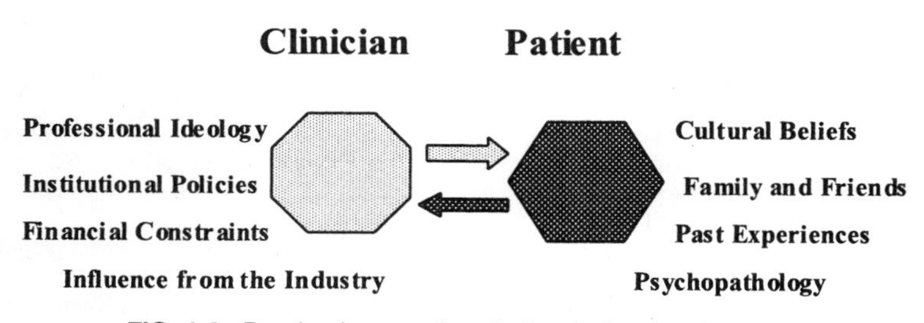

FIG. 1-9. Psychopharmacology in the sociocultural context.

X. CONCLUSION

As is apparent from the literature reviewed here, culture and ethnicity are powerful determinants of an individual's response to psychopharmacotherapy. Progress in this regard will vastly improve our current practice in using medications. However, it is necessary to remember that there are often very substantial interindividual variations within any defined cultural or ethnic group, and that ethnic variations in pharmacological responses should not be interpreted stereotypically.

It is likely that progress in pharmacogenomics will eventually lead to specific clinical applications useful for clinicians to guide their decisions in terms of choosing psychotropics, forming strategies for titration, as well as predicting likely side effects. These developments should result in the formulation of treatment strategies that are not only more effective but also more cost-effective than "traditional" approaches. Together, these exciting new developments should help to make psychopharmacotherapy increasingly rational, evidence based, and effective. In addition, progress in pharmacogenetics might also stimulate research on "nonbiological" issues, such as cultural influences on adherence and other factors that determine patients' perceptions and actions, which in turn contribute towards their sense of satisfaction and their being able to maximally benefit from treatment with antidepressants or other medications. With such an integrative approach, we would be best able to define elements of optimal pharmacotherapeutic practices that would take both cultural and biological diversity into consideration and tailor treatment to individual characteristics rather than relying on global guidelines.

REFERENCES

1. Lin KM, Poland RE, Nakasaki G. *Psychopharmacology and psychobiology of ethnicity.* Washington, DC: American Psychiatric Press, 1993.
2. Kaplan B. Use of race and ethnicity in biomedical publication. *JAMA* 2003;289:2709–2716.
3. McGoldrick M. Ethnicity and family therapy: an overview. In: McGoldrick M, Giordano J, Pearce JK, eds. *Ethnicity and family therapy,* 2nd ed. New York: Guilford Press, 1996.
4. Brislin R. *Cross cultural encounters.* New York: Pergamon Press, 1981.
5. Kalow W. *Pharmacogenetics of drug metabolism.* New York: Pergamon Press, 1992.
6. Lin KM, Finder E. Neuroleptic dosage for Asians. *Am J Psychiatry* 1983;140:490–491.
7. Potkin SG, Shen Y, Pardes H, et al. Haloperidol concentrations are elevated in Chinese patients. *Psychiatry Res* 1984;12:167–172.
8. Lin KM, Poland RE, Lau JK, et al. Haloperidol and prolactin concentrations in Asians and Caucasians. *J Clin Psychopharmacol* 1988;8:195–201.
9. Lopez SR. Patient variable biases in clinical judgment: conceptual overview and methodological considerations. *Psychol Bull* 1989;106:184–203.
10. Jibiki I, Kubota T, Fujimoto K, et al. Effective clinical response at low plasma levels of haloperidol in Japanese schizophrenics with acute psychotic state. *Jpn J Psychiatry* 1993;47:627–629.
11. Yang YY. Prophylactic efficacy of lithium and its effective plasma levels in Chinese bipolar patients. *Acta Psychiatr Scand* 1985;71:171–175.
12. Zhou HH, Koshakji RP, Siolberstein D, et al. Altered sensitivity to and clearance of propranolol in men of Chinese descent as compared with American white. *N Engl J Med* 1989;320:565–570.
13. Lin KM, Poland RE. Ethnicity, culture, and psychopharmacology. In: Bloom FE, Kupfer DI, eds. *Psychopharmacology: the fourth generation of progress.* New York: Raven Press, 1995.

14. Weber WW. *Pharmacogenetics.* New York: Oxford University Press, 1997.
15. Daly AK, Brockmoller J, Broly F, et al. Nomenclature for human CYP2D6 alleles. *Pharmacogenetics* 1996;6:193–201.
16. Leathart JB, London SJ, Steward A, et al. CYP2D6 phenotype-genotype relationships in African Americans and Caucasians in Los Angeles. *Pharmacogenetics* 1998;8:529–541.
17. Masimirembwa CM, Hasler JA. Genetic polymorphism of drug metabolising enzymes in African populations: implications for the use of neuroleptics and antidepressants. *Brain Res Bull* 1997;44: 561–571.
18. Wan YJ, Poland RE, Han G, et al. Analysis of the CYP2D6 gene polymorphism and enzyme activity in African Americans in Southern California. *Pharmacogenetics* 2001;11:489–499.
19. Wang SL, Huang JD, Lai MD, et al. Molecular basis of genetic variation in debrisoquin hydroxylation in Chinese subjects: polymorphism in RFLP and DNA sequence of CYP2D6. *Clin Pharmacol Ther* 1993;53:410–418.
20. Dahl ML, Yue QY, Roh HK, et al. Genetic analysis of the CYP2D locus in relation to debrisoquine hydroxylation capacity in Korean, Japanese and Chinese subjects. *Pharmacogenetics* 1995;5: 159–164.
21. Roh HK, Dahl ML, Johansson I, et al. Debrisoquine and S-mephenytoin hydroxylation phenotypes and genotypes in a Korean population. *Pharmacogenetics* 1996;6:441–447.
22. Mendoza R, Wan YJ, Poland RE, et al. CYP2D6 polymorphism in a Mexican American population. *Clin Pharmacol Ther* 2001;70:552–560.
23. Akullu E, Persson I, Bertilsson L, et al. Frequent distribution of ultrarapid metabolizers of debrisoquine in an Ethiopian population carrying duplicated and multiduplicated functional CYP2D6 alleles. *J Pharmacol Exp Ther* 1996;278:441–446.
24. Schulman RW, Ozdemir V. Psychotropic medications and cytochrome P450 2D6: pharmacokinetic considerations in the elderly. *Can J Psychiatry* 1997;42:4S–9S.
25. De Morais SM, Wilkinson GR, Blaisdell J, et al. The major genetic defect responsible for the polymorphism of S-mephenytoin metabolism in humans. *J Biol Chem* 1994;269:15419–15422.
26. Goldstein JA, Ishizaki T, Chiba K, et al. Frequencies of the defective CYP2C19 alleles responsible for the mephenytoin poor metabolizer phenotype in various Oriental, Caucasian, Saudi Arabian and American black populations. *Pharmacogenetics* 1997;7:59–64.
27. Branch RA, Salih SY, Homeida M. Racial differences in drug metabolizing ability: a study with antipyrine in the Sudan. *Clin Pharmacol Ther* 1978;24:283–286.
28. Fraser HS, Mucklow JC, Bulpitt CJ, et al. Environmental factors affecting antipyrine metabolism in London factory and office workers. *Br J Clin Pharmacol* 1979;7:237–243.
29. Anderson KE, Kappas A. Dietary regulation of cytochrome P450. *Annu Rev Nutr* 1991;11:141–167.
30. Oesterheld J, Kallepalli BR. Grapefruit juice and clomipramine: shifting metabolic ratios. *J Clin Psychopharmacol* 1997;17:62–63.
31. Fuhr U, Klittich K, Staib AH. Inhibitory effect of grapefruit juice and its bitter principal, naringenin, on CYP1A2 dependent metabolism of caffeine in man. *Br J Clin Pharmacol* 1993;35:431–436.
32. Allen JG, Rack P, Vaddadi K. Differences in the effects of clomipramine on English and Asian volunteers: preliminary report on a pilot study. *Postgrad Med J* 1977;53:79–86.
33. Skrabal MZ, Stading JA, Monaghan MS. Rhabdomyolysis associated with simvastatin-nefazodone therapy. *South Med J* 2003;96:1034–1035.
34. Jacobson RH, Wang P, Glueck CJ. Myositis and rhabdomyolysis associated with concurrent use of simvastatin and nefazodone. *JAMA* 1997;277:296–297.
35. Thompson M, Samuels S. Rhabdomyolysis with simvastatin and nefazodone. *Am J Psychiatry* 2002; 159:1607.
36. Desai HD, Seabolt J, Jann MW. Smoking in patients receiving psychotropic medications: a pharmacokinetic perspective. *CNS Drugs* 2001;15:469–494.
37. Gelernter J, Kranzler H, Cubells JF. Serotonin transporter protein (SLC6A4) allele and haplotype frequencies and linkage disequilibria in African- and European American and Japanese populations in alcohol-dependent subjects. *Hum Genetics* 1997;101:243–246.
38. Goldman D, Lappalainen J, Ozaki N. Direct analysis of candidate genes in impulsive behaviours. *Ciba Found Symp* 1996;194:139–152.
39. Hodge SE. What association analysis can and cannot tell us about the genetics of complex disease. *Am J Med Genet* 1994;54:318–323.
40. Dean M, Stephens JC, Winkler C, et al. Polymorphic admixture typing in human ethnic populations. *Am J Hum Genet* 1994;55:788–808.

41. Chang FM, Kidd JR, Livak KJ, et al. The world-wide distribution of allele frequencies at the human dopamine D4 receptor locus. *Hum Genet* 1996;98:91–101.
42. Greenberg BD, McMahon FJ, Murphy DL. Serotonin transporter candidate gene studies in affective disorders and personality: promises and potential pitfalls. *Mol Psychiatry* 1998;3:186–189.
43. Hariri AR, Mattay VS, Tessitore A, et al. Serotonin transporter genetic variation and the response of the human amygdala. *Science* 2002;297:400–403.
44. Yu YW, Tsai SJ, Chen TJ, et al. Association study of the serotonin transporter promoter polymorphism and symptomatology and antidepressant response in major depressive disorders. *Mol Psychiatry* 2002;7:1115–1119.
45. Smeraldi E, Zanardi R, Benedetti F, et al. Polymorphism within the promoter of the serotonin transporter gene and antidepressant efficacy of fluvoxamine. *Mol Psychiatry* 1998;3:508–511.
46. Pollock BF, Ferrell RE, Mulsant BH, et al. Allelic variation in the serotonin transporter promoter affects onset of paroxetine treatment response in late-life depression. *Neuropsychopharmacology* 2000;23:587–590.
47. Serretti A, Zanardi R, Rossini D, et al. Influence of tryptophan hydroxylase and serotonin transporter genes on fluvoxamine antidepressant activity. *Mol Psychiatry* 2001;6:586–592.
48. Rausch JL, Johnson ME, Fei YJ, et al. Initial conditions of serotonin transporter kinetics and genotype: influence on SSRI treatment trial outcome. *Biol Psychiatry* 2002;51:723–732.
49. Zanardi R, Serretti A, Rossini D, et al. Factors affecting fluvoxamine antidepressant activity: influence of pindolol and 5-HTTLPR in delusional and nondelusional depression. *Biol Psychiatry* 2001;50: 323–330.
50. Du L, Bakish D, Lapierre YD, et al. Association of polymorphism of serotonin 2a receptor gene with suicidal ideation in major depressive disorder. *Am J Med Genet* 2000;96:56–60.
51. Perlis RH, Mischoulon D, Smoller JW, et al. Serotonin transporter polymorphisms and adverse effects with fluoxetine treatment. *Biol Psychiatry* 2003;54:879–883.
52. Kim DK, Lim SW, Lee S, et al. Serotonin transporter gene polymorphism and antidepressant response. *Neuroreport* 2000;11:215–219.
53. Yoshida K, Ito K, Sato K, et al. Influence of the serotonin transporter gene-linked polymorphic region on the antidepressant response to fluvoxamine in Japanese depressed patients. *Prog Neuropsychopharmacol Biol Psychiatry* 2002;26:383–386.
54. Mcleod HL, Fang L, Luo X, et al. Ethnic differences in erythrocyte catechol-O-methyltransferase activity in black and white Americans. *J Pharmacol Exp Ther* 1994;270:26–29.
55. Li T, Vallada H, Curtis D, et al. Catechol-O-methyltransferase Val158 Met polymorphism: frequency analysis in Han Chinese subjects and allelic association of the low activity allele with bipolar affective disorder. *Pharmacogenetics* 1997;7:349–353.
56. Rivera-Calimlim L, Reilly DK. Difference in erythrocyte catechol-O-methyltransferase activity between Orientals and Caucasians: difference in levodopa tolerance. *Clin Pharmacol Ther* 1984;35: 804–809.
57. Egan MF Goldberg TE, Kolachana BS, et al. Effect of COMT Val108/158 Met genotype on frontal lobe function and risk for schizophrenia. *Proc Natl Acad Sci U S A* 2001;98:6917–6922.
58. Park TW, Yoon KS, Kim JH, et al. Functional catechol-O-methyltransferase gene polymorphism and susceptibility to schizophrenia. *Eur Neuropsychopharmacol* 2002;12:299–303.
59. Herken H, Erdal ME. Catechol-O-methyltransferase gene polymorphism in schizophrenia: evidence for association between symptomatology and prognosis. *Psychiatr Genet* 2001;11:105–109.
60. Woo J, Yoon K, Yu B. Catechol O-methyltransferase genetic polymorphism in panic disorder. *Am J Psychiatry* 2003;159:1785–1787.
61. Hwu HG, Yeh EK, Chang LY. Prevalence of psychiatric disorders in Taiwan defined by the Chinese Diagnostic Interview Schedule. *Acta Psychiatr Scand* 1989;79:136–147.
62. Aoki Y, Fujihara S, Kitamura T. Panic attacks and panic disorder in Japanese non-patient population: epidemiology and psychosocial correlates. *J Affect Disord* 1994;32:51–59.
63. Lee CK, Kwak YS, Yamamoto J, et al. Psychiatric epidemiology in Korea. Part I: gender and age differences in Seoul. *J Nerv Ment Dis* 1990;178:242–246.
64. Eaton WW, Kessler RC, Wittchen HU, et al. Panic and panic disorder in the United States. *Am J Psychiatry* 1994;151:413–420.
65. Smith M, Lin KM, Mendoza R. "Non-biological" issues affecting psychopharmacotherapy: cultural considerations. In: Lin Km, Poland R, Nakasaki G, eds. *Psychopharmacology and psychobiology of ethnicity.* Washington, DC: American Psychiatric Press, 1993:37–38.

66. Lin K, Elwyn TS, Smith M, et al. Culture and drug therapy. In: Tseng Ws, ed. *Clinician's guide to cultural psychiatry.* Amsterdam: Elsevier, 2004.
67. Wertheimer AI, Santella TM. Medication compliance research: still so far to go. *J Appl Res* 2003; 3:254–260.
68. Buckalew LW, Coffield K. Drug expectations associated with perceptual characteristics: ethnic factors. *Percept Mot Skills* 1982;55:915–918.

2

Illness Beliefs of Depressed Chinese American Patients in a Primary Care Setting

*†Albert Yeung and †‡Raymond Kam

**Depression Clinical and Research Program, Massachusetts General Hospital, Boston Massachusetts 02114; †South Cove Community Health Center, Boston, Massachusetts 02111; and ‡Department of Psychiatry, Children's Hospital, Boston, Massachusetts 02115*

I. INTRODUCTION

Asian Americans are the fastest growing minority population in the United States, with their population tripling in the past 20 years. During the last decade, it grew by 44% to the current 10.1 million (in 2000), comprising 4% of the US population (1). The growth rate is expected to continue, and by 2020, Asian Americans are projected to make up 6% of the nation's population. It is increasingly important for clinical practitioners to understand the illness beliefs regarding mental disorders of this group of diverse populations.

Early cross-national studies concluded that Asians tend to have lower rates of depression than other ethnic groups (2). However, more recent studies in Asian countries have provided evidence to suggest that depression is more prevalent among Asians than previously considered (3–5). Between 1998 and 1999, our group conducted a two-phase epidemiological survey in the primary care clinic of a community health center serving less acculturated Asian Americans in Boston, Massachusetts. The survey found that the estimated prevalence of major depressive disorder (MDD) among Asian Americans in this primary care setting was 19.6% ± 0.06%, suggesting that MDD is common among Asian Americans in urban, primary care settings (6).

In this chapter, we will focus on the illness beliefs of Chinese Americans, who comprise 24% (2.4 million) of the Asian American population and form its largest ethnic subgroup. In a recent study, our group investigated the illness beliefs of Chinese American immigrants with MDD in a primary care clinic, exploring their chief complaints, the labels they used for their illness, their experience of stigma, perceived etiologies, and the types of treatment sought for their depressive symptoms. These findings will help us understand the challenges of treating MDD among Asian Americans, and provide empirical evidence on possible approaches to improve the recognition and treatment of MDD among this population. We will also discuss the impact of culture on illness beliefs of depression, and assess whether the theoretical framework used by modern psychiatry is applicable to other cultures.

II. CONCEPTIONS OF ILLNESS AMONG DEPRESSED ASIAN AMERICANS

According to the Surgeon General's report (2001) (7), Asian Americans have the lowest rate of mental health service utilization of any ethnic group in the United States. The undertreatment of depression among the Asian American population has been attributed to a number of different causes, including the lack of recognition of depression among this population, stigma leading to nontreatment, and somatization (8).

In European and North American cultures, depressive symptomatology, when meeting certain criteria, are viewed as part of the psychiatric syndrome of MDD, characterized by specific affective, cognitive, behavioral, and somatic symptoms. However, the interpretation of depressive symptoms varies across cultures, and leads to different ways of understanding the experience of negative, sad feeling states. Arthur Kleinman, a psychiatrist who also trained as an anthropologist, asserts that different cultures have different "explanatory models" of distress that define what is considered illness, the nature of symptoms, the appropriate treatments for any given symptom, and the kind of relationships within which treatment takes place (9). It may surprise many Western-trained mental health clinicians that in many non-European cultural groups, including the Chinese, Japanese, Southeast Asians, and Canadian Eskimos, concepts of depressive disorders equivalent to MDD are not found (10).

When experiencing depressive symptoms, Chinese Americans typically do not describe their distress in terms easily recognized by Western mental health practitioners. Oftentimes, their complaints are seen as "somatizing," disregarding obvious depressive states. One reason for this apparent disregard may be the stigma that is attached to psychiatric symptoms in Chinese culture, compared to the relative acceptance of physical complaints. In a study of primary care patients in Hunan, China in the 1980s, Kleinman (9) found that depressed Chinese patients usually presented with somatic rather than mood symptoms. He suggested that somatic symptoms were the more appropriate "idioms of distress" in Chinese culture, in which the designation of mental illness usually refers only to stigmatized psychiatric disorders such as psychosis and mental retardation (11). Absent the psychodynamic influences of Freud and his successors in the West, there has been no tradition of treating depressive or anxious states within the purview of psychiatry amongst the Chinese. Being labeled as psychiatrically ill in China, whether for depression or another reason, risks being associated with those who are crazy or cognitively unsound, and being thought of in the same way.

Certainly, there is a powerful societal pressure in Chinese culture to suppress and disguise negative feeling states, and to avoid being associated with mental illness (12–14). Other reasons for the high prevalence of somatization in Chinese populations, besides avoiding stigma, have been proposed (15,16). One possibility is that patients from non-Western cultures and members of lower socioeconomic groups are less willing or able to express emotional distress (15,17,18). Another may be their lack of familiarity with the Western psychiatric classification system of mental disorders (3). From a study of primary care patients in Hong Kong, which also found that depressed Chinese patients complained primarily of somatic symptoms (19), Cheung (20) suggested an alternative hypothesis: that the presentation of somatic symptoms among depressed Chinese patients may be a learned behavior to adapt to the norms of primary care settings. With limited time for clinical encounters and practitioners' inclination toward a biomedical model, patients may surmise that physicians are more interested in physical, rather than psychological, symptoms. This is not surprising considering that a typical primary care visit lasts, on average, 5 to 10 minutes in many Asian countries. (One of the authors [RK] witnessed an orthopedic surgery clinic in small hospital in Taidong, Taiwan, in the summer of 1994. The surgeon had arrived for his twice monthly 2-hour clinic, and had over 100 patients waiting. Averaging just over 1 minute per patient, this intrepid surgeon was helped by two nurses, one bringing in patients and having each sit in one of three chairs spaced about 6 feet apart. Each patient would have a brief moment, seconds at most, to share his most pressing concern, after which the doctor would give his clinical impression—that the wound needed redressing, that an antibiotic was indicated, that the patient had been delinquent in his wound care, etc.—shouting over the clamor to be heard. The second nurse would then jump in, carry out any directives, and discharge the patient before stepping a few feet over to attend to the next patient. The clinic ended on time. As one might imagine, there was neither the context nor the expectation that the patient share anything other than pressing somatic concerns.)

III. ILLNESS BELIEFS OF DEPRESSED CHINESE AMERICANS IN A PRIMARY CARE SETTING

A. Methods

Our team at the Massachusetts General Hospital Depression Clinical and Research Program has recently performed a study using a structured instrument to examine the illness beliefs of depressed Chinese American patients in primary care (21). The study took place at the South Cove Community Health Center (South Cove) in Boston, Massachusetts between May 1998 and November 1999. South Cove is an urban community health center with wide-ranging clinical services that primarily serves low-income, Asian immigrants who face financial, linguistic, and cultural barriers to health care. In this collaboration with primary care physicians, 680 Chinese American patients who sought care at South Cove were randomly approached and screened for depression using the Chinese translation of the Beck Depression Inventory (CBDI), (22) which has been previously validated by our group (23). Fifty patients screened positive, and of these, MDD was formally diagnosed in 40 (8.0% of patients completing screening) using the Structured Clinical Interview for DSM-III-R, patient version (SCID-I/P) (24).

We approached those in whom depression had been diagnosed and asked them to participate in the next phase of the study, in which their illness beliefs would be elicited using the Explanatory Model of Interview Catalogue (EMIC) (25). The EMIC is a structured interview tool in which patients are probed about five dimensions of illness behaviors and beliefs: chief complaints, conceptualization and labeling of illness, perceptions of stigma, causal attributions, and help-seeking patterns. Twenty-nine (72.5%) of the 40 depressed patients agreed to be interviewed with the EMIC [see our published study for detailed methodology (21)]. They included 18 females and 11 males, with a mean age of 46 years (SD = 15, range = 8–84), and a mean length of stay in the United States of 6 years (SD = 5.0, range = 1–12).

B. Results

1. Chief Complaints

The majority (n = 22, 76%) of the depressed Chinese Americans complained chiefly of somatic symptoms. Among them, 12 (41%) presented with general physical symptoms, and 10 (34.5%) presented with neurovegetative symptoms that are used as criteria for diagnosing MDD (e.g. sleep disturbance, marked weight loss or weight gain). The most common presenting complaints were fatigue (17.0%), insomnia (17.0%), headache (14.0%), cough (7.0%), pain (7.0%), dizziness (7.0%), cervical problems (3.4%), and sexual dysfunction (3.4%). Four subjects (14.0%) complained of psychological symptoms of depression, including irritability (7.0%), ruminations (3.5%), and poor memory (3.5%) (Table 2-1). Two subjects (7.0%) described feelings of nervousness, but none complained spontaneously about depressed mood. One subject attended the primary care clinic for his annual physical examination and did not spontaneously report any health concerns. The profiles of depressive symptoms endorsed by patients based on the CBDI are described in Table 2-2. Interestingly, 27 patients (93%) endorsed depressed mood even though none of them reported depressed mood as their chief complaint.

2. Conceptualization and Labeling of Illness

When patients were asked to label their condition, over half (55%) reported "I don't know," five (17%) responded "not a (diagnosable medical) illness," and five (17%)

TABLE 2-1. *Chief complaints of depressed Chinese patients (N = 29)*

Chief complaints	n (%)
Physical symptoms	12 (41)
Headache	4 (14)
Cough	2 (7)
Pain	2 (7)
Dizziness	2 (7)
Others	2 (7)
Depressive neurovegetative symptoms	10 (34)
Insomnia	5 (17)
Fatigue	5 (17)
Depressive psychological symptoms	3 (14)
Irritability	2 (7)
Rumination	1 (3.5)
Poor memory	1 (3.5)
Nervousness	2 (7)
Depressed mood	0 (0)
No complaints	1 (3.5)

TABLE 2-2. *Frequency of CBDI symptoms among depressed Chinese-American patients (N = 29)*

Beck symptom	Frequency (%)
1. Feel sad	27 (93)
2. Hopelessness	17 (59)
3. Failure	23 (79)
4. No satisfaction	22 (76)
5. Guilt	21 (72)
6. Feel being punished	11 (38)
7. Disappointed	20 (69)
8. Blame self	25 (86)
9. Suicidal	12 (41)
10. Crying	19 (66)
11. Irritability	21 (72)
12. Loss of interest	19 (66)
13. Difficulty making decisions	23 (79)
14. Look ugly	21 (72)
15. Can't work	23 (79)
16. Insomnia	23 (79)
17. Fatigue	28 (97)
18. Appetite loss	15 (52)
19. Weight loss	6 (21)
20. Hypochondriasis	26 (90)
21. Lost interest in sex	21 (72)

CBDI, Chinese translation of the Beck Depression Inventory.

TABLE 2-3. *Labels used by depressed Chinese patients to describe their illness (N = 29)*

Name of the illness	n (%)
"Don't know"	16 (55)
"Not an illness"	5 (17)
Medical illnesses (hypertension 1, cold 2, poor health 1, injured arm 1)	5 (17)
Posttraumatic stress syndrome	1 (3.5)
Mental illness or "craziness"	2 (7)

attributed their symptoms to preexisting medical problems. Most of the patients (n = 26, 90%) did not ascribe their symptoms to depression or any other psychiatric condition. The remaining three patients (10%) thought that they suffered from a psychiatric disorder, including one who labeled himself as having "posttraumatic stress syndrome" (Table 2-3). When asked if they agreed with a diagnosis of MDD as indicated by the SCID-I/P, 14 (48%) reported that they had never heard of the diagnosis (Yeung AS. Effectiveness of cultural consultation on the willingness for treatment among depressed Chinese Americans. Personal Communication, 1999). When asked how the symptoms affected them, 26 patients (90%) felt that the symptoms affected their mind, and 23 patients (79%) felt the symptoms affected their body. Twenty-two patients (76%) felt that the symptoms affected both their mind and their body, which is consistent with an integrated mind/body concept used in traditional Chinese medicine (TCM).

3. Perceptions of Stigma

Most patients reported low levels of stigma (mean stigma score = 7.0, SD = 12, range = 0–36). More than half of them (n = 15, 52%) reported no stigma regarding their symptoms, and an additional eight patients (28%) scored less than 12 (Fig. 2-1 patients with high stigma scores tended to have severe depression and/or psychotic symptoms.

4. Perceived Causes

Subjects were asked to endorse all factors that they considered to be causal in their condition. Reported causes included psychological stress and/or psychological factors (93%), magico-religious-supernatural factors (45%), medical problems (17%), traditional beliefs (14%), hereditary (14%), toxicity (10.5%), and ingestion (7%)(Table 2-4).

5. Help-Seeking Patterns

Help-seeking strategies prior to seeking treatment at South Cove included using general hospital services (69%), seeking lay help (62%), using alternative treatments

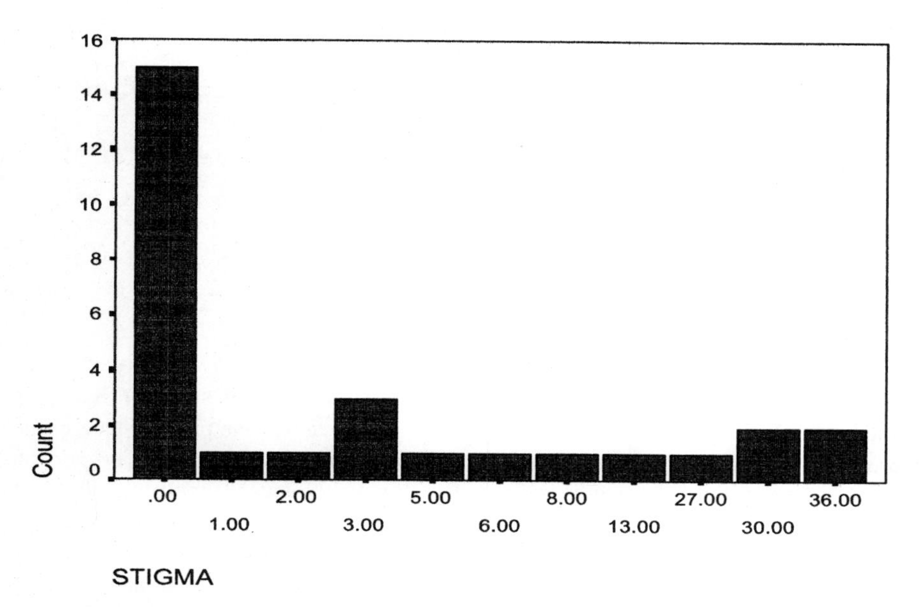

FIG. 2-1. Distribution of stigmatization scores among depressed Chinese American patients (N = 29).

administered by clinical providers (55%), seeking spiritual treatment (e.g., faith healers, astrologers/palmists, praying) (14%), and self-administering alternative treatments (10%). Only one subject in the sample reported seeking mental health services (3.5%)(Table 2-5).

C. Illness Beliefs about Somatic Symptoms and Depression

With the use of the structured instrument (EMIC), the South Cove Study generated informative data on the different dimensions of how Chinese Americans view depres-

TABLE 2-4. *Causes of illness perceived by Chinese patients (N = 29)*

Methods	Frequency (%)
Psychological stress	22 (76)
Psychological factors	20 (69)
Magico-religious-supernatural	13 (45)
Medical problems	5 (17)
Traditional beliefs	4 (14)
Hereditary	4 (14)
Toxicity	3 (10.5)
Ingestion	2 (7)
Sex	0 (0)

TABLE 2-5. *Methods of help-seeking by depressed Chinese patients (N = 29)*

Methods	Frequency (%)
General hospital	20 (69)
Lay help	18 (62)
Alternative treatment from others	16 (55)
Spiritual treatment	4 (14)
Alternative self-treatment	3 (10.5)
Mental health professionals	1 (3.5)

sion and seek help for it. Consistent with results from previous studies (13,26,27), a high proportion (76%) of depressed Chinese Americans in the primary care clinic presented physical symptoms as their chief complaints. Only a small proportion (14%) of patients in this study presented with psychological symptoms including irritability, rumination, and poor memory. It is intriguing that none of the depressed patients in this study considered depressed mood as their chief problem when they were asked about their depressive symptoms, yet the majority of them had no problems reporting psychological symptoms using a standardized instrument. When assessed with the CBDI, over 90% of the subjects in this study did endorse having depressed mood, showing that they were aware of their depressed mood though they did not consider it their main problem. In addition to endorsing "feel sad," the depressed patients also reported many of the affective symptoms in the CBDI, including "hopelessness" (59%), "failure" (79%), "no satisfaction" (76%), "guilt" (72%), "feeling being punished" (38%), "disappointed" (69%), "blame self" (86%), "suicidal" (41%), and "irritability" (72%). These findings argue against the hypotheses that Chinese patients suppress or are unable to express their feelings, are alexithymic (28), or are lacking in emotional differentiation (18).

Although depressed patients were able to recognize and report their sadness and other affective symptoms on the CBDI questionnaire, they did not consider affective symptoms their main problem or connect them with the label of a depressive illness. Over half of the subjects (n = 16, 55%) did not or could not give a name to describe their condition, and an additional five patients (17%) did not believe that they even had a diagnosable medical illness. Five patients (17%) attributed their symptoms to prior medical illnesses, including the vague cause of "poor health." Out of the 29 subjects, 26 (90%) did not consider themselves as having a psychiatric disorder. Of the remaining three patients (10%), one believed he had posttraumatic stress disorder and not depression, and the other two had unformed impressions of themselves as "crazy." Our findings suggest that Chinese Americans interpret their depression symptoms differently from the Western psychiatric conception. In our study, they predominantly attributed their affective and somatic symptoms to stress/psychological factors, and did not consider depression a distinct disease entity.

IV. CULTURAL FACTORS INFLUENCING THE CONCEPTUALIZATION OF DEPRESSIVE SYMPTOMS

Psychiatric disorders are highly stigmatized in Chinese society (29). Low stigmatization scores among many of the subjects from this study toward their symptoms provide further support that they did not consider their illness a psychiatric problem. In fact, when we asked the subjects about their understanding of depression, many of them reported that they had never heard of the term. Not conceptualizing their depressive symptoms as indicative of a psychiatric illness may be protective for depressed Chinese Americans in a cultural context where mental illness is highly stigmatized. In the discussion below, we will try to explore how social and cultural factors may shape the Chinese understanding of depression symptoms, and the possible reasons for the divergence of the concept of depression between health professionals and Chinese American patients.

Cross-cultural studies have informed us that each individual culture tends to have selective emphasis and presentation of emotional experiences. Based on an ethnographical literature review, Jenkins et al. (30) illustrated the dramatic degree to which certain cultures may contrast with one another in the expression of feeling states. For example, whereas Eskimos and Tahitians seldom display angry feelings, the Kaluli of New Guinea and the Yanamamo of Brazil use quite elaborate and complex means of expressing anger (30,31). In Western culture, emotional distress is thought of as separate from physical distress, and is often demarcated into relatively "pure forms" of anxiety and depression. As Tseng (32) notes, though, this differentiation into discrete "psych" and "soma" is arbitrary and not universal to all cultures. Many Chinese, for instance, manifest combined somato-mood presentations.

Culture also influences the definition of selfhood. Individuals in Western, industrialized populations often think of themselves as unique, separate, and autonomous, whereas individuals in non-Western populations usually define themselves in relational terms, as part of an interdependent collective, defined by kinship and myth (30). People in the latter populations understand themselves as part of a living system of social relationships (33). They are less likely to be introspective about feelings of subjective anguish or express individually oriented, decontextualized self-statements of dysphoria (e.g., "I feel blue," "These things no longer mean anything to me") and worry (e.g., "I am bothered by things that usually do not bother me.") (34). Under the predominant influence of Confucianism, traditional Chinese society is a typical collectivistic culture. According to Confucius, certain interpersonal relationships, called the Five Cardinal Relations (Wu-Lun), are of paramount importance: those between ruler and subject, father and son, elder and younger brother, husband and wife, and friend and friend. Of these five dyads, three belong to the family and the other two are based on the family model. In Confucian social theory, the family occupies a central position—it is not only the primary social group, it is also the prototype of all social organizations (35). In traditional Chinese society, there is no differentiation between social and political units, with the basic unit being not the individual but the family (36). During the socialization process, children learn early on that they are to develop a dependent social orientation toward authority, and a group orientation toward the family. Within a group orientation, harmony within the family and society is primary; negative affects, rightfully or not, are considered undesirable or harmful to the social fabric, and as something to be mastered and blocked from overt expression as one matures (9,37).

In tandem with Confucianism, Taoism is the other philosophy that has vastly influenced Chinese culture. Founded by the mythical figure of Lao-tzu, who may have been a contemporary of Confucius, Taoism avers that the essence of life is to learn to live with and imitate nature. Everything has its natural course. Distress is a part of life, not to be fought, but to be understood and to be harmonized with. This way of thinking has informed such Chinese practices as tai chi and acupuncture, as well as influenced the development of Buddhism. The Buddhist practice of meditation to isolate grief, fear, hostility, and negative affects, is readily understood within the Taoist framework. Meditation diminishes negative affects by facilitating the practitioner's becoming detached from them and transcending them in a mindfulness state. This is in sharp contrast with the Western psychological approach, which encourages emotional catharsis and intrapsychic exploration (9).

The Taoist theory of Yin–Yang has also had enormous influence on the Chinese understanding of physiological functioning, and forms the pillar of traditional Chinese medicine (TCM). In TCM, proper physiologic functioning is conceptualized in terms of balance and harmony, represented by the Yin–Yang schematic (the Yang is the strong, male essence; the Yin the yielding, female essence).

Every sign and symptom (including psychological ones because psych and soma are not split) is interpreted within Yin–Yang theory as an excess or deficiency of Yang, and the corresponding deficiency or excess of Yin; and every treatment modality is aimed at either enhancing Yang (or Yin), or eliminating excess Yang (or Yin) (38). TCM further characterizes physiological and pathological phenomena according to the Yin–Yang balance within the Five Phases (Wu Xing) of the body. The Five Phases and the corresponding organs are Wood (Liver), Earth (Spleen), Water (Kidney), Fire (Heart), and Metal (Lungs). The essences of each phase influence the functioning of various domains, from digestive functioning to emotional states, with each phase generating the succeeding phase (Fig. 2-2) (39). The interconnection of these phases implies the unity of the mind–body, so that disparate symptoms such as chest pain, headache, sadness, and even psychosis are all seen as extensions of the same physiological framework. Practiced in China for thousands of years, TCM has had a strong influence on lay and folk concepts of illness, and on the language used to describe them.

The combined influences of Confucianism, Taoism, and TCM-based folk medical concepts, therefore, help explain why depressed Chinese Americans selectively focus on and report somatic symptoms, minimize and underreport affective symptoms, and understand interpersonal tension as the cause of their distress. The reporting of physical symptoms is a more familiar and culturally appropriate way to communicate their distress than using psychological idioms to do so, which would be more familiar

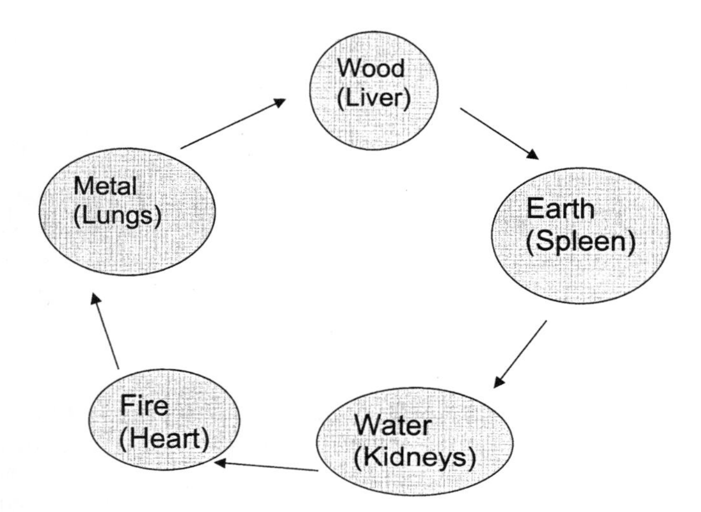

FIG. 2-2. Mutual control order of the five phases. (Adapted from Kaptchuk T. *The web that has no weaver: understanding Chinese medicine.* New York: Contemporary Books, 2000.)

to patients from Western cultures. Within Western medicine, psychologization has long been considered the norm for symptom conception and presentation, and somatization deviant and a barrier to both the diagnosis and treatment of psychiatric disorders. Even within Western medical systems, however, the appropriateness of marginalizing somatization has been questioned. Simon et al. (40) analyzed World Health Organization data on psychological problems in general health care and found that more than 40% of depressed patients in centers all over the world presented initially with somatic complaints.

Modern psychiatry is rooted in Western psychological existential idioms, and in disease classifications that are based on an intrapsychic orientation (9). Such an orientation suits middle-class populations in the West, yet it does not generalize well to non-Western cultures, including the Chinese culture, which tends to focus on physical symptoms and interpersonal relationships. This explains, in part, why ethnic minorities in the United States and people in non-Western countries underutilize mental health services. Depressed patients who do not articulate psychological symptoms tend to be underdiagnosed by practitioners. To many Chinese patients, depression is an unfamiliar concept that does not fit well with their indigenous illness beliefs. As a result of their differences in the conceptualizing and labeling of symptoms, Chinese Americans and other Asian Americans have limited access to mental health services. Educating people from non-Western cultures about the concept of depression would increase treatment and mental health care utilization, as would the broadening of current psychiatric classification systems to incorporate belief systems from other cultures. Cross-cultural research would be extremely helpful in providing empirical support for this goal, as well as the data needed to implement such changes.

V. IMPLICATIONS FOR TREATING DEPRESSED ASIAN AMERICANS

The findings of our study have practical implications for treating Chinese Americans with depression. The somatic presentation of depressive symptoms, so common among Chinese Americans, has important public health implications since it often leads to the underrecognition and inadequate treatment of psychiatric disorders. Physicians commonly perform numerous unnecessary diagnostic tests and medical treatment to work up these physical complaints, which result in patient suffering, frustration among health professionals, and wasted resources (41). Yet our study shows that when depressed Chinese Americans are asked explicitly, they readily report their depressive symptoms and have no difficulty doing so. Chinese Americans tend not to complain of affective symptoms spontaneously. It seems apparent, then, that to better serve this less acculturated population, practitioners need to explicitly ask about the presence of depressive symptoms.

Treating Chinese Americans, who often do not have an intuitive sense of depression as a clinically distinct diagnosis and often attach stigma to any psychiatric diagnosis, presents another clinical challenge: to treat the patients without explicitly telling them that they are being treated for a psychiatric disorder, or to openly inform patients that they have a depressive disorder. The former approach may decrease stigma and be more acceptable to some patients, but could be seen as paternalistic and possibly disrespectful under Western societal standards. The latter approach assumes a more egalitarian physician–patient relationship and allows patients to make their own informed decisions, but may run the risk of increasing stigma and lead the patient to deny the illness or refuse treatment.

In the United States, we do not have access to the diagnostic construct of "neurasthenia," a diagnosis embraced by patients and physicians in China during the 1980s as a way to avoid labeling patients with psychiatric diagnoses. Neurasthenia, much like the diagnoses of chronic fatigue syndrome and fibromyalgia, is a somatically conceived illness with psychological symptoms, and may be a more culturally appropriate diagnostic category for Chinese Americans than depression. Despite being limited to using depression as the only available diagnosis, however, we have not found it burdensome to introduce the concept of depression to less acculturated Chinese Americans at South Cove. Our experience suggests that if the practitioner shows acceptance of patients' illness beliefs, the diagnosis of major depressive disorder is usually well received by Chinese Americans. Furthermore, explaining depression using a more biologically based model of neurotransmitter imbalances seems to fit well with Chinese concepts of balance, harmony, and somatically based emotional symptoms. About half of the depressed patients in this study showed interest in receiving treatment for their depressive symptoms after we explained the Western understanding of depression and the treatments that are available (Yeung AS. Personal communication, 1999).

Although there may be advantages to introducing the Western concept of depression to patients, it is helpful to remain open to multiple explanatory models of illness. Although the majority of depressed Chinese American patients presented with physical symptoms, most of them considered their illness to be caused by psychosocial stress associated with personal responsibilities and interpersonal relationships. This highlights the importance of psychosocial treatment among depressed Asian Americans. Treatment with medication alone, without alleviating personal and family tension, is less likely to be successful. In addition to psychological stress, close to half of depressed Chinese American patients in this study considered magical-religious-supernatural factors (44.5%) and traditional explanations (14%) as causative factors. Many depressed Asian Americans have used alternative treatment, particularly herbal remedies (55% in our study) to treat their symptoms. Kirmayer et al. (42) suggest using multiple explanatory models, including biomedical, psychological, religious, and traditional ones, to enhance communication with ethnic minority patients. In practice, clinicians should be receptive to the use of traditional forms of treatment, while at the same time monitoring possible side effects due to interactions between herbs and pharmacological agents.

Another strategy for enhancing the treatment of Chinese American patients is working to integrate primary care and mental health services. The majority of patients in our study used general hospital outpatient services and lay help for treatment of their symptoms (Table 2-5). Only one subject (3.5%) in the study reported using mental health services for a chief complaint of depression. Although many depressed patients seek help at primary care clinics, most of them remained undiagnosed and untreated for depression (43). This is a serious public health problem that will only grow in magnitude, because Chinese Americans are one of the fastest-growing immigrant groups in the United States. We have been testing an integrative service model to increase detection and treatment of psychiatric disorders inside primary care. It may reduce the stigma and bureaucratic barriers that arise in using mental health services. The preliminary results of a study of integrating primary care and mental health services have been promising (44), yet much more needs to be done to improve the delivery of psychiatric services to this highly underserved population.

VI. CONCLUSION

Depressed Chinese Americans generally present with somatic symptoms in primary care. Nonetheless, when questioned explicitly about their symptoms, they often meet criteria for major depression. The lack of awareness of depression as a treatable illness, the influence of Asian philosophical and religious traditions, and the adoption of collectivistic social values may all contribute to their somatic presentation. Such illness beliefs may lead to the tendency of many depressed Chinese Americans to seek help in primary care, underreport their mood symptoms, and underutilize mental health services. It is important to keep an open mind and try to understand how they view their illness, and to accept their alternative explanatory models so that a mutually agreed upon treatment can be negotiated. Actively eliciting patients' mood symptoms, using culturally sensitive terminology in the explanation of MDD to minimize stigma associated with mental conditions, and integrating treatment of MDD into primary care settings may enhance recognition and treatment of MDD among Asian Americans. In addition, incorporating illness conceptions from other cultures into the current psychiatric classification system may broaden its theoretical basis, and facilitate delivery of mental health services to people from non-Western cultures.

REFERENCES

1. US Census Bureau, 2002. The Asian population: 2000. (C2KBR/01-16). Available at: http://www.census.gov/prod/2002pubs/c2kbr01-16.pdf. Accessed September 6, 2002.
2. Weissman MM, Bland RC, Canino GJ, et al. Cross-national epidemiology of major depression and bipolar disorder. *JAMA* 1996;276:29–299.
3. Cheng TA. Symptomatology of minor psychiatric morbidity: a cross-cultural comparison. *Psychol Med* 1989;1919:697–708.
4. Chong MY, Chen CC, Tsang HY, et al. Community study of depression in old age in Taiwan: prevalence, life events and sociodemographic correlates. *Br J Psychiatry* 2001;178:29–35.
5. Takeuchi DT, Chung RCY, Lin KM, et al. Lifetime and twelve-month prevalence rates of major depressive episodes and dysthymia among Chinese Americans in Los Angeles. *Am J Psychiatry* 1998;155:1407–1414.
6. Yeung AS, Chan R, Gresham RL, et al. Prevalence of major depressive disorder among Chinese Americans in primary care. *Gen Hosp Psychiatry* 2004;26:24–30.
7. US Department of Health and Human Services. Asian health care for Asian Americans and Pacific Islanders. In: *Mental health: culture, race, and ethnicity: a supplement to mental health: a report of the Surgeon General.* Rockville, MD: US Department of Health and Human Services, 2001: 107–126.
8. Atkinson DR, Gim RH. Asian American cultural identity and attitudes toward mental health services. *J Counsel Psychol* 1989;36:209–215.
9. Kleinman AM. *Patients and healers in the context of culture: an exploration of the borderland between anthropology, medicine and psychiatry.* Berkeley: University of California Press, 1980.
10. Marsella AJ, Sartorius N, Jablensky A, et al. Cross-cultural studies of depressive disorders: an overview. In: Kleinman A, Good B, eds. *Culture and depression.* Berkeley and Los Angeles, CA: University of California Press, 1985:299–324.
11. Kleinman AM. *Social origins of distress and disease.* New Haven: Yale University Press, 1986.
12. Hsu FLK. Suppression versus repression. *Psychiatry* 1949;12:223
13. Kleinman A. Neurasthenia and depression: a study of somatization and culture in China. *Cult Med Psychiatry* 1982;6:117–190.
14. Bui KV, Takeuchi DT. Ethnic minority adolescents and the use of community mental health care services. *Am J Commun Psychol* 1992;20:403–417.
15. Katon W, Kleinman A, Rosen G. Depression and somatization, a review: part I. *Am J Med* 1982; 72:127–135
16. Fisch RZ. Masked depression: its interrelations with somatization, hypochondriasis, and conversion. *Int J Psychiatry Med* 1987;17:367–379.
17. Lerner J, Noy P. Somatic complaints in psychiatric disorders: social and cultural factors. *Int J Soc Psychiatry* 1968;14:145–150.
18. Leff J. Culture and the differentiation of emotional states. *Br J Psychiatry* 1973;123:299–306.
19. Cheung FM, Lau BWK. Situational variations of help-seeking behavior among Chinese patients. *Comp Psychiatry* 1982;23:252–262.
20. Cheung FM. Conceptualization of psychiatric illness and help-seeking behavior among Chinese. *Cult Med Psychiatry* 1987;11:97–106.
21. Yeung AS, Gresham RL Jr, Mischoulon D, et al. Illness beliefs of depressed Chinese Americans in primary care. *J Nerv Ment Dis* 2004;192:324–327.
22. Zheng Y, Wei L, Goa L, et al. Applicability of the Chinese Beck Depression Inventory. *Comp Psychiatry* 1988;29:484–489.

23. Yeung AS, Howarth S, Chan R, et al. Use of the Chinese version of the Beck Depression Inventory for screening depression in primary care. *J Nerv Ment Dis* 2002;190:94–99.
24. First MB, Spitzer RL, Gibbon M, et al. *Structured Clinical Interview for Axis I DSM-IV Disorders (Version 2.0)—Patient Edition.* New York: Biometrics Research Department, New York State Psychiatric Institute, 1995.
25. Weiss MG, Doongaji DR, Siddhartha S, et al. The explanatory model interview catalogue (EMIC): contribution to cross-cultural research methods from a study of leprosy and mental health. *Br J Psychiatry* 1992;160:819–830.
26. Kirmayer LJ, Robbins JM. Patients who somatize in primary care: a longitudinal study of cognitive and social characteristics. *Psychol Med* 1996;26:937–951.
27. Cheng FM. Somatization among Chinese: a critique. *Bull Hong Kong Psychol Soc* 1982;Jan:27–35.
28. Taylor GJ. Alexithymia: concept, measurement, and implications for treatment. *Am J Psychiatry* 1984;141:725–732.
29. Sue S, Morishima JK. *The mental health of Asian Americans.* San Francisco, CA: Jossey-Bass Publishers, 1982.
30. Jenkins JH, Kleinman A, Good BJ. Cross-cultural studies of depression. In: Becker J, Kleinman A, eds. *Advances in mood disorders.* Hillsdale, NJ: Erlbaum, 1990.
31. Manson SM. Culture and DSM-IV: implications for the diagnosis of mood and anxiety disorders. In: Mezzich JE, Kleinman A, Fabrega H, et al, eds. *Culture and psychiatric diagnosis: a DSM-IV perspective.* Washington, DC: American Psychiatric Press, 1996.
32. Tseng WS. Cultural comments on mood and anxiety disorder: I. In: Mezzich JE, Kleinman A, Fabrega H, et al., eds. *Culture and psychiatric diagnosis: a DSM-IV perspective.* Washington, DC: American Psychiatric Press, 1996.
33. De Craemer W. A Cross-cultural perspective of personhood. *Milbank Q* 1983;61: 19–34.
34. Manson SM, Walker RD, Kivlahan DR. Psychiatric assessment and treatment of American Indians and Alaska Natives. *Hosp Comm Psychiatry* 1987;38:165–173.
35. King AYC, Bond MH. The Confucian paradigm of man: a sociological view. In: Tseng WS, Wu DYH, eds. *Chinese culture and mental health.* London: Academic Press, 1985.
36. Johnson RF. *Lion and dragon in northern China.* New York: Dutton, 1910.
37. Chih A. *Chinese humanism: a religion beyond religion.* Taipei: Chia Feng Printing Enterprise, 1981.
38. Maciocia G. *The foundations of Chinese medicine: a comprehensive text for acupuncturists and herbalists.* London: Churchill-Livingstone, 1989.
39. Kaptchuk T. *The web that has no weaver: understanding Chinese medicine.* New York: Contemporary Books, 2000.
40. Simon G, Gater R, Kisely S, et al. Somatic symptoms of distress: an international primary care study. *Psychosomatic Medicine* 1996;58:481–488.
41. Lipowski ZJ. Somatization and depression. *Psychosomatics* 1990;31:13–21.
42. Kirmayer LJ, Fletcher C, Corin E, et al. Inuit concepts of mental health and illness: an ethnographic study (working paper 4). Montreal: Culture and Mental Health Research Unit, Department of Psychiatry, Sir Mortimer B. David-Jewish General Hospital, 1994.
43. Yeung AS, Howarth S, Nierenberg AA, et al. Outcome of recognizing major depression among Chinese patients in primary care. Presented at the 153rd Annual Meeting of the American Psychiatric Association. Chicago, Illinois, 2000.
44. Yeung AS, Kung WW, Chung H, et al. Integrating psychiatry and primary care improves acceptability to mental health services among Asian Americans. *Gen Hosp Psychiatry* 2004 *(in press).*

3

Panic Attacks in Traumatized Southeast Asian Refugees

Mechanisms and Treatment Implications

*[†]Devon E. Hinton, [†]Vuth Pich, and *Mark H. Pollack

**Department of Psychiatry, Massachusetts General Hospital, Boston, Massachusetts 02114; and †Southeast Asian Clinic, Arbour Counseling Center, Lowell, Massachussetts 01852*

I. INTRODUCTION

A. Background: The Cambodian and Vietnamese Refugee Experience

During the Pol Pot regime (1975–1979), when the Khmer Rouge ruled the country, between 1 and 3 million of Cambodia's 7 million people died (1,2). Disease, starvation, slave labor, displacement, and sexual and physical violence (3–7) were constant assaults, with starvation killing the most people. As the well-nourished Khmer Rouge watched, the populace withered, forced to toil at producing crops while fed a watery gruel—crops that were immediately whisked away upon harvesting and sold by the Khmer Rouge to China for munitions and other products. This process was justified as a rite of purification by which the so-called effete capitalists, the members of the former regime and their sympathizers, would be eliminated. In starvation, the body grew thinner each day until it swelled because of a lack of protein, and then it soon shrank back down to a skeletal form, reduced to skin over bone; if the person didn't obtain larger daily rations of food, the cycle repeated itself two or three times before death occurred.

To reach the United States, a Cambodian had to pass through various horrific events that can categorized into five main periods: (i) the time of Khmer Rouge domination from 1975–1979, when so many Cambodians starved to death, died from illness, or—if deemed by the Khmer Rouge to be feigning illness, to be too slow in completing allotted work, or to be a representative of the former regime by virtue of social status or education—were brutally killed (most typically by a blow to the back of the head); (ii) the Vietnamese invasion in 1979, when many Khmer were caught in cross-fire, while others were killed in violence unleashed by the Khmer Rouge in a paranoid rage; (iii) traversing the country to the Thai border, which might take up to a month, during which many succumbed to illness and starvation; (iv) the actual border crossing into Thailand along a mined road patrolled by marauders, the road strewn with corpses in various stages of decay, dead from starvation, mine explosions, or murder; and (v) in Thailand, the hardship of a long stay in chaotic and dangerous refugee camps, awaiting permission to come to the United States (1). Upon arrival to the United States, Cambodians had to adjust to a completely new culture and language, facing poverty and urban violence.

Like the Cambodians, the Vietnamese people passed through years of civil war, although their experiences manifested significant differences (8). After the communists gained control of the country in 1975, former Southern Vietnamese officials were imprisoned, often for over 10 years; in prison, the political detainees were subjected to illness, torture, slave labor, and starvation. The detainee's property was seized, and his wife and children sent to jungle areas to face harassment, illness, overwork, and starvation.

Upon attempting escape by boat to the United States, most Vietnamese suffered dehydration, starvation, and seasickness, and many were raped, beaten, and robbed by pirates. Most Vietnamese attempted escape in a small boat, and there was the ever-present threat of becoming lost in the ocean, being capsized in a storm, or running out of fuel, left to float aimlessly on the waves until either death or rescue occurred. Like the Cambodians, Vietnamese refugees then confronted a long and difficult stay in refugee camps, and the often-painful transition to living in the United States.

B. Posttraumatic Stress Disorder and Panic Disorder in Southeast Asian Refugees

As would be expected, traumatized Cambodian and Vietnamese refugees have very high rates of posttraumatic stress disorder (PTSD)—over 70% in surveys of psychiatric clinic populations (6–8). These two Southeast Asian refugee groups also have elevated rates of panic disorder (PD)—in psychiatric clinic populations, 60% among Cambodians (9) and 50% among Vietnamese (10). In addition, they display unique panic attack subtypes: "orthostatic panic," that is, panic triggered by dizziness and other sensations experienced upon rising upright from a sitting or lying position; "gastrointestinal panic," that is, panic with prominent gastrointestinal distress (this subtype is much more common among Cambodian refugees); "sore neck" panic, that is, panic focusing on neck sensations (this subtype is found only among Cambodian refugees); and "headache panic," that is, panic with prominent head pain (9,10).

Panic attacks are a central aspect of both PD and PTSD (11,12). PTSD-type panic attacks are classifiable by trigger—a sudden noise, a flashback, or a trauma-related stimulus. PD-related panic attacks may be classified by the triggering situation (like a shopping mall), sensation (focusing, for example, on chest pain), and catastrophic cognition (such as fear of stroke, asphyxia, insanity, heart attack, or loss of bowel control). But how does one classify panic attacks that have characteristics of both PTSD and PD? How can one know whether a patient's so-called PD-type panic attack might also be classified as a PTSD-type panic attack? For it may be that some still-unidentified traumatic event acts as the source of the panic cues, or it may not have been realized that some known traumatic event was the source of the panic cue (11,12,18,19). And how does one classify a so-called PTSD-type panic attack—that is, a panic attack triggered by a trauma-related stimulus, as in a smell—if catastrophic cognitions, for example, fear of asphyxia, are also present? Given that PTSD-type panic attacks and PD-type panic attacks are physiologically similar—both resulting from the activation of amygdala-based fear networks (20–22)—and hybrid types often occur, the clinician should phenomenologically characterize these panic attacks by symptomatology and associated cognitions.

In certain traumatized groups—Cambodian and Vietnamese refugees being two examples—panic attacks are a central complaint. When treating members of these groups, panic attacks should therefore be a key area of clinical assessment and therapeutic intervention, with the clinician profiling symptomatology and identifying catastrophic cognitions and trauma associations. In this chapter we describe the *TCMIE model of panic attack generation,* in which "T" stands for trauma associations, "C" for catastrophic cognitions, "M" for metaphoric associations, "I" for interoceptive conditioning of an arousal-reactive sensation to psychological and somatic fear, and "E" for escalating arousal. After introducing the TCMIE model of panic attack generation, we will illustrate how it can be applied to the Southeast Asian population, focusing on Cambodian examples. We will demonstrate the model's application to the understanding and treatment of orthostatic panic attacks among Cambodian refugees, illustrating these principles with an extended case study, and conclude by outlining the broader treatment implications of the TCMIE model.

II. THE TCMIE MODEL OF PANIC ATTACK GENERATION

Why do Southeast Asian patients have such a high rate of panic disorder? What are the mechanisms that produce unique panic attack subtypes? In this section, we will try to answer these questions by exploring traditional models of panic attacks in PD and PTSD and introducing an approach that integrates and expands these theories, the TCMIE (multiplex) model.

A. Clark's Model of Panic Attack Generation in Panic Disorder

According to Clark's (23) model of how panic occurs in a patient with panic disorder, the patient initially experiences an arousal-reactive sensation—also called an anxiety-reactive sensation—namely, a symptom made worse by the biology of anxiety itself, as in dizziness or palpitations. The patient catastrophically cognizes about the arousal-reactive sensation and so becomes frightened. When the patient experiences fear, the arousal-reactive sensation may intensify by two mechanisms. In *attentional amplification,* the very act of seeking a symptom amplifies that symptom, like a camera focusing down on one object. In *physiological amplification,* the biology of fear worsens certain symptoms by the activation of the autonomic nervous system (ANS); sympathetic nervous system activation, for example, causes palpitations by a direct influence on the heart and produces cold hands and feet by vasoconstriction. When attentional and physiological amplification worsens the symptom, the patient becomes even more frightened. Then the increased fear leads to yet more attentional and physiological amplification of the symptom. In this way, the patient becomes caught in an escalating spiral of fear (see Figs. 3-1 and 3-2).

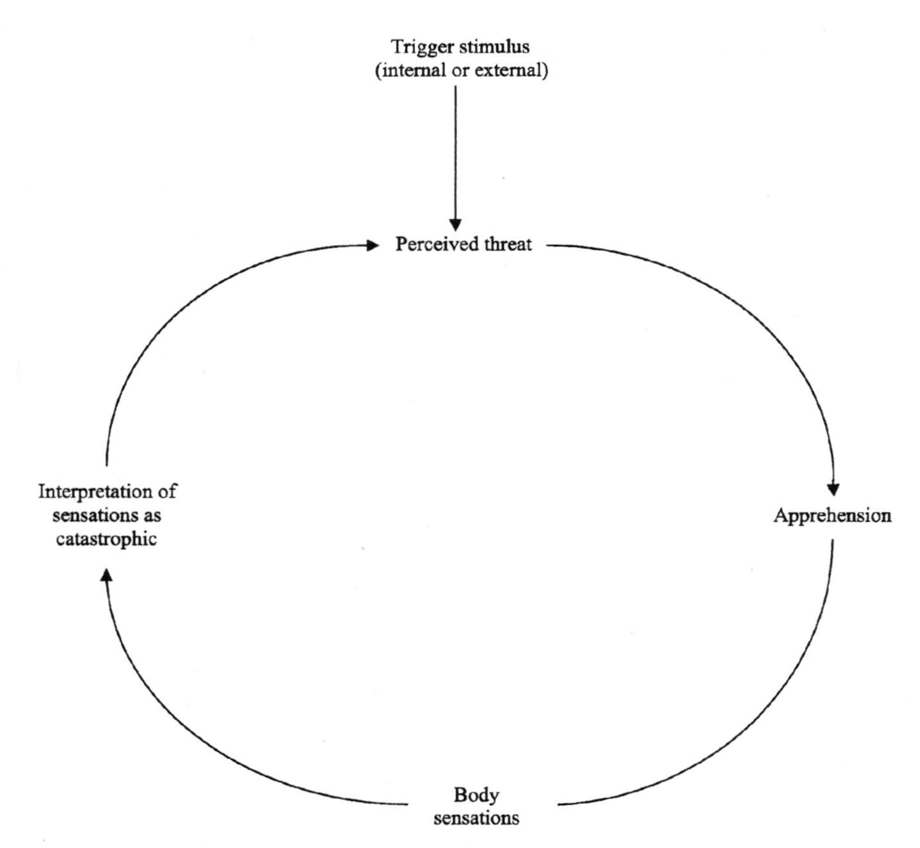

FIG. 3-1. A cognitive model of panic attack. (Adapted from Clark D. A cognitive approach to panic. *Behav Res Ther* 1986;24:461–470.)

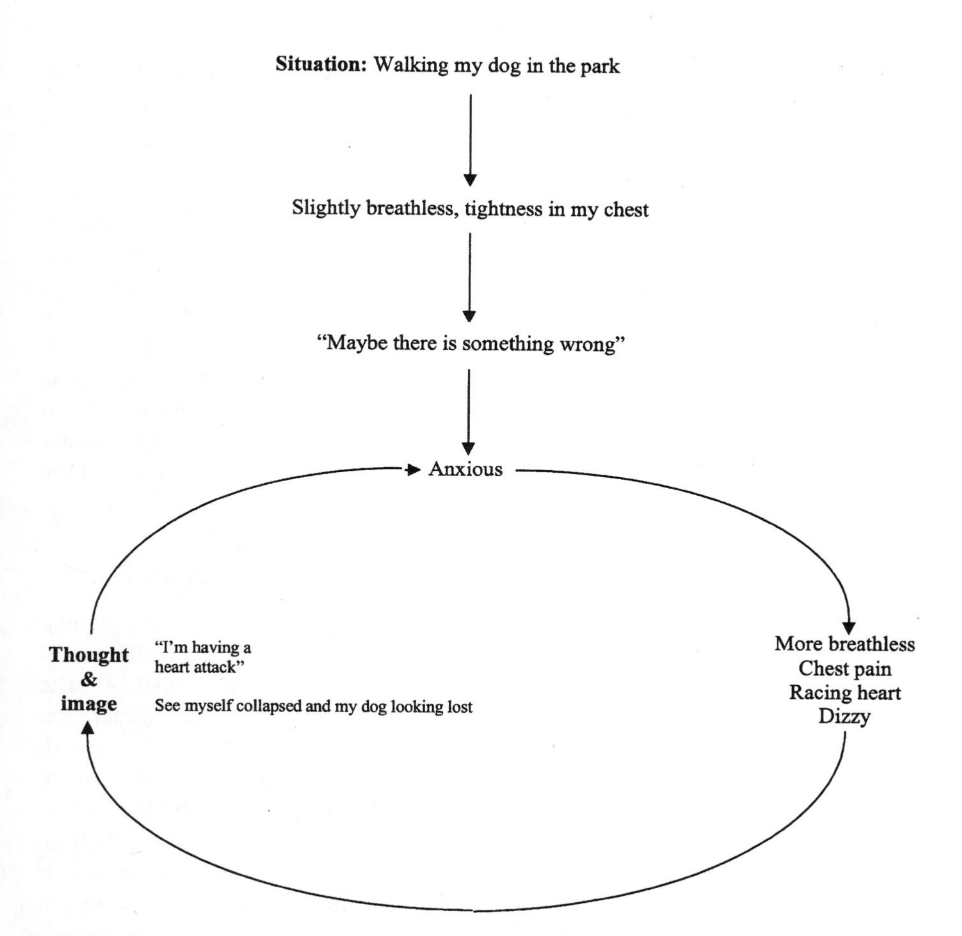

FIG. 3-2. A specific panic attack. (Adapted from Clark D, Wells A. Cognitive therapy for anxiety disorders. In: Dickstein L, Riba M, Oldham J, eds. *Review of psychiatry.* Washington, DC: APA Press, 1997:1–9.)

B. Typical Model of Panic Attack Generation in PTSD

PTSD-type panic attacks may be triggered by an external stimulus if the following conditions are met: (i) a person underwent a traumatic event, (ii) an external stimulus present during the trauma became encoded into the memory of the traumatic event, (iii) the person now encounters the external stimulus that was encoded into the trauma memory, and (iv) this encounter with the external stimulus activates the trauma memory. For example, the person may either meet someone who resembles the perpetrator or smell an odor that was present during the trauma, and then this exterior stimulus causes fear and dysphoria and possibly a vivid recall of the event. Alternatively, the panic-attack trigger may be a stimulus not related to the trauma—for example, a loud noise—that activates fear circuits in a hyperexcitable amygdala.

C. Clark's Model Applied to PTSD-Type Panic Attacks

Clark's model for PD-type panic attacks can be applied to PTSD-type panic attacks. If an arousal-reactive sensation becomes encoded into a traumatic memory network, then later, when this trauma-related arousal-reactive sensation is experienced (e.g., dizziness as a result of hyperventilation), a *positive feedback loop* may lead to an escalating spiral of arousal (see Fig. 3-3). For example, if dizziness, as in the vertigo experienced upon encountering maggot-infested corpses, becomes a prominent node of that fear network, then when dizziness is experienced, it may activate this memory—of the maggot-infested corpses—and cause an increase of fear, and the increase of fear will lead to yet more dizziness, which in turn leads to yet more activation of the memory network, and so on, until panic occurs.

D. The TCMIE (Multiplex) Model of Panic Attack Generation

To explain the high rate of panic attacks—and unique panic attacks—among trauma-exposed Cambodian and Vietnamese refugees, we have proposed the TCMIE model of panic generation, or *multiplex model of panic attack generation* (9,10,24). The multiplex model is based on the psychological theory of panic attack generation (23,25)—in particular, Clark's model, as described earlier (23)—and fear network theory (26). According to the multiplex model, a trigger—anger, exertion, a worry episode, orthostasis, overeating, head rotation, hyperventilation, or thinking about a traumatic event—causes the patient to experience an arousal-reactive symptom, such as dizziness. The arousal-reactive sensation then activates one or more of four different types of dysphoria networks: catastrophic cognitions, trauma associations, metaphoric resonances, and interoceptive conditioning.

Earlier, we discussed the structure of catastrophic cognitions and trauma associations. The term *metaphoric resonances* refers to how certain sensations, like a feeling of dizziness, may bring to mind existential and social issues: a confrontation with life's meaning, or a sense of confused anger with circling thoughts about a personal dilemma. Put another way, a sensation may evoke metaphor-encoded distress. Interoceptive conditioning designates the following process: If a patient endures repeated panic attacks, then by a process of conditioning, the patient's neural networks construct an associative link between interoceptive sensations—that is, some internal bodily sensation, as in dizziness—and somatic and psychological fear (25).

A patient feels mounting anxiety when one or more of the four types of dysphoria networks—catastrophic cognitions, trauma associations, metaphoric resonances, and interoceptive conditioning—is activated by the arousal-reactive sensation. As anxiety increases, it aggravates the arousal-reactive symptom by attentional and physiological amplification. When the arousal-reactive symptom worsens, dysphoria networks become even more activated. Through this positive feedback loop, the patient

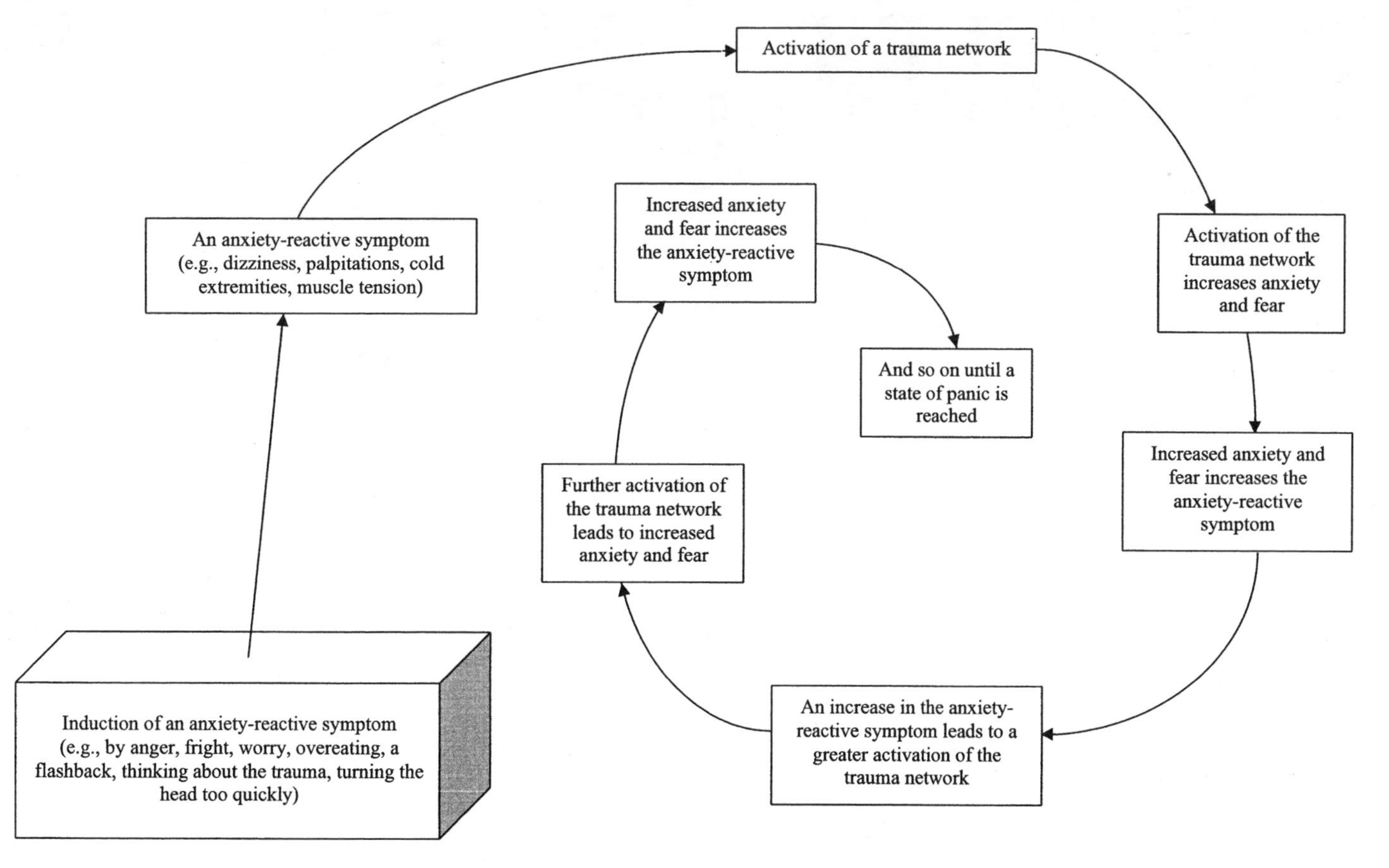

FIG. 3-3. An anxiety-reactive symptom triggering a spiral of panic: the activation of trauma networks.

experiences an escalating spiral of arousal that leads to a panic attack. If all four types of fear networks are simultaneously activated, we refer to this as a TCMIE panic attack (see Fig. 3-4) (10,24).

The TCMIE model provides a way to classify panic attacks. Although one could alternatively use the categories of PTSD-type panic attacks, PD-type panic attacks, and PTSD–PD-type panic attacks, or hybrid panic attacks, this terminology is imprecise. In the TCMIE model, a patient may experience a *traumatic memory panic attack,* i.e., a panic attack driven by the activation of a trauma-related fear network; a *catastrophic cognitions* (CC) panic attack, i.e., a panic attack driven by catastrophic cognitions concerning arousal-reactive symptoms; a *metaphoric resonances* (MR) panic attack, i.e., a panic attack driven by metaphoric resonances to the sensation; or an *interoceptive conditioning* (IC) panic attack, i.e., a panic attack driven by the interoceptive conditioning of an arousal-reactive symptom directly to the affect and physiology of fear. Moreover, patients may experience panic attacks that consist of various combinations of the above: a *traumatic memory/catastrophic cognitions/ escalating arousal* (TCE) panic attack; a *traumatic memory/catastrophic cognitions/ metaphoric resonances/escalating arousal* (TCME) panic attack; or a *traumatic memory/catastrophic cognitions/metaphoric resonances/interoceptive conditioning/ escalating arousal* (TCMIE) panic attack.

III. THE SOUTHEAST ASIAN UNDERSTANDING OF ANXIETY SYMPTOMS: AN ETHNOPHYSIOLOGY OF WIND

Cambodians and Vietnamese consider anxiety symptoms to be generated by the effects of wind on the body. This interpretation of physiological arousal leads to frequent CC panic attacks. Below, we will only discuss the Cambodian ethnophysiology of wind; for a discussion of these same processes among Vietnamese patients, see our previous work (10,27).

A. An Ethnophysiology of *Khyâl:* The Cambodian Understanding of Anxiety Symptoms

"Why am I dizzy? What is causing my dizziness? Does this dizziness indicate a serious medical problem?" These are the types of questions that a person asks upon first noticing a bodily symptom. Cambodians interpret somatic sensations in terms of a pathomechanics of *khyâl* (28,29). *Khyâl* refers not only to "wind," the air that sweeps over the external environment, but also to a key part of bodily physiology, an air that courses along the inner conduits of the body alongside blood. Cambodians immediately attribute somatic anxiety sensations to the complex pathomechanics of an ethnophysiology of *khyâl;* consequently, somatic anxiety symptoms generate great fear. Cambodians refer to any anxiety episode, especially a panic attack, as a "*khyâl* attack" ("wind attack," or *kaeut khyâl*). [For a discussion of related Vietnamese ideas about *gió,* a term that, like *khyâl,* refers both to an external and bodily wind, see Hinton et al. (27).]

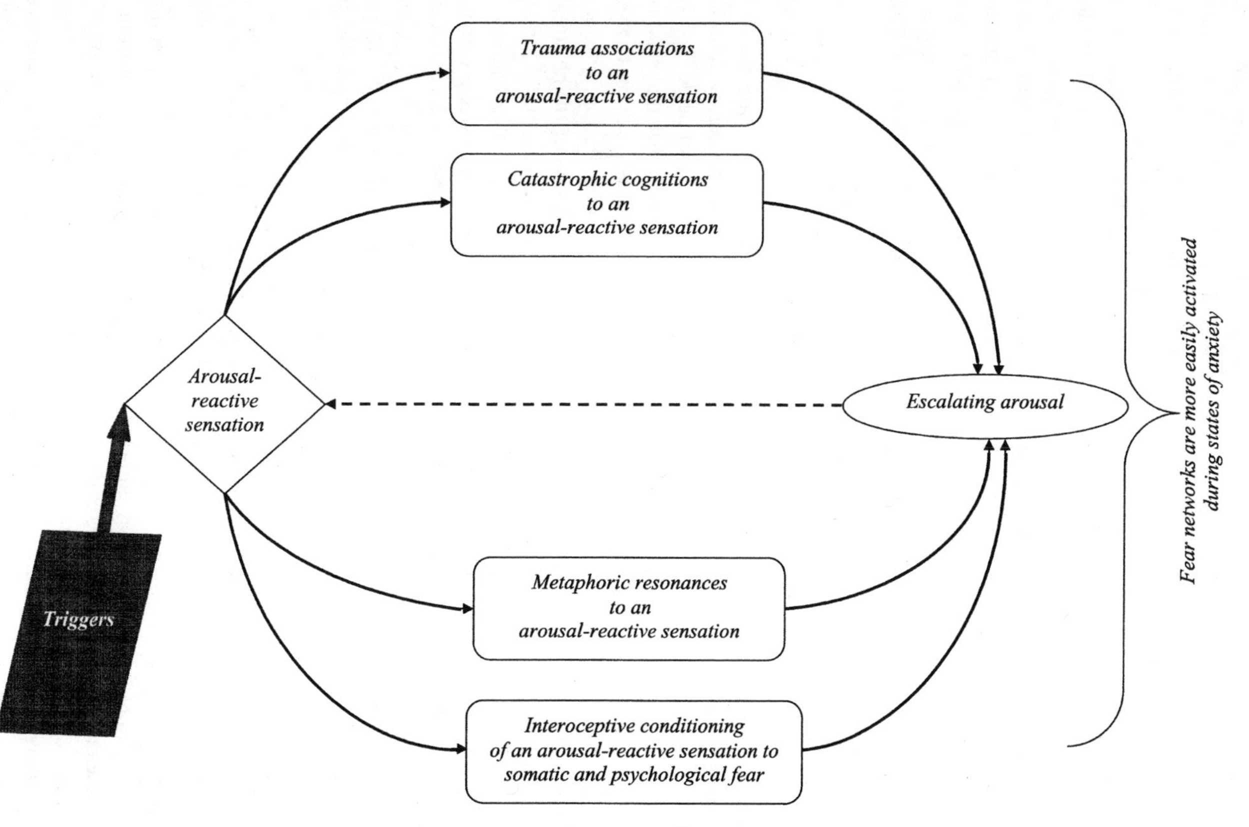

FIG. 3-4. The generation of a TCMIE panic attack.

Let us further examine how the Cambodian understanding of how what we call "somatic anxiety symptoms" is generated. When healthy, the person's blood and *khyâl* ("inner air") run unimpeded through conduits in the body (28,29). Symptoms of joint discomfort or cold hands and feet result from the blockage of the flow of blood and *khyâl* through the vessels, with the knee and elbow being considered the locations of most frequent blockage. If not corrected, this blockage leads to the "death" of the limb distal to the blockage as a result of insufficient blood. If blood and *khyâl* cannot flow outward along the limb, they ascend upwards in the body, bringing about various disturbances: Blood and *khyâl* (i) enter the thorax, causing palpitations and shortness of breath—possibly resulting in cardiac arrest and fatal asphyxia; (ii) distend the neck vessels, causing neck soreness—and possibly neck-vessel rupture; or (iii) enter the head, causing dizziness, tinnitus (*khyâl* exiting from the ears), and blurry vision (*khyâl* exiting the eyes)—and possibly syncope, deafness, and blindness.

B. The Self-Treatment of a *Khyâl* Attack

Because Cambodians consider anxiety attacks to be generated by *khyâl,* they self-treat anxiety attacks through *khyâl*-extraction techniques, most frequently "coining" and "cupping." Coining is performed on the arms, chest, back, and neck. To coin, a Cambodian dips the edge of a coin in "*khyâl* oil," a menthol substance that promotes *khyâl*'s escape from the body. He or she next places the coin edge upon the skin, and then drags the coin along the skin in a proximal-to-distal direction, producing a linear mark upon the epidermis. Patients worriedly assess the color of the streaks: A red color denotes minimal *khyâl* accumulation; a darker hue, especially a purple color, indicates excessive bodily *khyâl.* Upon noting a purple color, a Cambodian becomes much more concerned, immediately initiating more coining and often another second-line "*khyâl*-removal" technique, almost always cupping. To cup, Cambodians apply a warmed glass to the skin, most usually to the back or to the forehead. When the glass cools, the contained air contracts, and the resulting vacuum pulls the skin into the glass, purportedly pulling *khyâl* through the skin pores and into the glass.

C. The Cambodian Ethnophysiology of *Khyâl* and the Predisposition to Catastrophic Cognitions Panic Attacks

As shown in the previous section, the Cambodian's pathophysiology of somatic anxiety symptoms, based on an ethnophysiology of blood and *khyâl,* profoundly influences the interpretation of anxiety states and gives rise to fears of dire physical outcomes caused by a pathomechanics of blood and *khyâl.* Although *khyâl* may be a culture-specific concern, these thoughts fit the same form as the catastrophic cognitions in Western cultures that often increase anxiety symptoms to the point of panic; in the West, these include fear of death and disability ("Am I having a stroke?" "Is this a heart attack?") and fear of insanity ("Am I having a nervous breakdown?")

(23,30,31). The natural result of such catastrophic thinking—about *khyâl* concerns or other catastrophic explanations of symptoms—is increased anxiety. Panic intensity is correlated with the severity of associated catastrophic cognitions (32). The Cambodian refugee's complex explanatory models for anxiety symptoms, the *khyâl* ethnophysiology, provide one source of catastrophic fears that may drive panic responses to anxiety-related and other somatic sensations.

IV. THE TCMIE MODEL OF PANIC GENERATION IN CULTURAL CONTEXT

In this section, we will explore how the catastrophic cognitions, trauma associations, and metaphoric resonances of Cambodian patients to specific arousal-reactive sensations generate a TCMIE panic attack. [For a discussion of these same processes among Vietnamese patients, see our previous work (10,27).] Each section also begins with a short description of how the sensation is generated by physiological mechanisms according to current Western scientific understanding. Each arousal-reactive symptom may be produced by the physiology of general anxiety, chronic anxiety, or acute fear, most usually by means of an activation of the sympathetic and parasympathetic branches of the autonomic nervous system—what we called above "physiological amplification." In addition, attentional amplification—produced, for example, by concerns that the symptom has important health consequences—plays an important role in the initial generation of the symptom. In each culture, during anxiety states, anxiety-mediated effects on bodily physiology generate certain symptoms that then become a sort of Rorschach to which persons of a specific culture and personal history react. This reaction is in large part generated by the local understanding of physiology that gives rise to catastrophic cognitions about somatic and psychological anxiety symptoms, by trauma associations, and by metaphoric meanings.

A. Dizziness Dysphoria Networks

The Production of Dizziness

Dizziness may be produced by the ANS or by such mechanisms as hyperventilation. Other complex mechanisms of dizziness generation include increased vestibular sensitivity (hence motion sickness) and decreased baroreceptor sensitivity (hence an excessive decrease in blood pressure upon standing and dizziness). Several authors have noted the prominence of dizziness as a dysphoric response among Cambodian and Vietnamese refugees (33,34); and Asians more generally may be unusually susceptible to dizziness, particularly motion sickness and orthostatic dizziness (10,33). Usually the Cambodian patient's dizziness occurs during episodes of worry (including worry about somatic symptoms such as sore neck), orthostasis, and agoraphobia (e.g., when in a mall or riding in a car) (9,10,28,29), with dizziness and other symptoms often increasing to the point of panic.

Catastrophic Cognitions about Dizziness

Cambodians consider dizziness to be the key indicator of an upward rise of blood and *khyâl.* As discussed earlier, dizziness indicates that *khyâl* has risen upwards in the body all the way to the head, a severe state called a "*khyâl* attack" (or "wind attack," *kaeut khyâl*). Upon experiencing dizziness, the patient will search the body for other signs of excessive inner wind and a dysregulation of blood and wind flow—cold hands and feet, shortness of breath, palpitations, sore neck, tinnitus—and will fear all the various catastrophes associated with excessive inner wind: stroke, asphyxia, heart arrest, deafness, vision loss, syncope, rupture of the neck vessels. Also, Cambodians believe that moving to the upright position from a sitting or lying position may cause a sudden surge of blood and *khyâl* towards the head, called "*khyâl* overload," or "wind overload" (*khyâl ko*), that may cause syncope and even death. Upon standing, a Cambodian anxiously assesses for the presence of bodily symptoms indicative of a pressurized upward rise of blood and *khyâl* toward the head—of an event of "*khyâl* overload." Dizziness will be attributed to a sudden surge of blood and *khyâl* into the head; a sore neck, to distension of the neck vessels by blood and *khyâl;* blurry vision, to *khyâl* exiting the eyes; tinnitus (called "*khyâl* exiting from the ears," *khyâl ceuny pii treujieu*), to the forceful exiting of *khyâl* from the auditory canal. Cold feet and hands are attributed to the blockages of blood flow along the limbs, which will cause an upward surge of blood and *khyâl; khyâl* is considered a cold substance that can cause blood to coagulate, most particularly at the knee and elbow joint, thereby preventing blood flow to the feet and hands.

Trauma Associations to Dizziness

In the Pol Pot period, a combination of starvation and overwork caused Cambodians to often stand up and feel dizzy. During the transplanting of rice seedlings, Cambodians bent over and rose up again and again during the course of a day; the ceaseless digging during dam construction required similar motions. Malarial episodes produced yet another dizziness-encoded fear network. Malaria tormented almost all Cambodians during the Pol Pot period. Many Cambodians died of malaria; others recovered in 6 months or so. Attacks typically occurred once a day, with an initial hour-long period of chills followed by an hour-long period of intense fever accompanied by nausea, anxiety, palpitations, shortness of breath, and a severe, retch-inducing dizziness. The dizziness is made far more severe should the person attempt to stand before the complete cessation of the attack. A malarial attack is thus very similar to a cold-type panic attack followed by a hot-type panic attack with extreme vertigo. Malaria predisposes to panic disorder by forming trauma associations—and interoceptive conditioning—to symptoms of autonomic arousal such as chills, dizziness, and palpitations (27). Certain Pol Pot traumas resulted in dizziness by vagal-type mechanisms: seeing blood (e.g., from shrapnel injury), execution eviscerations, and decaying bodies. Exposure to these images most likely caused not only a sensation of dizziness but also an actual deceleration of heart rate and decrease in blood pressure (35).

Metaphoric Resonances of Dizziness

Cambodians frequently utilize dizziness images to describe distress. As an example, if a child acts out and causes distress, a patient often says, "my son shakes me" (*goun greulok knyom*). The very word for being busy is "to be spinning rapidly" (*rewuel*). Worry itself is configured as a kind of spinning of the mind, a turning of the head from one problem to another: "I think here and then I think there, I think up and then I think down" (*kut nih, kut nuh, kut anjeh anjoh*). Patients often string together these expressions when explaining why they currently feel dizzy: "My son shakes me. He makes me dizzy."

B. Palpitations Fear Networks

The Production of Palpitations

Palpitations are produced by attentional amplification and the biology of fear.

Catastrophic Cognitions about Palpitations

Cambodians greatly fear palpitations because of concerns about a cultural syndrome called "weak heart" (36). Palpitations, resulting, for example, from anger or a loud noise, indicate a "weak heart" (*ksaoy beh doung*). It is believed that a weak heart may suddenly stop functioning, especially during episodes of palpitations.

Trauma Associations to Palpitations

During a trauma, seized by fear, one becomes suddenly aware of the heart, a rapid pounding in the chest. Trauma triggered by sudden loud noises is particularly likely to have this effect. Airplane bombs, grenades, mines, and mortar shells killed many Cambodians during the years leading up to the Khmer Rouge takeover in 1975, and again in 1979 during the Vietnamese invasion of the country. For this reason, various trauma memories, encoded by vigorous palpitations, are recalled by unusual movements of the heart.

Metaphoric Resonances of Palpitations

To be offended is "to have pain in the heart" (*chuu ceut*).

C. Abdominal Sensations Dysphoria Networks

The Production of Abdominal Sensations

Acute and chronic anxiety produce abdominal bloating, discomfort, and other sensations; for example, acute fear causes a decrease of blood in the stomach and sense of lightness and cold in that area. In American populations, anxiety-mediated gastrointestinal distress often causes such functional disorders as irritable bowel syndrome; but in the Cambodian population, abdominal sensations trigger multiple dysphoria networks, leading to panic.

Catastrophic Cognitions about Abdominal Sensations

During anxiety states, North American PD patients commonly experience a sudden "sinking sensation in the stomach" or "butterflies in the stomach" (37,38), but these sensations do not commonly give rise to catastrophic cognitions of dangerous bodily dysfunction—at most, patients experience embarrassment and fear of loss of bowel control. In contrast, Cambodians interpret a tight or gaseous abdomen as evidence of "upwards hitting *khyâl" (khyâl theau laeung leu*). This upwardly ascending *khyâl* may impede breathing, inhibit normal heart motion, and produce neck soreness, tinnitus, and dizziness. The fears of "upwards hitting *khyâl*" become more severe should the Cambodian remark any corporal signs of excessive *khyâl,* for example, a sore neck or tinnitus.

Trauma Associations to Abdominal Sensations

In the Pol Pot period, prolonged starvation caused abdominal pain and intestinal cramps. Desperate to find any means of nourishment, Cambodians ate indigestible foodstuffs including leaves, rice husks, and the roots of the banana tree, precipitating severe abdominal cramps. Also, gastrointestinal distress was caused by such illnesses as cholera, malaria, and typhoid; by traumatic sights; and by certain accidental ingestions—most particularly, the common event of unknowingly taking water from a pond in which a corpse or corpses floated, the mistake immediately noted upon bringing the water to the lips, the person first detecting a fatty taste and a foul odor, a mistake confirmed by the visual confirmation of the taste's origin, increasing distress even more.

Metaphoric Associations to Abdominal Sensations

Cambodians often speak in idioms—like the English idioms "fed up" or "can't stomach it"—to express that they are no longer able to endure a certain situation: "overfull of a situation" (*ceuaet*) or "fed up in the heart" (*ceuaet ceut*). Also, hate is often cast in images of disgust, as in "he makes me nauseated" (*gpeum*), meaning, "I detest him."

D. Limb-Sensations Fear Networks

The Production of Limb Sensations

Cold hands and feet result from vasoconstriction produced by the sympathetic branch of the ANS and from hyperventilation-caused vasoconstriction. Joint discomfort is produced by excessive muscle tension on the tendons at the joints. Numbness and tingling arise from hyperventilation. Among Americans, such symptoms as joint discomfort give rise to functional syndromes, in particular fibromyalgia; however, as we will see—and as was suggested in the ethnophysiology section—Cambodians react to joint discomfort with great fear owing to various cultural beliefs.

Catastrophic Cognitions about Limb Sensations

According to the Cambodian understanding of bodily physiology, various limb sensations—such as cold hands and feet, muscular and joint pain—signal the pressurized build-up of *khyâl* at the knees and elbows. Lacking nurturing blood, the limb may "die," and the *khyâl* and blood may ascend upward toward the trunk and the head (28,29). Thus cold extremities and joint soreness warn of possible "limb death" (*slap day slap ceung;* i.e., stroke) and the *khyâl*'s imminent upsurge toward the trunk, neck, and head.

Trauma Associations to Limb Sensations

During the Pol Pot period, because of starvation, even though ambient temperature remained high, a chill took hold of the body. The intolerable feeling of cold sharpened whenever a Cambodian was forced to work in inclement weather. With the rain pounding down, a cold winter wind striking the body, and the feet in mud and legs up to the knees in water, a Cambodian transplanted rice seedlings, continually pulling leeches from the body—with the cold, the leeches, and the forced labor seemingly conspiring to drain the body of the last inner supplies of energy and warmth. Limb sensations also encode the trauma of malarial attacks; the malarial attack is preceded by muscular pain and soreness; and the attack itself begins with body-shaking chills (like "cold" panic attacks) (27).

Metaphoric Associations to Limb Sensation

Many Cambodian idioms express personal connectedness as a sense of bodily warmth: a good relationship is described as "warm" (*kâ kdaw*). A feeling of blockage at the limb serves as a metaphor of blocked flow, of life and relationship lacking a sense of smooth progression.

E. Neck Tension Fear Networks

The Production of Neck Discomfort

Anxiety states—in particular, panic—increase tension in shoulder and neck musculature, primarily the trapezius muscle, which may cause pain (38–41). And anxiety and panic increase the tension of the frontalis muscle, producing a feeling of pressure in the head (42).

Catastrophic Cognition about Neck Tension

Cambodians attribute neck tension to excessive *khyâl,* and they fear that blood pressure may rupture the neck vessels. Cambodians consider neck sensations to be caused by a pressurized rise of blood and *khyâl* upward into the confines of the cranium. "Sore neck" sensations cue panic attacks among Cambodian refugees by conjuring to mind catastrophic scenarios, most particularly, the bursting the neck vessels by blood and *khyâl,* rising blood and *khyâl* setting the cranial contents to spinning, and *khyâl* shooting forth from the ears and eyes (43).

Trauma Associations to Neck Tension

Cambodians worked up to 15 hours a day during the Pol Pot period. One of the most difficult of the imposed tasks was dam building, consisting of a repeated corvée: Digging enough dirt to fill two buckets and carrying the dirt up the earthen slopes of the growing dam to deposit the contents at the ridge. And if a certain quantity of dirt—that contained in a hole 3 m deep, wide, and long—was not dug out and transported in a given day, then no food was given. Climbing up the side of the dam, the person balanced a pole at the shoulder; at either end of the pole oscillated a bucket filled with dirt. Soon the neck and shoulders ached; long before, these areas had become calloused. Here in the United States, if a Cambodian has a sore neck, it may evoke vivid flashbacks of this labor. Or if it does not evoke a vivid flashback, it evokes a dolorous recall of those events. And if it does not trigger a pained recall of those events, it usually causes the patient to cite those labors as the pain's origin (43). In the Pol Pot period, Khmer Rouge killed Cambodians by striking the back of the victim's head with a wooden club, an execution technique that was called "bursting the neck vessels" (*dac sosai go*). In a common but less used method, Khmer Rouge executed by severing the victim's throat with the serrated edges of a palm-tree frond. And in the Pol Pot period, the constant straining of the neck and shoulder musculature caused soreness, the soreness sensations becoming part of the memory network of all Pol Pot events, so that now, here in the United States, a twinge of the shoulder or neck discomfort brings back to mind Pol Pot events, a sudden sense of dysphoria.

Metaphoric Associations to Neck Tension

In English, we have a multiplicity of metaphors concerning posture and weight carrying that seemingly reflect and contribute to the commonness of back pain as a somatic idiom of distress: overburdened, slouch, "Can't bear any more," shirker, a pillar of the community, upright, rectitude. In Cambodian, many distress expressions are based on the neck. For example, one may say, "*tnguen go,*" meaning "heavy in the neck," to describe a state of being overwhelmed by financial or other problems. You may tell someone, "Don't carry that pole at your neck, with its heavy load, all by yourself" (*gom reek khluen aeng*), meaning, let me help with your burden. Or, if one gives a little money to someone in financial distress, one "helps to carry the pole at the neck, with its heavy load" (*juey reek*).

V. ORTHOSTATICALLY INDUCED PANIC IN CAMBODIANS

Culture-specific dysphoria networks about sensations result in Cambodian patients' experiencing unique panic attack subtypes. Let us now examine orthostatic panic attacks in more detail.

A. Orthostatic Phobia: A TCMIE Panic Subtype

Many Cambodians experience "orthostasis phobia" that may generate panic by mechanisms similar to those that produce *situationally predisposed* panic attacks (44). An agoraphobic may anticipate panicking because of the particularities of a situation, including weather conditions (e.g., a cloudy day), locations marked by sensory complexity and intensity (e.g., a busy traffic intersection), and assessment of bodily state, as in a self-perceived state of bodily vulnerability (e.g., during fatigue). This expectation leads to both increased bodily attention and actual physiological arousal (23,44). Similarly, in a specific situation and bodily state, a Cambodian will consider panic to be more probable. Upon arising from bed in the morning, if a Cambodian slept poorly and is worrying about some problem—with worry and poor sleep both being considered processes that weaken the body—the Cambodian will anticipate feeling dizzy upon standing (36). This self-perceived state of weakness and vulnerability induces anticipatory anxiety that then leads to increased bodily surveillance and actual physiological arousal. Subsequently, upon standing, dizziness may result through attentional amplification (45) and physiological mechanisms [e.g., anxiety causes decreased baroreceptor sensitivity that causes a greater blood pressure fall upon standing (46)]. Then the dizziness sensations, along with other autonomic arousal symptoms, activate dysphoria networks, including trauma associations, metaphoric resonances, catastrophic cognitions, and interoceptive conditioning. This activation of fear networks results in greater anxiety. Next, because dizziness sensations and other autonomic arousal symptoms are arousal reactive, dizziness intensifies. Subsequently, escalating dizziness and other autonomic sensations cause more activation of fear networks. This spiral ultimately may result in panic (23,25). If a patient's neural networks contain all four types of fear networks, and if all four types of fear networks are simultaneously activated, the patient experiences a TCMIE panic attack, involving trauma associations, catastrophic cognitions, metaphoric resonances, interoceptive conditioning, and escalating arousal (see Fig. 3-4) (24).

B. A Case of Orthostatic Dizziness in a Cambodian Man

Upon initial presentation to the psychiatric clinic, the 59-year-old Chan was having orthostatic panic attacks three times a week. During the attacks, he experienced severe dizziness, along with cold hands, palpitations, and neck soreness upon standing. He would immediately sit down, fearing "*khyâl* overload," cardiac arrest, neck-vessel rupture, and "death of the hands and legs" (*ngoeup day ngoeup ceung*). Chan's panic attack would last about an hour. During about a third of the orthostatically induced panic attacks, Chan had a visual flashback of either his brother's execution or of stacks of body parts, the body parts being the butchered bodies of two Cambodians who had attempted escape from his village during the Pol Pot period. Chan's dizziness, neck tension, and palpitations were particularly severe. To relieve the symptoms, Chan immediately began to "coin" his neck and limbs in order to remove excessive inner *khyâl*.

In the Khmer Rouge period, Chan had to work 12 hours a day; twice a day, he was fed a watery broth that contained but a few grains of rice. The work was mainly of two types: rice transplantation and dam building, the latter entailing digging up and then carrying dirt in a bucket in order to help construct a dam. During those tasks—all the while hit by a scorching sun above, undermined by a gnawing hunger, and sapped by chronic malaria—he often felt dizzy, especially after bending over. Many people collapsed while working. In the Pol Pot period, Chan, like most Cambodians, suffered from severe malaria. Chan had malarial attacks every day for 6 months. Each episode essentially formed a cold-type panic attack, usually lasting 45 minutes, marked by rigors and palpitations. This was followed by a hot-type panic attack lasting half an hour, marked by palpitations, headache, extreme dysphoria, and severe dizziness. He was forced to continue working even after a malarial attack commenced. He would struggle to accomplish his task, but when the malarial attack intensified, Chan experienced extreme dizziness and collapsed to the ground; lying vertiginous and helpless, he would be dragged to the side of the field. During the Pol Pot regime, Chan, like most Khmer, was accused by his Khmer Rouge captors of feigning illness; they claimed his malarial attacks were simulated, and he was threatened with execution.

In the Khmer Rouge period, just before the Vietnamese invasion of his village, Chan and his two brothers were transplanting rice about an hour's walk from the village. Suddenly, six Khmer Rouge arrived at the rice field; they arrested both Chan and his brothers. The soldiers had learned that Chan's two brothers were government soldiers prior to the Khmer Rouge invasion. The Khmer Rouge routinely hunted down and executed all former soldiers. Though Chan had worked as a rice farmer his entire life, he was also arrested. Chan was charged with two crimes: being related to a soldier and not revealing his brothers' identities to the authorities. Three Khmer Rouge soldiers escorted Chan's brothers to a distance of about 50 yards while another three Khmer Rouge soldiers remained behind to guard Chan. One of the guards lit a cigarette, and while exhaling smoke directly into Chan's face, told him that they intended to kill and to eviscerate his two brothers and later consume their livers and drink the bile of their gall bladders—in this way, they would assimilate the brothers' vital essence and power, thought to reside in those body parts. Chan's heart pounded against his rib cage, his chest tightened, and his face flushed with blood; his head was sent into a whirling spiral of fear and rage and cigarette fumes. He watched as the Khmer Rouge bound his brothers' hands behind their backs and then fired a rifle into each brother's chest. The soldiers escorted Chan to his dead brothers and forced him to watch as they cut open the abdomens with a long knife, cut out the livers—the gall bladder still attached—and placed them on a banana leaf. Chan was overcome with panic, nausea, dizziness, and leg weakness; he thought himself about to collapse. (The sight of blood may have triggered a vagal response.) The soldiers let him go, loudly announcing that he would experience a similar fate if he committed any errors.

A few weeks later, the Khmer Rouge commanded the villagers to assemble before the leader's house. Chan and his fellow villagers were forced to view the butchered corpses of two people who had tried to escape the village. The body parts were placed in orderly heaps arranged by body part: eight limbs (four lower and four upper limbs); two heads, severed at the neck; two eviscerated trunks, the flaps of skin draping to either side like small flexible doors, revealing an abdominal cavity from which the liver had been extricated and eaten. Weak-kneed, dizzy, and nauseated, Chan stared at the horrifying image of his own likely fate. (Note the prominence of blood in this trauma memory.) A month later, Vietnamese invaded his village; he seized the moment to escape and managed to reach the Thai border.

Recent events had caused Chan to become more anxious. His 18-year-old son had stopped school, stayed out until late at night, and acted very disrespectfully towards him, often using foul language. Thinking about his son made Chan angry, anxious, and dizzy. When he stood up and felt dizzy, thoughts about this son circled through his mind, increasing distress and dysphoria. For Chan, dizziness encoded memories of specific social problems and conflicts, and if he became distressed for any reason, by worrying, for example, that standing up may cause him to collapse, the resulting dizziness activated these memory networks. Also, when he thought about a current social or financial problem, such as his son, dizziness and other symptoms were evoked that then predisposed him to panic upon standing. Sometimes, if he thought about his conflicts with this son just before standing, dizziness and panic upon rising became severe. Chan was concerned that worry about his son "weakened" him (directly and by decreasing sleep and appetite), predisposing to dizziness upon standing. In addition, he and his wife were having conflicts, many of their fights centering on issues of how to deal with the son. (For a summary of Chan's case in terms of the TCMIE model, see Fig. 3-5.)

VI. TREATMENT IMPLICATIONS OF THE TCMIE MODEL OF PANIC ATTACK GENERATION

The TCMIE model of panic attack generation has therapeutic implications. During the treatment of a Southeast Asian with panic, catastrophic cognitions concerning orthostasis should be specifically addressed, as is standard in panic treatment protocols (48). The trauma networks associated with arousal symptoms experienced during the panic attack need to be explored (11,16), and the metaphoric resonances of the prominent symptoms to current social and financial duress must be investigated. If symptoms persist despite the modifying of catastrophic cognitions, the exploring

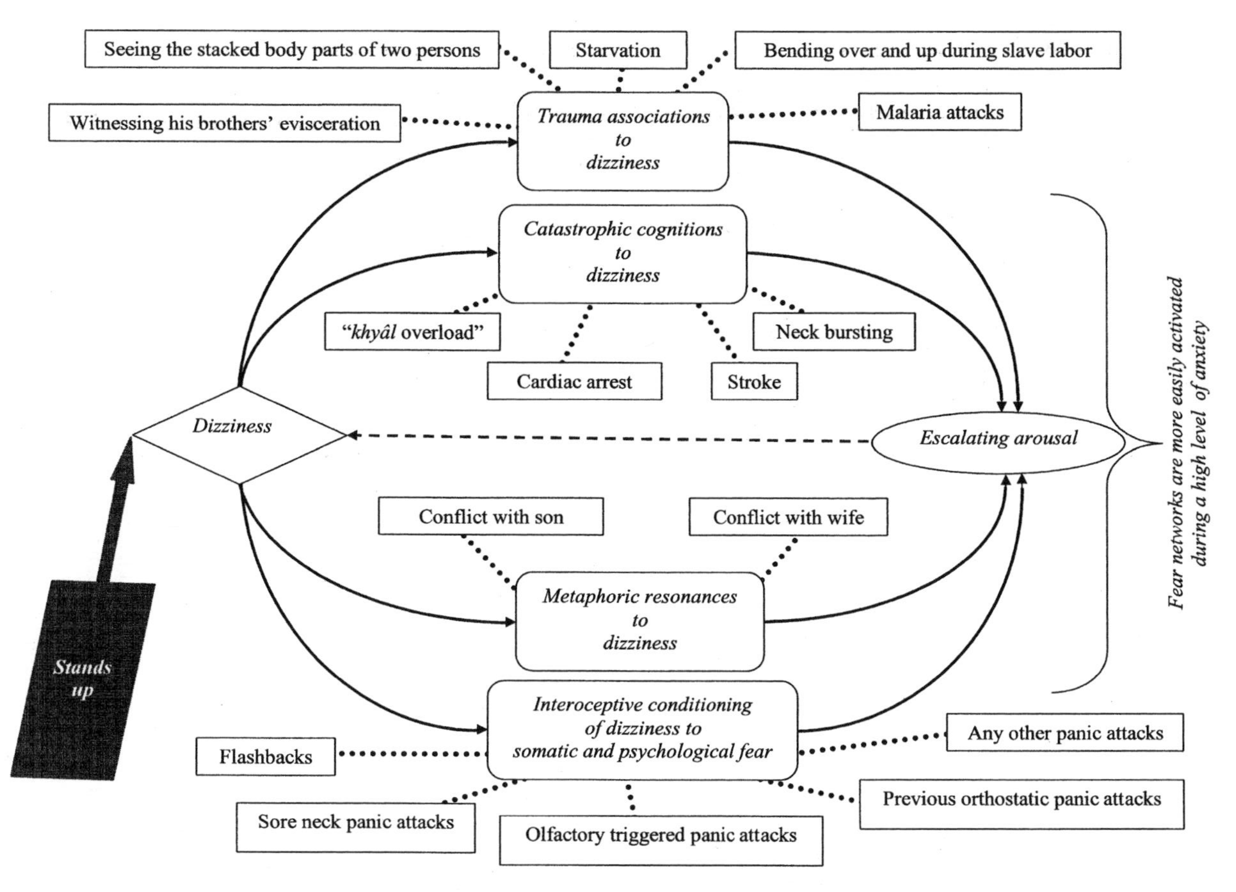

FIG. 3-5. The generation of an orthostatic panic attack (a TCMIE panic attack): the case of Chan.

of trauma networks, and the investigating of metaphoric resonances of prominent sensations, the clinician should consider utilizing interoceptive exposure (13,48)—most particularly, interoceptive exposure that includes reassociation of pleasant events to the problematic sensation; for example, reassociation of dizziness to such pleasurable activities as being on a carousel or roller coaster, to having drunk a little wine, to dancing a traditional whirling dance (*lam lieu*), or playing a traditional game that involves much rapid running in a circle (*leu geunsaeng*). We have found these techniques—modifying catastrophic cognitions, exploring sensation-related trauma networks and sensation-based metaphoric resonances to current social and interpersonal distress, interoceptive exposure, and reassociation—to be effective in the treatment of panic and PTSD among Cambodian refugees (49). Nine general therapeutic principles follow (some of these are illustrated in Fig. 3-6).

1. Provide information about the nature of PTSD and panic disorder, such as how trauma reminders and catastrophic cognitions generate panic attacks (13,50).
2. Train the patient in muscle relaxation and diaphragmatic breathing procedures, including the use of applied relaxation techniques (51).
3. Instruct the patient in a culturally appropriate visualization—a lotus bloom that spins in the wind at the end of a stem (an image encoding key Asian cultural values of flexibility)—while having the patient perform analogous rotational movements at the neck after each relaxation of the neck and head musculature; these rotational movements also serve as an introduction to dizziness interoceptive exercises (52).
4. Frame relaxation techniques as a form of mindfulness (53), that is, attending to specific sensory modalities (e.g., muscular tension and the kinesthetics of breathing).
5. Work toward cognitive restructuring of fear networks, especially trauma memories and catastrophic misinterpretations of somatic sensations, including culture-related fears (50,52).
6. Determine social, economic, and other current concerns that may trigger worry episodes that precede panic episodes and that may be evoked by sensations experienced during panic (i.e., metaphoric resonances to panic-related sensations).
7. Conduct interoceptive exposure to anxiety-related sensations (including reassociation to positive images) to treat panic attacks generated by catastrophic cognitions, interoceptive conditioning, and trauma associations to those sensations (13,24,54).
8. Provide an emotional processing protocol (52, 55) to utilize during times of trauma recall, as during flashbacks; such a protocol can bring about a shift from an attitude of pained acceptance to one of mindfulness, with multisensorial awareness of the present moment.
9. Explore panic attacks by investigating firing sequences—the sensations, activities, and thoughts that initiate the sequence leading to panic—and associated catastrophic cognitions and trauma associations (10,13,24).

Let us examine how some of these treatment principles were applied in Chan's case. Chan was educated about the ANS, with an explanation of how fright could generate

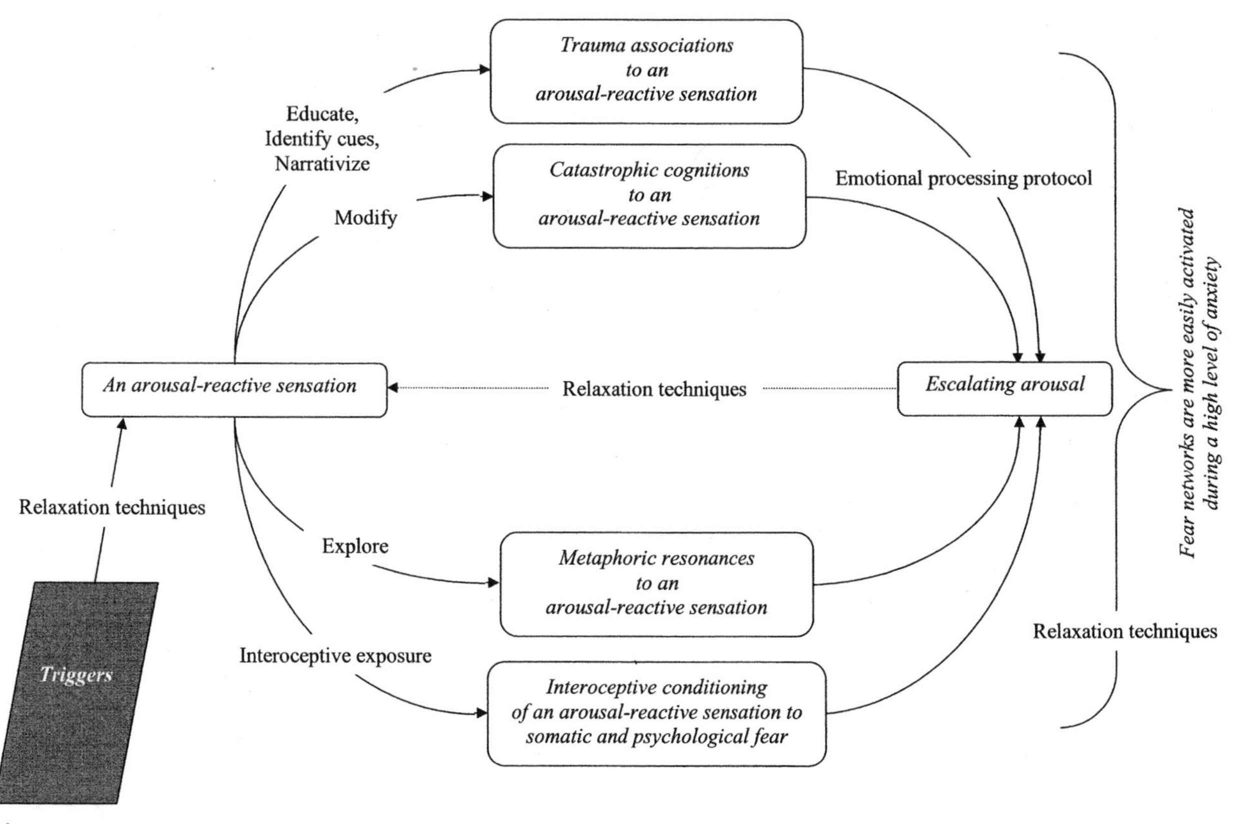

FIG. 3-6. Therapeutic interventions that decrease the probability of a TCMIE panic attack.

such symptoms as cold extremities or dizziness. Chan was educated about trauma-related disorder, including a discussion of TCMIE panic attacks. His catastrophic cognitions about somatic symptoms were addressed. In addition, the trauma associations to dizziness and other symptoms elicited by standing were explored. The metaphoric resonances of dizziness to his current life situation—and their power to evoke and intensify distress about current social and financial issues—were discussed, and we explored how he might better handle conflicts with his son and wife. Muscle relaxation decreased his general level of arousal. A selective serotonin reuptake inhibitor (paroxetine) and a benzodiazepine were given to further manage panic and promote sleep. Following these interventions, orthostatic panic decreased to once a week, and the episodes were less severe.

VII. CONCLUSION

In designing the treatment for a particular cultural group, one must initially identify the main patterns of distress. One should then ascertain how that stress is generated in order to be able to design effective and culturally sensitive treatments. For Southeast Asian refugees, various types of panic attack subtypes—noise induced, flashback associated, orthostatic induced, sore-neck centered—form a key aspect of trauma-related disorder. For effective treatment, the clinician should identify and assess the severity of the panic attacks that afflict the Southeast Asian patient. In our experience, therapeutic intervention using the nine techniques outlined in section VI reduces the distress of traumatized Southeast Asian refugees. Two outcome studies by our group, one of Cambodian refugees (49) and another of Vietnamese refugees (56), have yielded encouraging results. To further investigate efficacy, we are conducting a large, National Institutes of Mental Health–sponsored cognitive-behavioral outcome study of Cambodian refugees with comorbid panic attacks based on a manualized treatment. Continued ethnographic work and systematic treatment studies should enable our field to further refine efforts to alleviate the suffering of Southeast Asian refugees.

REFERENCES

1. Chung R. Psychosocial adjustment of Cambodian refugee women: implications for mental health counseling. *J Ment Health Counsel* 2001;23:115–126.
2. Kiernan B. *The Pol Pot regime: race, power, and genocide in Cambodia under the Khmer Rouge, 1975–79.* New Haven, CT: Yale University Press, 1996.
3. Kinzie JD, Fredrickson RH, Ben R, et al. Posttraumatic stress disorder among survivors of Cambodian concentration camps. *Am J Psychiatry* 1984;141:645–650.
4. Kroll J, Hebenicht M, Mackenzie T, et al. Depression and posttraumatic stress disorder in Southeast Asian refugees. *Am J Psychiatry* 1989;146:1592–1597.
5. Mollica R, Wyshak G, Marneffe D, et al. Indochinese version of the Hopkins Symptom Checklist-25: a screening instrument for the psychiatric care of refugees. *Am J Psychiatry* 1987;144:497–500.
6. Mollica R, Mcinness K, Poole C, et al. Dose-effect relationships of trauma to symptoms of depression and post-traumatic stress disorder among Cambodian survivors of mass violence. *Br J Psychiatry* 1998;173:482–488.
7. Kinzie J, David J, Boehnlein P, et al. The prevalence of posttraumatic stress disorder and its clinical significance among Southeast Asian refugees. *Am J Psychiatry* 1990;147:913–917.

8. Mollica R, McInnes K, Pham T, et al. The dose-effect relationships between torture and psychiatric symptoms in Vietnamese ex-political detainees and a comparison group. *J Nerv Ment Dis* 1998;186: 543–553.
9. Hinton D, Ba P, Peou S, et al. Panic disorder among Cambodian refugees attending a psychiatric clinic: Prevalence and subtypes. *Gen Hosp Psychiatry* 2000;22:437–444.
10. Hinton D, Nguyen L, Nguyen M, et al. Panic disorder among Vietnamese refugees attending a psychiatric clinic: prevalence and subtypes. *Gen Hosp Psychiatry* 2001;23:337–344.
11. Ehlers A, Clark D. A cognitive model of posttraumatic stress disorder. *Behav Res Ther* 2000;38: 319–345.
12. Jones JC, Barlow D. The etiology of posttraumatic stress disorder. *Clin Psychol Rev* 1990;10: 299–328.
13. Falsetti S, Resnick H. Cognitive-behavioral treatment for PTSD with panic attacks. *J Contemp Psychother* 2000;30:163–179.
14. Bouton M. Conditioning, remembering, and forgetting. *J Exp Psychol* 1994;20:219–231.
15. Bouton M, Mineka S, Barlow D. A modern learning theory perspective on the etiology of panic disorder. *Psychol Rev* 2001;108:4–32.
16. Brewin C, Dalgleish T, Joseph S. A dual representation theory of posttraumatic stress disorder. *Psychol Rev* 1996;103:670–686.
17. Keane T, Barlow DH. Posttraumatic stress disorder. In: Barlow DH, ed. *Anxiety and its disorders.* 2nd ed. New York: Guilford Press, 2002:418–454.
18. Bouwer C, Stein D. Association of panic disorder with a history of traumatic suffocation. *Am J Psychiatry* 1997;154:1566–1570.
19. Kellner M, Yehuda R. Do panic disorder and posttraumatic stress disorder share a common psychoneuroendocrinology? *Psychoneuroendocrinology* 1999;24:485–504.
20. Ledoux J. *The emotional brain.* New York: Simon and Schuster, 1996.
21. Gorman J, Kent J, Martinez J, et al. Physiological changes during carbon dioxide inhalation in patients with panic disorder, major depression, and premenstrual dysphoric disorder: evidence for a central fear mechanism. *Arch Gen Psychiatry* 2001;58:125–131.
22. Gorman J, Kent J, Sullivan G, et al. Neuroanatomical hypothesis of panic disorder, revisited. *Am J Psychiatry* 2000;157:493–505.
23. Clark DM. A cognitive approach to panic. *Behav Res Ther* 1986;24:461–470.
24. Hinton D, So V, Pollack M, et al. The psychophysiology of orthostatic panic in Cambodian refugees attending a psychiatric clinic. *J Psychopathol Behav Assess* 2004;26:1–13.
25. Barlow DH. *Anxiety and its disorders: the nature and treatment of anxiety and panic.* 2nd ed. New York: Guilford Press, 2002.
26. Foa E, Kozak MJ. Emotional processing of fear: exposure to corrective information. *Psychol Bull* 1986;99:20–35.
27. Hinton D, Pham T, Chau H, et al. "Hit by the wind" and temperature-shift panic among Vietnamese refugees. *Transcultural Psychiatry* 2003;40:342–376.
28. Hinton D, Um K, Ba P. *Kyol goeu* ("wind overload") part I: a cultural syndrome of orthostatic panic among Khmer refugees. *Transcultural Psychiatry* 2001a;38:403–432.
29. Hinton D, Um K, Ba P. *Kyol goeu* ("wind overload") part II: prevalence, characteristics and mechanisms of *kyol goeu* and near-*kyol goeu* episodes of Khmer patients attending a psychiatric clinic. *Transcultural Psychiatry* 2001b;38:433–460.
30. Clark DM. Panic disorder: from theory to therapy. In: Salkovskis PM, ed. *Frontiers of cognitive therapy.* New York: Guilford Press, 1996:318–344.
31. Harvey JM, Richards JC, Dziadosz T, et al. Misinterpretation of ambiguous stimuli in panic disorder. *Cogn Ther Res* 1993;17:235–248.
32. Hedley L, Hoffart A, Dammen T, et al. The relationship between cognitions and panic attack intensity. *Acta Psychiatr Scand* 2000;102:300–302.
33. Hinton D, Hinton S. Panic disorder, somatization, and the new cross-cultural psychiatry; or, the seven bodies of a medical anthropology of panic. *Culture Med Psychiatry* 2002;26:155–178.
34. Mollica R, Donelan K, Tor S, et al. The effect of trauma and confinement on functional health and mental health status of Cambodians living in Thailand-Cambodian border camps. *JAMA* 1993;270: 581–586.
35. Wenzel A, Golden S. Situation-specific scripts for threat in blood fearful and nonfearful individuals. *J Psychopathol Behav Assess* 2003;25:213–219.

36. Hinton D, Hinton S, Um K, et al. The Khmer "weak heart" syndrome: fear of death from palpitations. *Transcultural Psychiatry* 2002;39:323–344.
37. Chambless D, Caputo C, Bright P, et al. Assessment of fear of fear in agoraphobics: the body sensations questionnaire and the agoraphobic cognitions questionnaire. *J Counsel Clin Psychol* 1984; 6:1090–1097.
38. Noyes R, Hoehn-Saric R. *The anxiety disorders.* Cambridge: Cambridge University Press, 1998.
39. Beck G, Scott S. Physiological and symptom response to hyperventilation: a comparison of frequent and infrequent panickers. *J Psychopathol Behav Assess* 1988;10:117–127.
40. Arena J, Bruno G, Hannah S, et al. A comparison of frontal electromyographic biofeedback training, trapezius electromyographic biofeedback training, and progressive muscle relaxation therapy in the treatment of tension headache. *Headache* 1995;35:411–419.
41. Hazlett R, Mcleod R, Hoehn-Saric R. Muscle tension in generalized anxiety disorder: elevated muscle tonus or agitated movement. *Psychophysiology* 1994;31:189–195.
42. Hoehn-Saric R, Mcleod D, Zimmerli W. Psychophysiological response patterns in panic disorder. *Acta Psychiatr Scand* 1991;83:4–11.
43. Hinton D, Um K, Ba P. A unique panic disorder presentation among Khmer refugees: the sore-neck syndrome. *Culture Med Psychiatry* 2001;25:297–316.
44. Anthony M, Swinson R. *Phobic disorders and panic in adults.* Washington, DC: American Psychological Association, 2000.
45. Salkovksis P, Warwick M. Making sense of hypochondriasis: a cognitive model of health anxiety. In: Asmundson J, Taylor S, Cox B, eds. *Health anxiety.* West Sussex: Wiley, 2001:46–64.
46. Roy-Byrne P, Cowley D, Stein M. Cardiovascular and catecholamine response to orthostasis in panic and obsessive-compulsive disorder and normal controls: effects of anxiety and novelty. *Depress Anxiety* 1997;6:159–164.
47. McNally RJ, Lukach BM. Are panic attacks traumatic stressors? *Am J Psychiatry* 1992;149:824–826.
48. Barlow D, Craske M. *Mastery of your anxiety and panic: client workbook for anxiety and panic.* 3rd ed. San Antonio, TX: Graywind Publications Inc, the Psychological Corporation, 2000.
49. Otto M, Hinton D, Korbly N, et al. Treatment of pharmacotherapy-refractory posttraumatic stress disorder among Cambodian refugees: a pilot study of combination treatment with cognitive-behavior therapy vs. sertraline alone. *Behav Res Ther* 2003;41:1271–1276.
50. Resick P, Schnicke M. *Cognitive processing therapy for rape victims.* London, New Delhi: Sage Publications, 1996.
51. Öst L-G, Westling B. Applied relaxation vs. cognitive behavior therapy in the treatment of panic disorder. *Behav Res Ther* 1995;33:145–158.
52. Hinton DH, Pich V, Pollack MH. The treatment of neck focused panic attacks among Cambodian refugees. *Cognitive Behav Prac* 2004 (in press).
53. Borkovec T. Life in the future versus life in the present. *Clin Psychol Sci Pract* 2002;9:76–80.
54. Otto M, Penava S, Pollack R, et al. Cognitive-behavioral and pharmacologic perspectives on the treatment of post-traumatic stress disorder. In: Pollack M, Otto M, Rosenbaum J, eds. *Challenges in clinical practice: pharmacologic and psychosocial strategies.* New York: Guilford Press, 1996: 219–260.
55. Rachman S. Emotional processing. *Behav Res Ther* 1980;24:685–688.
56. Hinton DE, Pham T, Tran M, et al. CBT for Vietnamese refugees with treatment-resistant PTSD and panic attacks: a pilot study. *J Traum Stress* 2004 *(in press).*

4

Ataque de Nervios

Anthropological, Epidemiological, and Clinical Dimensions of a Cultural Syndrome

*†‡Roberto Lewis-Fernández, §Peter J. Guarnaccia, *†Sapana Patel, ¶Dana Lizardi, and ¶Naelys Díaz

**Hispanic Treatment Program, New York State Psychiatric Institute, New York, New York 10032; †Department of Psychiatry, Columbia College of Physicians and Surgeons; New York, New York 10032; ‡Department of Social Medicine, Harvard Medical School, Boston, MA 02115; §Institute for Health, Health Care Policy and Aging Research, Rutgers, The State University of New Jersey, New Brunswick, New Jersey 08901; and ¶Graduate School of Social Service, Fordham University, New York, New York 10019*

I. INTRODUCTION

Psychiatric practice relies on a process of translation from patients' own experiential language into professional nosological categories. Valid diagnosis, positive therapeutic alliance, appropriate intervention, and treatment adherence all depend on the accuracy of this process of translation. Medical anthropologists use the terms *idioms of distress* and *popular illness categories* to describe locally diverse ways of expressing suffering—including mental and emotional illness—that reflect cultural understandings of emotion, causality, physiology, and meaning (1–3). Clinical awareness of the rich variety of these popular categories has increased recently as part of the growing psychiatric attention to ethnocultural diversity. The inclusion of a glossary of "culture-bound syndromes" in the *Diagnostic and Statistical Manual of Mental Disorders, Fourth Edition* (DSM-IV) provides a vital opportunity to highlight existing studies on these cultural categories as well as the need to expand research on valid cross-cultural diagnostics (4). The publication of this book now, based on a series of lectures at the Massachusetts General Hospital, is further indication of the growing role of cultural research in mainstream psychiatric practice. In this chapter, we summarize the anthropological, epidemiological, and clinical dimensions of *ataques de nervios* (attacks of nerves) as a model of the translational process between cultural categories and professional nosologies.

Ataque de nervios is a cultural syndrome particularly prominent among Latinos from the Caribbean, but recognized among many Hispanic groups. Commonly reported elements of *ataques* include: screaming/shouting uncontrollably, attacks of crying, trembling, heat in the chest rising into the head, and becoming verbally and physically aggressive. Dissociative experiences, seizurelike or fainting episodes, and suicidal gestures are prominent in some *ataques* but absent in others. Attacks frequently occur as a direct result of a stressful event relating to the family, such as news of the death of a close relative, separation or divorce from a spouse, conflicts with a spouse or children, or witnessing an accident involving a family member. For a minority of individuals, no particular social event triggers their *ataques*; instead, their vulnerability to losing control comes from the accumulated experience of suffering (5,6). We will further explore the phenomenological dimensions of *ataque* in a later section.

Cultural research on emotional affliction goes beyond the study of emotions as specific to the individual or as symptoms of disorder to reveal their characteristic as experiences taking place in a cultural framework (6). Bodily expressions of distress are more than individual experience; they are commentaries on the broader social and political world (7). Popular syndromes, such as *ataque,* are even forms of praxis—social practices in real-world settings of power. They constitute emotions presented with transformative force into a field of social relations in which things are at stake biographically, morally, and politically. These syndromes not only pattern and express distress, they also seek to affect the local moral world in which the distress occurs (8–11). Our chapter on *ataque de nervios* takes account of this perspective while providing a thumbnail sketch of its epidemiological and clinical dimensions for the benefit of clinicians and biomedical researchers.

II. OVERVIEW OF RESEARCH ON *ATAQUE DE NERVIOS*

Early psychiatric descriptions of *ataque de nervios* in the 1950s and 1960s focused on nosological questions and psychoanalytic explanations, while paying limited attention to the social context of *ataque* experience (12–16). Much of this early work was carried out by US military psychiatrists stationed in Puerto Rico, or by local clinicians responding to their writings. It primarily concerned young Puerto Rican men being treated in Veterans Administration clinics on the Island after having been inducted into the US Armed Services. These men responded to induction, basic training, weapons familiarization, and word of overseas shipment with *ataques* that frequently resulted in their removal from active duty. Most of the early articles looked to defective child-rearing patterns as the key to understanding *ataques de nervios,* rather than analyzing the current social situations facing these young men.

In keeping with psychoanalytic theory of the time, pathological personality patterns linked to proposed Puerto Rican cultural practices involving young infants (e.g., extended bottle feeding; "almost constant" fondling, caressing, and handling) were blamed for the *ataque* behavior (14,16). The power relationships embodied in the military, and the colonial situation represented by the presence of the US Armed Forces in Puerto Rico, were left unanalyzed. When acknowledged at all, the praxis aspect of the attacks—e.g., relief from active duty—was discussed unreflexively and dismissively as "malingering" (15).

Work in the 1970s and 1980s by Latino mental health professionals and medical anthropologists working in Latino communities began to apply a sociocultural and clinical perspective to understanding *ataques de nervios* (17–21). Latino mental health professionals argued that the *ataque* is a culturally recognized and sanctioned expression of emotion that should be understood as a form of communication about family relationships. Women in particular were seen as protesting the effects of economic disenfranchisement and male domination on their and their relatives' lives in the form of *ataques*. This indirect and relatively accepted form of resistance substituted for more direct and challenging types of protest. De la Cancela and colleagues (20) extended this argument to look at how the colonial experience has shaped the forms of expression among Puerto Ricans. They argued that *ataques* should be understood as a culturally specific form of expressing resistance to, and anger at, oppression.

Harwood (22), Garrison and Thomas (23,24), Guarnaccia et al. (21), Oquendo et al. (25), and Lewis-Fernández (26) provided rich case studies of experiences of *ataque* among Puerto Ricans and Dominicans in the United States and of their help-seeking strategies. The case studies identified the differences between family definitions of *ataques* as related to family conflicts; definitions in *espiritismo* that focus on the influence of spiritual forces; and psychiatric interpretations that focus on personality and disease processes underlying the *ataque*. What these detailed individual case studies attained in contextual and biographical depth, however, was balanced with what remained to be known about the epidemiological and broader clinical dimensions of this popular syndrome.

Taken together, the work of these early decades set the stage for the research summarized in this chapter, carried out since the late 1980s. This new, largely empirical turn in *ataque* research reflects the corresponding shift in psychiatric investigative practice during the same period. It also highlights a contemporary direction in cultural psychiatry. By incorporating the methods of epidemiological and clinical studies, this component of the field aims to communicate the importance of cultural factors in the empirical language of biomedical clinicians and researchers (4).

III. PHENOMENOLOGY OF *ATAQUE DE NERVIOS*

Guarnaccia and colleagues (6,27) went beyond existing case studies by collecting qualitative and quantitative data on the experiences of much larger samples of *ataque* sufferers. In collaboration with the Behavioral Sciences Research Institute of the

University of Puerto Rico, directed by Glorisa Canino, they surveyed a representative community sample of Island residents (N = 912) for the presence of *ataques*. This constituted one of the first epidemiological studies of a cultural syndrome, extending the pioneering work of Carstairs and Kapur (28) and Rubel et al. (29) in previous decades.

From general descriptions of *ataques de nervios* and the recounting of specific *ataque* episodes among a subsample of 145 respondents in this larger study—of whom 77 were *ataque* sufferers—a "prototype" of the *ataque* experience emerged (6). A prototype is the cultural representation that links collective and individual experiences of the syndrome (30). In this case, the term refers to a core image or description of a person who has *ataques de nervios;* a description which includes not only a set of symptoms the person experiences but also provides a view of the person and the social context within which *ataques de nervios* occur (31–33). The *ataque* prototype consists of an overriding sense of loss of control; emotions of sadness and anger; and expressions of distress in the form of physical symptoms, aggressive outbursts, and loss of consciousness. The prototype also includes a trigger, usually in the form of a threat to the order of the person's social world. Examples in the case of the family are the news of the death of a relative, rupture of family bonds such as through divorce, or serious conflicts with one's children (6). Each episode of *ataque* varies in the details of these experiences.

Qualitative coding of the first and most recent episodes of *ataque de nervios* among the 77 sufferers of the syndrome in this subsample revealed four domains of *ataque* experience: emotional expressions, bodily sensations, action dimensions, and alterations in consciousness (6). A core feature of the *ataque* is a sense of being out of control; this reflects a social world that is experienced as similarly out of control (34). The main emotional expressions of *ataque de nervios* are sadness, fear, and anger/rage. These emotions are often so powerful that they "resist language" (35) and are expressed through uncontrollable screaming, attacks of crying, and other bodily sensations, such as trembling and heart palpitations. Aggressiveness towards self, other people, or things exemplify the action dimension of the *ataque* experience. Especially in situations of family conflict, sufferers find extreme physical strength and describe breaking things or striking out at other people. Frank suicidality, which arises during a minority of *ataque* episodes (see Table 4-1), constitutes one of the more dangerous aspects of this syndrome. Finally, during an *ataque de nervios,* some people experience a marked change in consciousness. For these individuals time slows down, they cannot remember what happened and are stunned when others tell them what they did, and they feel dissociated from their bodies and selves. Although sufferers generally return rapidly to their normal level of functioning after an *ataque,* some may describe long-lasting amnesia for their behavior during the episode (36). The most frequent symptoms of respondents' first *ataque de nervios* are listed in Table 4-1. Biomedical practitioners will remark on the phenomenological overlap between *ataques* and panic attacks. We will take up this point in detail later in the chapter.

TABLE 4-1. *Most frequent symptoms of first* ataque de nervios *in Puerto Rico community study (N = 77)*

Symptom	Percentage of respondents	Symptom	Percentage of respondents
Became nervous	90	Afraid of going crazy	53
Attacks of crying	88	Felt anger	52
Trembled a lot	77	Blurred vision	43
Heart beat hard	75	Fainted	43
Chest pressure	75	Body felt unreal	42
Had headache	70	Afraid of dying	39
Hysterical	69	Dizzy	35
Frightened	65	Lost consciousness	35
Afraid of losing control	64	Aggressive	31
Suffocating	61	Period of amnesia	29
Heat in chest	56	Broke things	26
Screamed out of control	56	Suicidal thoughts	26
Out of breath	56	Fell to floor	21
Surroundings seemed unreal	53	Suicide attempt	14

(Adapted from Guarnaccia PJ, Rivera M, Franco F, et al. The experiences of *ataques de nervios*: towards an anthropology of emotions in Puerto Rico. *Cult Med Psychiatry* 1996; 20:343–367.)

Assessment of the phenomenological features of *ataques de nervios* experienced by the 77 respondents with at least one lifetime *ataque* revealed that the largest number (28%) had suffered only one such episode over the course of their life. Thirteen percent had a history of two *ataques*, 8% had experienced three, 9% had four, and 4% had five. The second largest number (23%) comprised those who had more than five lifetime *ataques*, whereas 15% were unsure about the total. The bimodal distribution of *ataque* frequency (one versus six or more) suggests that persons with frequent episodes constitute a minority of *ataque* sufferers. This raises the question whether having an isolated *ataque* in response to a markedly stressful event represents a relatively normal expression of distress in some Latino communities.

In this sample, the first experience of an *ataque* was closely tied to a triggering event. In 92% of cases, the *ataque* was directly provoked by a distressing situation, and 73% of the time it began within minutes or hours of the event. A majority of first *ataques* (81%) occurred in the presence of others, as opposed to when the sufferer was alone, and led to the person receiving help (67%). Finally, unlike the typical experience of persons with panic disorder, most respondents reported feeling better (71%) or feeling relieved (81%) after their first *ataque*. These findings suggest that first episodes of *ataque de nervios* are closely tied to the interpersonal world of the sufferer and that they result in an unburdening (*desahogarse*) of one's life problems, at least temporarily.

From the perspective of the sufferer and those around him/her, the *ataque* is experienced not as a collection of symptoms or domains, but as a seamless whole. It emerges directly from the force of social dislocation that provokes sadness, fear, or anger and explodes in a flood of feelings, expressions, and actions. The *ataque de nervios* momentarily remakes the self by taking the self out of time, place, and social role, and creates a new persona who is responding to the changes and rush of emotion that major family dislocations and other disruptions of the social world produce in many Latino communities.

IV. PREVALENCE, RISK FACTORS, AND PSYCHIATRIC COMORBIDITY

Guarnaccia et al. (27) conducted epidemiological research on *ataque de nervios* as part of the Puerto Rico Disaster Study (N = 912). This was a representative community-based study of the psychological consequences of the 1985 floods and mudslides that caused considerable damage and death in Puerto Rico (37,38). To estimate the lifetime prevalence and risk factors of *ataque de nervios,* a single question concerning this syndrome was added to the Diagnostic Interview Schedule/Disaster Supplement (DIS/DS) (39). On this basis, 16% of the sample (n = 145) reported experiencing an *ataque de nervios* at some point in their life. Of these 145 respondents, 109 (12% of the community sample) met DIS/DS criteria for a positive psychological symptom—that is, the *ataque* met severity criteria (consulting a physician or other professional, taking medications, or reporting some functional impairment) and could not be explained as resulting from physical illness or substance use. When the data were analyzed on the basis of sampling weights that permit an approximation to the total population of Puerto Rico, the lifetime prevalence of *ataque de nervios* became 13.8% of the population. This makes *ataque de nervios* one of the most frequently reported syndromes in the Puerto Rico Disaster Study (27,37).

Risk factors for *ataque de nervios* span a range of social, demographic, and psychiatric characteristics (27). People reporting an *ataque de nervios* in Puerto Rico were more likely to be female, over the age of 45, with less than a high school education, formerly married (i.e., divorced, widowed or separated), and out of the labor force (see Table 4-2). However, it is important to note that 10% of the men in the sample reported an *ataque de nervios,* which indicates that some men do express their distress through this cultural syndrome.

Ataque sufferers also reported less satisfaction in their social interactions generally, and specifically with their spouses. In addition, people who experienced an *ataque de nervios* were more likely to describe their health as only fair or poor, to seek help for an emotional problem, and to take medications for this purpose. Persons with *ataque* also reported deriving less satisfaction from leisure time activities and feeling overwhelmed more often. The social class dimensions of who experiences an *ataque* are important here. Persons of lower socioeconomic status, as compared with more advantaged persons, lack the time and resources for leisure and experience an increase in social problems leading to a feeling of being overwhelmed (27).

Overall, 63% of people who reported an *ataque de nervios* met diagnostic criteria for one or more psychiatric disorders measured in the DIS/DS, with *ataque* sufferers being 4.35 times more likely to meet criteria for a psychiatric diagnosis than those who did not report an *ataque* (see Table 4-3). The strongest association was found

TABLE 4-2. *Relationship between* ataques de nervios *and sociodemographic variables in the Puerto Rico Disaster Study (N = 912)*

Demographic variables	No *ataque* N = 767 (84%)	*Ataque de nervios* N = 145 (16%)
Sex		
Male	348 (45%)	41 (28%)[a]
Female	419 (55%)	104 (72%)
Age (y)		
17–24	189 (25%)	22 (15%)[a]
25–44	344 (45%)	61 (42%)
45–88	234 (30%)	62 (43%)
Education		
< High School	372 (48%)	96 (66%)[a]
High School +	395 (52%)	49 (34%)
Marital Status		
Married	379 (49%)	67 (46%)[a]
Formerly married	134 (18%)	43 (30%)
Never married	254 (33%)	35 (25%)
Employment Status		
Out of labor force	392 (52%)	91 (36%)[b]
Unemployed	140 (18%)	26 (18%)
Employed	225 (30%)	28 (19%)

[a] $p < 0.01$.
[b] $p < 0.05$.
Data are number (percentage) of respondents. Chi-square was used to establish if differences were significant for each demographic variable.
(Adapted from Guarnaccia PJ, Canino G, Rubio-Stipec M, et al. The prevalence of *ataques de nervios* in the Puerto Rico Disaster Study. *J Nerv Ment Dis* 1993;181:157–165.)

TABLE 4-3. *Relationship between* ataques de nervios *and psychiatric diagnosis in the Puerto Rico Disaster Study (N = 912)*

Psychiatric diagnosis	No *ataque*	*Ataque de nervios*	Odds ratio
Depression (5%)	19 (2%)	29 (20%)	9.84
Dysthymia (12%)	67 (9%)	40 (28%)	3.63
Generalized anxiety disorder (18%)	108 (14%)	55 (38%)	3.73
Panic disorder (2%)	3 (0.4%)	13 (9%)	25.08
PTSD (6%)	29 (4%)	25 (17%)	5.30
Any affective disorder	49 (6%)	43 (30%)	6.18
Any anxiety disorder	109 (14%)	58 (40%)	4.02
Any DIS Diagnosis	214 (28%)	91 (63%)	4.35
Total	N = 767 (84%)	N = 145 (16%)	

The numbers in parentheses after each psychiatric variable indicates the percentage of that diagnosis in the total sample.
PTSD, posttraumatic stress disorder; DIS, Diagnosis Interview Schedule.
(Adapted from Guarnaccia PJ, Canino G, Rubio-Stipec M, et al. The prevalence of *ataques de nervios* in the Puerto Rico Disaster Study. *J Nerv Ment Dis* 1993;181:157–165.)

with panic disorder. Significant associations were also found with major depression, dysthymia, generalized anxiety disorder, and posttraumatic stress disorder (PTSD), but not the alcohol use disorders (odds ratio [OR] = 1.15). Of particular concern was the strong relationship with suicidal ideation (OR = 6.22) and attempts (OR = 8.08). Trautman (40) also noted a relationship between *ataque* and suicide attempts in the early psychiatric literature.

These findings suggest that experiencing an *ataque de nervios* is often associated with a level of distress that biomedical practitioners would label a psychiatric disorder. Specifically, a strong association was found between having experienced an *ataque* and meeting criteria for depressive and anxiety disorders. It is also clear that *ataque* did not correlate exclusively with one psychiatric diagnosis and could not be treated as simply a culturally shaped version of a specific psychiatric disorder. We will take up the relationship between *ataque* and certain specific disorders, including panic, in subsequent sections. At the same time, 37% of *ataque* sufferers did not fulfill DIS/DS criteria. This suggests that a substantial proportion of respondents with this syndrome are either describing milder levels of distress or reporting forms of frank psychopathology not assessed by the study instrument.

Logistic regression analysis revealed that female gender, lower level of formal education, and disrupted marital status are the strongest independent demographic predictors of *ataque* status. After adjusting for other factors, assessing one's physical health as fair or poor made a report of an *ataque de nervios* 2.7 times more likely. Respondents who met criteria for an anxiety disorder were 3.5 times more likely to experience an *ataque,* whereas meeting criteria for a depressive disorder made one almost 3 times as likely to report an *ataque.* The picture that emerges from this risk factor analysis is that those individuals who suffer from a combination of social disadvantage, psychiatric disorder, and poor perceived physical health are at higher risk for experiencing an *ataque de nervios* (27).

Lewis-Fernández and colleagues (36,41) estimated the lifetime prevalence of *ataque de nervios* in two clinical settings serving Puerto Rican psychiatric outpatients. This "clinical epidemiology" approximates the expected presentation of the syndrome in this type of mental health service. The prevalence rate of *ataque* was remarkably similar across sites in the United States and Puerto Rico. In a Latino mental health clinic of an urban New England medical center, the lifetime prevalence of *ataque* was 55.1% among 89 consecutive Puerto Rican outpatients. The rate was 51.5% among 97 consecutive patients accessing an outpatient psychiatric consultation-liaison program serving three government-run primary care clinics in rural Puerto Rico. The comparability of the settings is increased because of the demographic parallels between the two patient samples. Nearly all the US-based respondents were first-generation migrants from rural areas such as the ones served in the Puerto Rico clinics. Moreover, the samples shared demographic characteristics to a striking degree, in terms of mean age (45 years in New England vs. 47 years in Puerto Rico), gender (71% female in both sites), unemployment (90% vs. 88%), and level of education (eighth grade or less: 50% vs. 54%) (34).

In both sites, the gender distribution of *ataque* sufferers was also very similar (56.3% female in New England vs. 54.8% in Puerto Rico). This suggests that among users of mental health services, the likelihood of having an *ataque* is nearly equivalent for men and women. However, women were more likely to seek this kind of care in both settings: in New England, female patients outnumbered male patients by 2.5 to 1, whereas the ratio was 1.8 to 1 in Puerto Rico. It is possible to put these study results in the context of the epidemiological findings in the Puerto Rico Disaster Study. In the community, *ataques* are more common among women. Once the severity of a man's psychopathology leads him to overcome the gender barrier to mental health services and present for care, however, clinicians should perceive his risk of *ataque* to be the same as that of a female patient. Finally, in these rural clinics for low-income residents in Puerto Rico, *ataque* rates also did not differ by age cohort or level of education. All social groupings among this disenfranchised sector of the population appear equally at risk for *ataque* episodes.

In terms of psychiatric research settings, Liebowitz and colleagues (42) found high rates of *ataque* (69.9%) among 156 mostly Dominican and Puerto Rican patients accessing a research program on mood and anxiety disorders at the New York State Psychiatric Institute (NYSPI). Some of these subjects were recruited purposefully for *ataque*-related research, artificially increasing the rate of the syndrome in this sample. Nevertheless, this study is notable for finding an equivalent *ataque* rate across Dominican and Puerto Rican patients, after adjusting for gender differences in prevalence. In this research setting, *ataque* was more common among women, but patients' age did not significantly affect the likelihood of having an *ataque* (42). More research in clinical and research settings with diverse Latino subpopulations is needed to help guide mental health professionals regarding the likelihood of presentation and demographic correlates of *ataque de nervios.*

V. *ATAQUE DE NERVIOS,* PANIC ATTACK, AND PANIC DISORDER

The potential overlap between *ataque de nervios* and panic disorder found in the Puerto Rico Disaster Study (Table 4-1) stimulated additional research to differentiate between these experiences. In order to perform a valid comparison with *ataque,* it is important at the outset to distinguish between panic attacks and panic disorder, since these two psychiatric entities are likely to bear different relationships to *ataque de nervios.*

A separate category for panic attacks was first established in DSM-IV, based on the recognition that these episodes can occur in the context of several psychiatric diagnoses, not just panic disorder (43). For example, persons suffering from social phobia often experience panic attacks when confronted with a dreaded social situation, such as public speaking. Because these panic attacks are not unexpected in that person, they are considered "cued," and do not merit a separate panic disorder diagnosis. Thus, the main characteristic of panic disorder as defined in DSM-IV is the presence of panic attacks that arise recurrently and unexpectedly, that is, in more than one unexpected situation. This is an important distinction in terms of *ataque,* because by popular definition (as confirmed by Guarnaccia et al.'s empirical research described earlier), most *ataques* arise in direct response to a distressing experience (i.e., are "cued"). These episodes may therefore meet criteria for panic attacks but not panic disorder, already suggesting a partial overlap between the cultural and professional categories.

The Puerto Rico Disaster Study revealed that persons reporting an *ataque* were 25 times more likely to receive a DIS/DS diagnosis of panic disorder than those without *ataques* (27). This elevated OR was due to the very low prevalence of panic disorder among respondents who did not report *ataques* (0.4%) (see Table 4-1) rather than to a clear one-to-one correspondence between *ataque* and panic. This finding indicates that it is rare to find panic disorder in Puerto Rico among community residents who do not self-identify as suffering from *ataque.* However, the converse is not true: only 9% of individuals with *ataques* met criteria for panic disorder, and there were strong associations between *ataques de nervios* and other anxiety and depressive disorders.

In their clinical study at the NYSPI, Liebowitz and colleagues (42) also demonstrated a partial overlap between *ataque de nervios* and panic disorder. Of the 109 patients with at least one lifetime *ataque,* panic disorder could be diagnosed in 45 (41%). However, this also meant that most (59%) patients with *ataques* in this specialty clinic did not fulfill criteria for this diagnosis.

More fine-grained phenomenological distinctions emerged when the investigators compared *ataques* that arose in persons with panic disorder, depression, or other anxiety disorders (44). *Ataques* in persons with panic (n = 45) resembled panic episodes more closely than in the other groups. These *ataques* were characterized by significantly more reports of panic symptoms than *ataques* in depressed subjects or in the other anxiety group. By contrast, *ataques* in persons suffering from depression (n = 33) were characterized by more anger and emotional lability than *ataques* in the other clinical groups, including significantly more reports of screaming, crying, anger, becoming aggressive, and breaking things. *Ataques* in the subgroup of subjects with other anxiety disorders (n = 24) were not characterized by a particular set of symptoms. These findings suggest that the phenomenology of *ataque* is intimately connected with the specific form of psychopathology associated with the episode. One possible interpretation is that a proportion of respondents are labeling panic disorder episodes as *ataques*, but other possibilities include that common vulnerabilities underlie both panic and *ataque,* or that the appearance of one disorder predisposes to developing the other (44).

In order to further untangle the nosological relationship between *ataque* and panic, Lewis-Fernández and colleagues (45) assessed key phenomenological features of the *ataque* experience. Sixty-six Dominican (73%) and Puerto Rican (27%) outpatients seeking care at the NYSPI Anxiety Disorder Clinic who reported a history of *ataque* were enrolled in the study. The age range of the sample was 18 to 72 years, 77% were women, and 96% were first-generation migrants. In a semistructured interview following a mixed clinical/ethnographic methodology (46), respondents were asked to describe their best-remembered *ataque de nervios* in terms of the symptom architecture of panic attacks and panic disorder. That is, for panic attacks, patients were asked whether their *ataque* was characterized by (i) a discrete period of intense fear or discomfort; (ii) the presence of four or more out of the DSM-IV list of 13 panic symptoms; and (iii) rapid peaking of symptoms (crescendo), defined as occurring within 10 minutes (DSM-IV). *Ataques* that fulfilled all of these criteria were judged to be likely panic attacks from a biomedical perspective.

Results are presented in Figure 4-1. These indicate that only a third of *ataques* fulfilled all three DSM-IV criteria for panic attacks. This includes subjects who reported either being "very afraid" or feeling "nervous" during their *ataque,* in order to approximate the inclusive features of the panic attack fear criterion ("intense fear or discomfort"). The phenomenological element that most distinguished *ataques* from panic attacks was a crescendo lasting longer than 10 minutes, which occurred in 15 subjects who otherwise met panic attack criteria, or 23% of the sample. This degree of overlap indicates that even at the level of panic attacks, many *ataques* display a distinct phenomenology from panic episodes. At the same time, there is a distinct subset of *ataques* that shares the symptom architecture of panic attacks.

The same procedure was then repeated for panic disorder. According to DSM-IV, panic disorder episodes must fulfill the criteria for panic attacks and in addition: (i) must occur more than once when not expected; and (ii) at least one attack must be followed by one month (or more) of at least one of the following sequelae: persistent concern about having a future attack, worry about the implications or the consequences of the attack, and/or behavior change as a result of the attack. Figure 4-2 shows the proportion of best-remembered *ataques* that fulfilled each of these criteria.

One in six patients (17%) had *ataques* whose symptom architecture met criteria for panic attacks and in addition fulfilled criteria for panic disorder. Patients who reported that at least some of their *ataques* were unprovoked (35%) were included in this number, rather than only those whose best-remembered *ataque* was unprovoked (26%), in order to cast the widest possible net for an overlap with panic disorder.

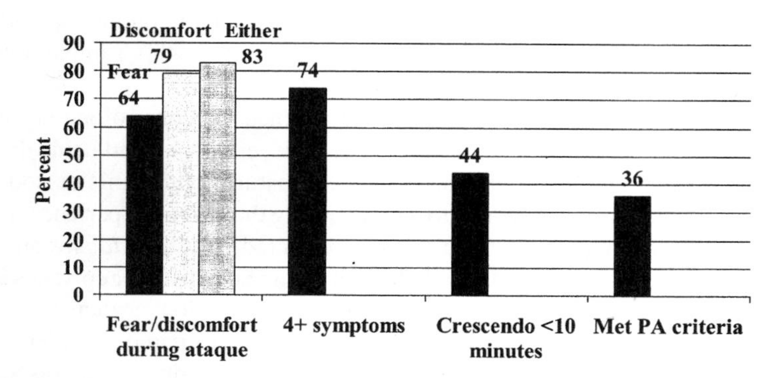

FIG. 4-1. Formal panic attack criteria met during best-remembered *ataque* episode (n = 66). (Adapted from Lewis-Fernández R, Guarnaccia PJ, Martínez, IE, et al. Comparative phenomenology of *ataques de nervios,* panic attacks, and panic disorder. *Cult Med Psychiatry* 2002;26: 199–223.)

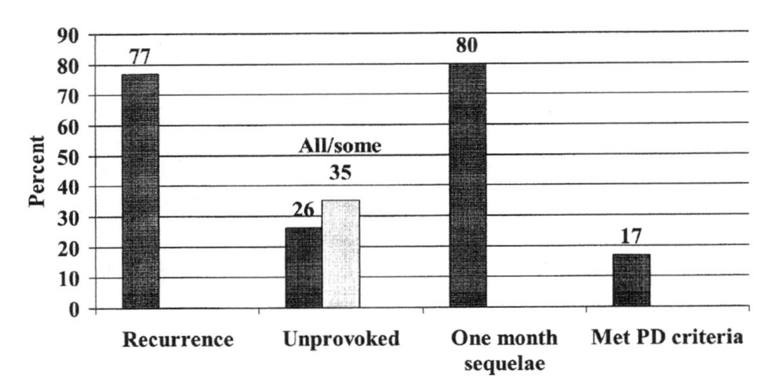

FIG. 4-2. Formal panic disorder criteria met during best-remembered *ataque* episode (n = 66). (Adapted from Lewis-Fernández R, Guarnaccia PJ, Martinez IE, et al. Comparative phenomenology of *ataques de nervios,* panic attacks, and panic disorder. *Cult Med Psychiatry* 2002;26: 199–223.)

(An example of a provoked attack was a woman who developed an *ataque* during an argument with her husband over his infidelity, whereas an example of an unprovoked *ataque* was a person whose *ataque* occurred during an otherwise uneventful bus ride to another city.)

In order to check the concurrent validity of these findings, the investigators also estimated the overlap between *ataque de nervios* and panic disorder by means of blinded structured clinical interview for DSM-III-R (SCID) assessments. The SCID is a clinician-administered, semistructured instrument that yields DSM diagnoses, including panic disorder (47). SCID interviews administered blind to the results of the clinical/ethnographic instrument revealed that 33% of patients with *ataque* met panic disorder criteria. Comparison of the two ways of reaching a panic disorder diagnosis found that both methods were identifying essentially the same subgroup of patients (Pearson chi-square = 3.84; p = 0.05). Depending on the method used, the range of overlap between *ataque* and panic disorder in this sample was thus 17% to 33% (45).

This degree of overlap clearly confirms the absence of a one-to-one correlation between *ataque de nervios* and panic attacks, or between *ataque* and panic disorder. *Ataques* often share individual phenomenological features with panic episodes, but these features do not necessarily "run together" during the *ataque* experience. Figures 4-1 and 4-2 help distinguish the features that are shared between *ataques* and panic disorder from those that are not. *Ataques* distinct from panic disorder episodes appear to be provoked by some important life event and to peak in longer than 10 minutes. However, features that seem common to both *ataque* and panic disorder include recurrence of attacks, the experience of fear or nervousness during an episode, and anticipatory or behavioral sequelae afterwards. In addition, patients who described "feeling relieved" after their *ataque* also reported significantly fewer panic symptoms than those without this feeling. This suggests that a postattack sense of relief, rather than intense fear or dread, is another feature of *ataques* that do not fulfill panic phenomenology (45). These indicators confirm some of the distinctions included in the Glossary of Culture-Bound Syndromes that appeared in Appendix I of DSM-IV (5) and provide some guidance to clinicians on how to diagnose patients presenting with *ataques de nervios.* Treatment implications of these findings are discussed in a later section.

VI. *ATAQUE DE NERVIOS,* DISSOCIATION, AND CHILDHOOD TRAUMA

In addition to the overlap between *ataque de nervios* and panic disorder, a second nosological relationship that has been specifically investigated is that between *ataque,* the dissociative disorders, and PTSD (36). Case reports over several decades (48) and Guarnaccia et al.'s (6) phenomenological research had suggested that dissociative symptoms are a primary feature of *ataque* episodes. These symptoms include depersonalization, amnesia, identity alteration, and trancelike states. *Ataques* have also been linked to childhood traumatic exposure in a clinical sample in New York City (49) and to higher rates of PTSD in the Puerto Rico Disaster Study (27). These findings raised the possibility that *ataque* could be understood from the biomedical perspective as a culturally-patterned dissociative reaction to stress arising in persons predisposed by childhood exposure to trauma (36).

Lewis-Fernández and colleagues (36) studied 29 female Puerto Rican outpatients in a New England medical center, assessing their *ataque* status, dissociative symptoms and disorders, childhood traumatic exposure, PTSD status, and general psychopathology. The number of lifetime *ataque* episodes was used as a proxy measure of *ataque* syndrome severity. All of the women had migrated from Puerto Rico. Nine had never experienced *ataque de nervios,* 12 had experienced one to five *ataque*s, and eight had experienced more than five *ataques* over their lifetime. No significant differences were found between the groups in age, years of education, or age at migration, facilitating their comparability for diagnostic purposes.

Ataque frequency was assessed as a function of several factors: self-reported dissociative symptoms, measured with the Dissociative Experiences Scale (DES) (50); clinician-rated dissociative symptoms and disorders, based on the SCID for Dissociative Disorders (SCID-D) (51); childhood traumatic exposure, assessed with the Traumatic Antecedents Questionnaire (TAQ) (52); and SCID-diagnosed PTSD and other anxiety and depressive disorders.

Figure 4-3 presents the results. Self-reported and clinician-rated dissociative symptoms and SCID-diagnosed dissociative disorders showed a significant positive association with number of *ataques.* SCID interview also yielded partial evidence of a relationship between *ataque* frequency and PTSD. Although a diagnosis of PTSD was 2.5 times more likely among persons with frequent *ataques* than those without, sample size limitations resulted in a nonsignificant association. However, TAQ total score, as well as measures for specific kinds of traumatic exposure (i.e., physical abuse, sexual abuse), were clearly not significantly associated with *ataque*

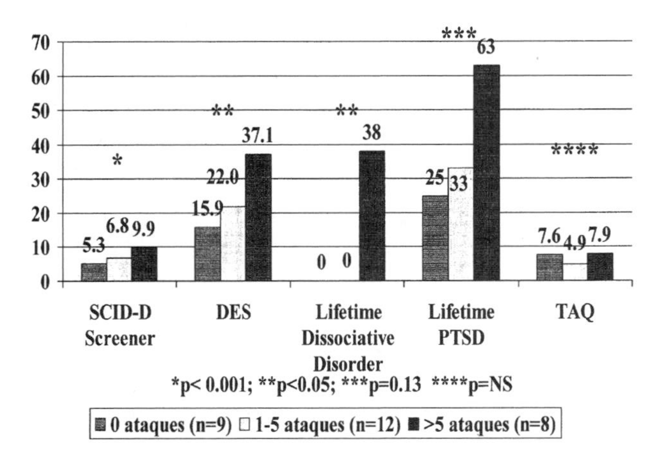

FIG. 4-3. Dissociative symptoms and disorders, posttraumatic stress disorder, and childhood trauma by number of *ataques* in female Puerto Rican patients (n = 29). (Adapted from Lewis-Fernández R, Garrido-Castillo P, Bennasar MC, et al. Dissociation, childhood trauma, and *ataque de nervios* among Puerto Rican psychiatric outpatients. *Am J Psychiatry* 2002;159:1603–1605.)

frequency, dissociative symptoms, or PTSD rates. Finally, lifetime diagnosis of panic disorder was also positively associated with *ataque* frequency, but lifetime major depression, dysthymia, and generalized anxiety disorder were not (36).

Contrary to the expected relationship, these findings indicate that childhood trauma per se was not associated with *ataque* frequency, dissociation, or PTSD. Rather, traumatic exposure was uniformly high across cohorts (52), suggesting that, in this sample, factors in addition to childhood trauma accounted for these conditions. This contradicts previous findings with a different clinical population and trauma scale that showed an association between *ataque* and childhood trauma (49), but is consistent with a multifactorial model of dissociation, *ataque,* and PTSD (53). Traumatic exposure was not sufficient to cause frequent *ataques*, but whether it is necessary remains unclear. The same patients who developed frequent *ataques* in the context of childhood trauma appeared to also be at higher risk for the dissociative disorders and PTSD. The presence of mood and anxiety psychopathology in the subgroup without *ataques* highlights the specificity of the association between *ataques* and dissociation, since this association is not solely attributable to the correlation between general psychopathology and dissociation (54).

Taken together, these findings suggest that frequent *ataques* are, in part, a marker for psychiatric disorders characterized by dissociative symptoms. This further confirms the diagnostic heterogeneity of this cultural syndrome. In the community—at least in Puerto Rico—*ataques* are associated more generally with mood and anxiety disorders. In clinical settings serving Puerto Ricans and Dominicans in Manhattan and New England, *ataques* appear to be particularly associated with panic disorder, the dissociative disorders, and possibly PTSD. The relationship with other depressive and anxiety disorders was nonspecific. Clinicians should be particularly aware of the specific diagnostic associations found for *ataques* in clinical settings. However, research with larger and more diverse Latino samples is needed to further clarify these associations.

Additional evidence of the relationship between *ataque de nervios* and dissociation comes from the association between *ataque* and other Latino idioms of distress that have strong dissociative characteristics. These are the idioms known as *celajes* (glimpses) and "hearing one's name," which are common forms of expressing distress in Puerto Rican and other Hispanic communities (55,56). *Celajes* are characterized by the visual perception of fleeting shapes or shadows that have no material basis, while "hearing one's name" refers to auditory perceptions usually involving one's name or other everyday noises (e.g., steps) that occur when the person is alone (57). These experiences can occur without producing undue distress, but in the context of emotional problems the sufferer and the community often take them as signs of worsening dysfunction.

In a sample of 132 Spanish-speaking Latino outpatients seeking care at the Anxiety Disorders Clinic of NYSPI, Lewis-Fernández (57) found an elevated positive correlation (Pearson $r = 0.8$) between DES scores and the frequency of these idioms. This strongly suggests that these experiences constitute culturally shaped forms of dissociative capacity.

Lewis-Fernández (57) also assessed the prevalence of these idioms and of self-reported *ataque de nervios* in a sample of 81 consecutive psychiatric referrals in rural Puerto Rico primary care clinics. The rate of *celajes* was 70.4%, that of "hearing one's name" was 76.5%, and that of *ataque* was 58.7%. Seeing *celajes* and hearing one's name when alone were each significantly more likely among patients reporting *ataque* than among those without this syndrome ($p < 0.05$). Given the dissociative character of these perceptual idioms, evidenced by their correlation with DES scores, the association of these idioms with *ataque* confirms the relationship between *ataque* and the dissociative scales that was found in the New England patient sample.

Moreover, the distribution of *celajes* and "hearing one's name" across demographic groups in these low-income rural settings in Puerto Rico was very similar to that of *ataque*. Both idioms were evenly distributed across gender and level of education. Only older age showed a trend association (chi-square = 3.52, df = 1, $p = 0.06$) with "hearing one's name", with patients 45 years or older more likely than younger respondents to report this experience (84% vs. 67%). Older age had a smaller impact on the rate of *celajes* (76% vs. 64%; chi-square = 1.31, df = 1, $p = 0.25$). These results suggest that rural background and low-income status exert a stronger influence on the experience of these idioms of distress than the other sociodemographic variables tested.

VII. *ATAQUE DE NERVIOS* IN THE CONTEXT OF POPULAR NOSOLOGY

The complex relationship between *ataque de nervios* and psychiatric diagnosis may be further clarified by examining this syndrome in the larger context of the popular nosology to which it belongs (34,58). For Caribbean Hispanics and several other Latino groups, *ataque* forms part of an overall popular nosology of *nervios* (nerves), composed also of other related categories (58,59). This nosology links experiences of adversity to ensuing "alterations" of the nervous system. The functioning of the nervous system is understood to be consequently impaired, including the peripheral nerves, and this quasi-anatomical damage is evidenced in emotional and physical symptoms. Examples of the emotional aspects of *nervios* illness include interpersonal susceptibility, anxiety, and irritability, while examples of the associated physical damage are trembling, palpitations, and decreased concentration (58). Certain people are considered at greater risk for *nervios* when confronted with adversity, such as those with an inherited predisposition or with stressful perinatal experiences (e.g., mother's alcoholism). But in all cases, the possibility that sufficient adversity will result in an alteration of the nervous system leads to the popular view that persons faced with experiences of suffering should "control" their reactions to avoid nervous system damage. This usually takes the form of dampening the emotional impact of the experience, so that the nerves will not be substantially "altered" (34,58).

Clinical and popular discussions about *nervios* and *ataques* in Latino communities thus typically reference views about the importance of remaining in control, and of facing the world with *tranquilidad* (equanimity) regardless of the severity of the stressor. What is at stake in these discussions is how to behave in contexts of adversity. In its more extreme form, this worldview posits that "uncontrolled" reactions to suffering can result not only in individual illness, but also in communal disintegration through expressions of violence and chaos (60). In this sense, it is useful for clinicians to realize that this popular nosology has even more of an explicit moral purpose than the professional classification system.

The salience of this perspective for *ataque* sufferers may be seen in the frequent mention of the term "control" when discussing their experience. Among Puerto Rican and Dominican psychiatric patients interviewed by the senior authors, references to the need for additional "control" are nearly ubiquitous. Most common is the view that the person has "tried to control him/herself" and has been unable to do so, resulting in the *ataque*. *Ataque de nervios* thus has a strong communicative function: it is an outburst with a message. In effect, the person is letting others know that his or her ability to cope has been overwhelmed by adversity. This is evidenced by the common statement before an *ataque*: "*ya no me aguanto más* (I cannot/will not hold it in [or, hold myself back] anymore)" (6,34,58).

A mature social actor, however, is not supposed to stay in an uncontrolled state for any substantial length of time. Rather, the outburst should end and the person should regain control, at least until the next overwhelming situation, when the outburst may recur. Nevertheless, in the presence of too many overwhelming stressors or an excess of vulnerability, the sufferer eventually may express *ataques* even after minor precipitants. It is the pattern of holding in, blowing up, and holding in, that makes up the *ataque* syndrome.

This should help clarify why *ataques* do not have a one-to-one relationship with any single psychiatric disorder. *Ataque de nervios* constitutes instead a behavioral syndrome stemming from general cultural notions and practices about how to behave, rather than a peculiar cultural expression of a particular diagnosis. It is a marker of being overwhelmed that can be associated with various forms of psychopathology (58). This explains why *ataques* would occur in persons in whom psychopathology develops in response to traumatic stress, because the *ataque* constitutes a statement about the suffering of the person. Persons faced with traumatic events in whom psychopathology does not develop would be less overwhelmed by the exposure and thus less likely to have recurrent *ataques*. But the *ataque* itself cannot be reduced to just the psychiatric disorder; rather it is a marker of the severity of the stressor, of the person's reaction style, of his or her level of support, and of the resulting distress and pathology (6,34).

The predisposition to *ataque* is thus more like the predisposition to dissociation that characterizes various disorders that have a strong relationship to traumatic exposure, such as the dissociative disorders, PTSD, and even panic disorder (61): Not a disorder per se necessarily, but a behavioral repertoire associated with several disorders (62). The association between *ataque* frequency and dissociation described earlier in the chapter in fact suggests that both of these behavioral reactions may be mediated by related vulnerabilities, because they "run together" in clinical samples.

Caribbean Latino culture may promote this association, because the appearance of dissociation during the *ataque* may be enhanced by the cultural perception that a mature social actor needs to be always in control. Dissociation may be particularly promoted by the popular view that when out of control the person is no longer him or herself ("*ése no era yo* [that was not me]"). The uncontrolled behavior is disavowed as not being part of the self. This may facilitate the emergence of dissociative splits that allows the person to distance him/herself from the moral consequences of the *ataque* episode (34).

Thus, some types of cultural factors could predispose to the appearance of *ataques* among certain trauma sufferers and not others within the same ethnic group. The key cultural variables would be the extent to which a person adheres to the cultural code of "control" and the related idea that uncontrolled behavior is ego-alien. This leads to the testable hypothesis that individuals faced with adversity who hold these cultural notions and thus embody such practices are more vulnerable to the appearance of *ataques* than those who do not hold or embody these notions. The role of these local views in the etiology of *ataque* highlights the importance of intraethnic cultural factors in the study of popular syndromes, as opposed to variables that represent ethnic background as a more monolithic construct.

VIII. ASSESSMENT AND TREATMENT OF *ATAQUE DE NERVIOS*

A. Assessment

Research on *ataque* illustrates for clinicians how being informed about the popular nosology of Latino patients not only decreases the chances of misdiagnosis, but also facilitates the formulation of an effective treatment plan. In light of the clinical heterogeneity of *ataque de nervios* evidenced in this chapter and the diversity of life contexts in which the syndrome emerges, clinicians must be prepared to perform a case-by-case mental health evaluation of each *ataque* sufferer. As this chapter shows, a generic translation of *ataque* episodes into professional categories (e.g., as panic disorder) in the absence of individual clinical information is very likely to result in misdiagnosis and a compromised therapeutic alliance. It also robs the patient of the possibility of "telling the story" of what led to the *ataque* in a safe, supportive environment as part of the evaluation process. This process of *desahogarse* (unchoking or unburdening oneself) is considered in the popular view to be the best therapeutic intervention for this syndrome (6).

One method that has been operationalized in recent years for the systematic, individual assessment of cultural factors when conducting a clinical evaluation is the Cultural Formulation (CF) model. This method supplements the biopsychosocial approach by highlighting the effect of culture on the patient's symptomatology, explanatory models of illness, etiological views, levels of support, help-seeking preferences, and outcome expectations (63–66). It is described in Appendix I of DSM-IV. Clinicians are encouraged to apply the CF model during an evaluation of an *ataque* sufferer in order to obtain the necessary cultural and clinical information for an individual diagnosis and treatment plan. Lewis-Fernández and Díaz (67) illustrate a case scenario of a Puerto Rican woman suffering from *ataque de nervios* whose care was markedly improved by the implementation of a cultural evaluation using the CF approach.

Application of the CF model should include a detailed account of family relationships and conflicts, because these are usually central to the *ataque* story. The role of traumatic exposure is also particularly important, given the very high prevalence of this risk factor among female users of psychiatric services suffering from *ataques* (36). Often, recurrent *ataques* are a sign of severe and enduring trauma, which necessitates specialized intervention. Other potential sources of stress, such as migration- or poverty-related issues, should also be assessed.

Ataque evaluations should elicit the person's and the family's expectations regarding the role in the assessment process of a medical workup, such as physical examination and laboratory or imaging tests. Particularly when *ataques* have become recurrent, many Caribbean Hispanics question whether the nervous system has been "altered" by repeated stress, and this understanding leads them to desire biomedical confirmation of physical normalcy. Statements by clinicians about "not needing" these workups may be perceived as inattention, negligence, or even active discrimination, unless they are accompanied by careful explanation of biomedical views about the current status of the patient's nervous system. A process of negotiation is required between the participants in the clinical encounter. Patients and relatives may be quite relieved about not needing further tests, as long as they are convinced that the clinician has thoroughly assessed the possibility of *nervios* damage. However, some sufferers may not have contemplated the possibility of physical "alteration" and may be shocked by what they perceive as suggestions of abnormality.

Clinicians are advised to inquire about the person's explanatory models of the *ataque* syndrome using the CF model during the early phases of the evaluation (67).

The process of psychiatric diagnosis should obviously include consideration of the *ataque* episode, but not be overly determined by its appearance. As discussed earlier, *ataques* constitute a behavioral marker of being overwhelmed, which may indicate the presence of various disorders. In the case of single or occasional *ataques*, no psychopathology may be evident. Only about a third of *ataque* sufferers merit a diagnosis of panic disorder, for which the phenomenology of the attack itself and its sequelae are the principal elements of the nosological decision. The appearance of *ataques* should help guide the diagnostician toward certain likely disorders, but the differential should be determined by the full clinical picture.

B. Treatment

No treatment studies of *ataque* have ever been conducted. However, certain clinical suggestions may be advanced when formulating a treatment plan for an *ataque* sufferer.

Acutely, the first priority is to ensure the safety of the person and those around her/him. During an *ataque,* suicidal and violent gestures should be prevented, but inadvertent injury may also result from the uncontrolled behavior (e.g., falls). However, involuntary restraints should be avoided unless absolutely necessary, since these may cause the *ataque* to escalate. The main intervention is to attempt to "talk the person through" the *ataque.* Acknowledgment of the stressors that overwhelmed the sufferer tends to defervesce an acute *ataque* fairly quickly and to help restore the *status quo ante.* Clinicians will be aided in this process by the cultural emphasis on returning to a "controlled" state as soon as possible. Relatives may provide assistance by rubbing the person with *alcoholado* (rubbing alcohol) during the nonaggressive phases of the episode in order to help reduce the agitation and communicate support (58).

"Telling the story" of what led to the *ataque* also constitutes the principal therapeutic approach in subsequent stages of treatment. Because one of the main functions of the attack is to communicate a feeling of being overwhelmed, indicating receipt of the message and the desire to offer support are usually perceived as therapeutic. The person should be allowed to set the pace of disclosure and to give enough details and circumstances to feel "unburdened" (*desahogado[a]*) (6).

It can be very useful to couch all interventions within the popular paradigm of remaining "in control." This requires individual assessment of the centrality of this value for each patient. In our experience, most *ataque* sufferers will respond to inquiries on this topic by detailing how they have tried and been unable to control their reactions. Treatment can then initially be described as a way of increasing the person's ability to "control themselves" (*controlarse*). Psychotherapy and medications are amenable to this description. Once trust is established over time, clinicians may choose to gently problematize the person's need to remain strictly "in control" in the face of any stressor. If this view is challenged too early in the treatment, however, the person may feel that the clinician does not understand his or her reality. Often, *ataque* sufferers see themselves as barely hanging on to their sense of control as it is and resent suggestions to "let go."

In the case of single or occasional *ataques* in the absence of a psychiatric diagnosis, brief follow-up visit is usually sufficient. This may be discussed with the patient and the family as a way of ensuring the full return to a previous healthy state. For recurrent *ataques*, treatment depends on several factors. These include the associated psychopathology, the nature of the precipitants, including traumatic exposure, the degree of family conflict or support, the social context, the previous treatment experiences, and the patient's and family's expectations, among other factors.

Psychotherapy is typically the mainstay of treatment, given the usual source of the overwhelmed behavior in the interpersonal milieu. A family or systems approach is particularly helpful, in order to provide a setting for verbal decoding of the *ataque* behavior and negotiation of subsequent relationships and actions among the participants in the story. Specialized psychotherapies may be required for particular disorders signaled by the *ataque,* such as cognitive behavioral therapy for panic disorder or prolonged exposure for PTSD.

It is desirable for the clinician to adopt a social activist stance, since the distress that precipitates *ataques* among low-income Latinos is often rooted in experiences of socioeconomic disenfranchisement or ethnic/racial discrimination. Helping the patient and the family identify the social origins of their suffering and decide on possible interventions at a community level may be long-lasting therapeutic activities. These may include, for example, discussing the social roots of drug abuse among urban youth or of the violent behavior of an unemployed spouse (68).

Finally, psychopharmacological agents may also be very useful in the treatment of *ataque*-related psychopathology. Primary emphasis should be placed on treating the underlying disorder, such as by using antidepressants and other agents in the case of panic disorder. Judicious use of short-acting benzodiazepines also has a role in helping abort an impending *ataque.* The slower crescendo of most *ataques* typically affords sufferers the opportunity to prevent the episode through medication taken only as needed. However, this should not be the main form of treatment for recurrent *ataques*, because it only forestalls the principal function of the syndrome as a mode of communication. Instead, psychotherapy and social activism are usually required to address the interpersonal and sociocultural roots of *ataque de nervios.*

IX. CONCLUSION

This chapter examined the anthropological, epidemiological, and clinical dimensions of *ataque de nervios.* In Caribbean Latino communities, *ataque* is a prevalent popular syndrome that signals a sufferer's strong feeling of loss of control in the face of interpersonal and communal adversity. Individuals who suffer from a combination of social disadvantage, psychiatric disorder, and poor perceived health and interpersonal support are at higher risk for experiencing an *ataque de nervios.* However, *ataque* clearly does not represent a cultural version of a single psychiatric diagnosis.

Instead, these attacks are associated in community studies with several depressive and anxiety disorders, as well as with normal and transient reactions to stress. Research to date suggests that *ataque* sufferers who present to clinical settings may be more likely to meet criteria specifically for panic disorder, the dissociative disorders, and PTSD. The paroxysmic nature of the syndrome may relate to the cultural value placed on emotional and social "control" in various Latino groups. Attention to this and other cultural interpretations and expectations is central to the process of clinical assessment and treatment. The *ataque* label adds important clinical information on the precipitating causes of the distress, the social context, and the expected interventions from the perspective of the sufferer and his or her community.

REFERENCES

1. Nichter M. Idioms of distress: alternatives in the expression of psychosocial distress. A case study from South India. *Cult Med Psychiatry* 1981;5:379–408.
2. Good BJ, Delvecchio-Good MJ. Toward a meaning-centered analysis of popular illness categories: "fright-illness" and "heart distress" in Iran. In: Marsella AJ, White GM, eds. *Cultural conceptions of mental health and therapy.* Dordrecht: D. Reidel, 1982:141–166.
3. Guarnaccia PJ. *Ataques de nervios* in Puerto Rico: culture-bound syndrome or popular illness? *Med Anthropol* 1992;15:1–14.
4. Guarnaccia PJ,Rogler LH. Research on culture-bound syndromes: new directions. *Am J Psychiatry* 1999;156:1322–1327.
5. American Psychiatric Association. *Diagnostic and statistical manual of mental disorders, fourth edition (DSM-IV).* Washington, DC: American Psychiatric Association, 1994.
6. Guarnaccia PJ, Rivera M, Franco F, et al. The experiences of *ataques de nervios:* towards an anthropology of emotions in Puerto Rico. *Cult Med Psychiatry* 1996;20:343–367.
7. Lock M, Scheper-Hughes N. A critical-interpretive approach in medical anthropology: rituals and routines of discipline and dissent. In: Johnson TM, Sargent CF, eds. *Medical anthropology: contemporary theory and method.* New York: Praeger, 1990:47–72.
8. Farmer P, Kleinman A. AIDS as human suffering. *Daedalus* 1989,118:135–160.
9. Kleinman A, Kleinman J. Suffering and its professional transformation: toward an ethnography of experience. *Cult Med Psychiatry* 1991;15:275–301.
10. Desjarlais R. *Body and emotion: the aesthetics of illness and healing in the Nepal Himalayas.* Philadelphia: University of Pennsylvania Press, 1992.
11. Farmer P. *AIDS and accusation: Haiti and the geography of blame.* Berkeley: University of California Press, 1992.
12. Robert de Ramírez de Arellano MI, Ramírez de Arellano M, García L, et al. '*Ataques*,' hyperkinetic type: the so-called 'Puerto Rican Syndrome': its medical, psychological, and social implications. Presented at the annual meeting of the Puerto Rico Medical Association, Puerto Rico, 1954.
13. Rubio M, Urdaneta M, Doyle JL. Psychopathologic reaction patterns in the Antilles Command. *US Armed Forces Med J* 1955;6:1767–1772.
14. Fernández-Marina R. The Puerto Rican Syndrome: its dynamics and cultural determinants. *Psychiatry* 1961;24:79–82.
15. Mehlman RD. The Puerto Rican Syndrome. *Am J Psychiatry* 1961;118:328–332.
16. Rothenberg A. Puerto Rico and aggression. *Am J Psychiatry* 1964;120:962–970.
17. Abad V, Boyce E. Issues in the psychiatric evaluations of Puerto Ricans: a socio-cultural perspective. *J Oper Psychiatry* 1979;10:28–39.
18. Bird HR. The cultural dichotomy of colonial people. *J Am Acad Psychoanal* 1982;10:195–209.
19. Rendón M. Myths and stereotypes in minority groups. *Int J Soc Psychiatry* 1984;30:297–309.
20. De la Cancela V, Guarnaccia PJ, Carrillo E. Psychosocial distress among Latinos: a critical analysis of *ataques de nervios. Humanity Soc* 1986;10:431–447.
21. Guarnaccia PJ, De la Cancela V, Carrillo E. The multiple meanings of *ataques de nervios* in the Latino community. *Med Anthropol* 1989;11:47–62.
22. Harwood A. *Rx: spiritist as needed.* New York: Wiley, 1977.

23. Garrison V, Thomas CS. A case of a Dominican migrant. In: Boyce-Laport RS, Thomas CS, eds. *Alienation in contemporary society.* New York: Praeger, 1976:216–260.
24. Garrison V. The "Puerto Rican Syndrome" in psychiatry and espiritismo. In: Crapanzano V, Garrison V, eds. *Case studies in spirit possession.* New York: Wiley 1977:383–448.
25. Oquendo M, Horwath E, Martínez A. *Ataques de nervios:* proposed diagnostic criteria for a culture specific syndrome. *Cult Med Psychiatry* 1992;16:367–376.
26. Lewis-Fernández R. Diagnosis and treatment of nervios and *ataques* in a female Puerto Rican migrant. *Cult Med Psychiatry,* 1996;20:155–163.
27. Guarnaccia PJ, Canino G, Rubio-Stipec M, et al. The prevalence of *ataques de nervios* in the Puerto Rico Disaster Study. *J Nerv Ment Dis* 1993;181:157–165.
28. Carstairs GM, Kapur RL. *The Great Universe of Kota: social change and mental disorder in an Indian village.* Berkeley: University of California Press, 1976.
29. Rubel AJ, O'Nell CW, Collado-Ardón R. *Susto: a folk illness.* Berkeley: University of California Press, 1984.
30. Kleinman A, Kleinman J. How bodies remember: social memory and bodily experience of criticism, resistance, and deligitimation following China's Cultural Revolution. *New Lit Hist* 1994;25:707–723.
31. Young A. The anthropologies of illness and sickness. *Ann Rev Anthropol* 1982;11:257–285.
32. Good BJ. Culture and psychopathology: directions for psychiatric anthropology. In: Schwartz T, White GM, Lutz CA, eds. *New directions in psychological anthropology.* Cambridge: Cambridge University Press, 1992:181–205.
33. Good BJ. *Medicine, rationality, and experience: an anthropological perspective.* Cambridge: Cambridge University Press, 1994.
34. Lewis-Fernández R. "That was not in me . . . I couldn't control myself": control, identity, and emotion in Puerto Rican communities [in Spanish]. *Rev Cien Soc* 1998;4:268–299.
35. Scarry E. *The body in pain: the making and unmaking of the world.* New York: Oxford University Press, 1985.
36. Lewis-Fernández R, Garrido-Castillo P, Bennasar M, et al. Dissociation, childhood trauma, and *ataque de nervios* among Puerto Rican psychiatric outpatients. *Am J Psychiatry* 2002;159:1603–1605.
37. Canino GJ, Bravo M, Rubio-Stipec M, et al. The impact of disaster on mental health: prospective and retrospective analyses. *Int J Ment Health* 1990;19:51–69.
38. Bravo M, Rubio-Stipec M, Canino GJ, et al. The psychological sequelae of disaster stress prospectively and retrospectively evaluated. *Am J Commun Psychol* 1990;18:661–680.
39. Robins LN, Helzer JE, Croughnan J, et al. National Institute of Mental Health Diagnostic Interview Schedule. *Arch Gen Psychiatry* 1981;38:281–389.
40. Trautman EC. The suicidal fit. *Arch Gen Psychiatry* 1961;5:76–83.
41. Lewis-Fernández R, Canino G, Ramírez R, et al. Latino perspectives on mental health in primary care. Presented at the 49th Institute on Psychiatric Services, American Psychiatric Association, Washington, DC, 1997.
42. Liebowitz MR, Salmán E, Jusino CM, et al. *Ataque de nervios* and panic disorder. *Am J Psychiatry* 1994;151:871–875
43. Liebowitz MR. Anxiety disorders. In: Widiger TA, Frances AJ, Pincus HA, et al., eds. *DSM-IV sourcebook.* Washington, DC: American Psychiatric Association, 1996;2:397–410.
44. Salmán E, Liebowitz MR, Guarnaccia PJ, et al. Subtypes of *ataques de nervios:* The influence of coexisting psychiatric diagnoses. *Cult Med Psychiatry* 1998;22:231–244.
45. Lewis-Fernández R, Guarnaccia PJ, Martínez IE, et al. Comparative phenomenology of *ataques de nervios,* panic attacks, and panic disorder. *Cult Med Psychiatry* 2002;26:199–223.
46. Weiss M. Explanatory Model Interview Catalogue (EMIC): framework for comparative study of illness. *Transcult Psychiatry* 1997;34:235–263.
47. Spitzer RL, Williams JBW, Gibbon M, et al. The Structured Clinical Interview for DSM-III-R (SCID): history, rationale, and description. *Arch Gen Psychiatry* 1992;49:624–629.
48. Lewis-Fernández R. Culture and dissociation: a comparison of *ataque de nervios* among Puerto Ricans and possession syndrome in India. In: Spiegel D, ed. *Dissociation: culture, mind, and body.* Washington, DC: American Psychiatric Press 1994:123–167.
49. Schechter DS, Marshall R, Salmán E, et al. *Ataque de nervios* and history of childhood trauma. *J Traum Stress* 2000;13:529–534.
50. Bernstein EM, Putnam FW. Development, reliability, and validity of a dissociation scale. *J Nerv Ment Dis* 1986;174:727–735.

51. Steinberg M, Rounsaville B, Cicchetti DV. The Structured Clinical Interview for DSM-III-R Dissociative Disorders: preliminary report on a new diagnostic instrument. *Am J Psychiatry* 1990;147:76–82.
52. Herman JL, Perry JC, Van der Kolk BA. Childhood trauma in borderline personality disorder. *Am J Psychiatry* 1989;146:490–495.
53. van Ijzendoorn MH, Schuengel C. The measurement of dissociation in normal and clinical populations: meta-analytic validation of the Dissociative Experiences Scale (DES). *Clin Psychol Rev* 1996; 16:365–382.
54. Mulder RT, Beautrais AL, Joyce PR, et al. Relationship between dissociation, childhood sexual abuse, childhood physical abuse, and mental illness in a general population sample. *Am J Psychiatry* 1998;155:806–811.
55. Guarnaccia PJ, Guevara-Ramos LM, Gonzáles G, et al. Cross-cultural aspects of psychotic symptoms in Puerto Rico. *Res Commun Ment Health* 1992;7:99–110.
56. Olfson M, Lewis-Fernández R, Weissman MM, et al. Psychotic symptoms in an urban general medicine practice. *Am J Psychiatry* 2002;159:1412–1419.
57. Lewis-Fernández R. Assessing psychosis screeners among underserved urban primary care patients. Presented at the NARSAD 15th Annual Scientific Symposium, New York, New York, 2003.
58. Guarnaccia P, Lewis-Fernández R, Marano MR. Toward a Puerto Rican popular nosology: nervios and *ataques de nervios. Cult Med Psychiatry* 2003;27:339–366.
59. Davis DL, Guarnaccia PJ. Health, culture, and the nature of nerves. *Med Anthropol* 1989;11:1–95.
60. Benítez-Rojo A. *The repeating island: the Caribbean and the postmodern perspective.* Durham, NC: Duke University Press, 1992.
61. Stein MB, Walker JR, Anderson G, et al. Childhood physical and sexual abuse in patients with anxiety disorders and in a community sample. *Am J Psychiatry* 1996;153:275–277.
62. Carr JE, Vitaliano PP. The theoretical implications of converging research on depression and the culture-bound syndromes. In: Kleinman A, Good B, eds. *Culture and depression.* Berkeley: University of California Press, 1985:244–266.
63. Lu FG, Lim RF, Mezzich JE. Issues in the assessment and diagnosis of culturally diverse individuals. In: Oldham JM, Riba MB. *APA review of psychiatry, vol. 14.* Washington, DC: APA Press, 1995: 477–510.
64. Mezzich JE. Cultural formulation and comprehensive diagnosis: clinical and research perspectives. *Psychiatr Clin North Am* 1995;18:649–657.
65. Lewis-Fernández R. Cultural formulation of psychiatric diagnosis. *Cult Med Psychiatry* 1996;20: 133–144.
66. Group for the Advancement of Psychiatry, Committee on Cultural Psychiatry. *Cultural assessment in clinical psychiatry.* Washington, DC: American Psychiatric Publishing, 2001.
67. Lewis-Fernández R, Díaz N. The Cultural Formulation: a method for assessing cultural factors affecting the clinical encounter. *Psychiatr Q* 2002;73:271–295.
68. Singer M, Valentín F, Baer H, et al. Why does Juan García have a drinking problem? The perspective of critical medical anthropology. *Med Anthropol* 1992;14:77–100.

5

Psychiatric Treatment of Hispanic Patients*

David Mischoulon

Department of Psychiatry, Harvard Medical School, Boston, Massachusetts 02115; and Depression Clinical and Research Program, Massachusetts General Hospital, Boston, Massachusetts 02114

I. INTRODUCTION: THE HISPANIC-AMERICAN POPULATION

There are approximately 32.8 million Hispanic people in the United States, representing over 12% of this country's population (1). Hispanics have been the fastest growing ethnic group in the United States in the past decade, and now constitute the largest minority in the United States (2). There is much diversity in this population, which comprises individuals from Mexico, Puerto Rico, Cuba, and Central and South America (3,4), and it is therefore important not to use the term "Hispanic" or "Latino" too broadly (5).

Psychiatrists and other mental health professionals can expect to see increasing numbers of Hispanic patients, either on a regular basis in their practices, or by serving as consultants to general internists who manage depression in the primary care setting. Clinicians should therefore be familiar with effective approaches to working with this population. In this chapter, we will review different challenges faced by clinicians who treat Hispanics, including cultural factors and differing beliefs and attitudes about mental health; difficulties in diagnosis, including the impact of culture-bound syndromes; and different approaches to treatment, including the role of natural remedies and folk healing. We will also review basic

*Portions of this chapter were adapted from Mischoulon D. Management of major depression in Hispanic patients. *Directions Psychiatry* 2000;20:275–285. Permission from the Hatherleigh Company is acknowledged.

concepts in ethnopsychopharmacology as it relates to the Hispanic population. Three selected vignettes will be included to illustrate some of the concepts put forth in the chapter.

II. CULTURAL FACTORS THAT MAY AFFECT TREATMENT

A. Language Barrier

Many Hispanic Americans have limited English skills. This can become an obstacle to effective communication if the treating clinician does not speak Spanish (6). In many clinics, translators may be available to assist, but this can still result in discomfort on the part of the patient and the clinician. Misunderstanding or miscommunication of clinical information can occur regardless of the availability of translators (6–8). Even if the clinician speaks Spanish, he or she needs to appreciate the colloquialisms and slang of the patient (7), because these colloquialisms may differ among Hispanics from different nations. To give some examples, the word *coger* (to take) is a slang term for sexual intercourse in certain Latin American countries. The word *coraje* (courage) may be used by some Hispanics to refer to anger attacks.

B. Cultural Factors and Concepts of Mental Illness

Hispanics may present with different beliefs about mental health compared to other ethnic groups. Hispanics in general may be resistant to the idea of mental illness, in part because of fear of stigmatization (9). Disorders such as depression and anxiety may be viewed as a sign of weakness or madness (10). Consequently, Hispanics presenting with psychiatric illness may not describe themselves as depressed or anxious per se, or endorse the classic neurovegetative symptoms of these disorders. They may instead somatize mental anguish, and present with physical complaints, which upon medical workup do not appear to have a clear physiologic cause (3).

Some Hispanics also have different views about the causes of disease. For example, the "hot and cold theory" is based on the notion that the body contains four humors or liquids: blood (hot and wet), phlegm (cold and wet), black bile (cold and dry), and yellow bile (hot and dry) (11). This theory suggests that disease is caused by a humoral imbalance that can be cured with foods and medications designed to restore the balance. A typical strategy might involve treating a "hot" illness with a "cold" food or medication. Some Hispanics may express skepticism about "Western" medicine in general, and/or perceive Anglo-American clinicians as insincere and lacking warmth (12). These patients may prefer to consult with spiritual healers, participate in rituals aimed at alleviating their condition, and self-medicate with natural remedies (9). Many Hispanics, however, are comfortable going to both "Western-trained" clinicians as well as folk healers (11), particularly if they feel that their practitioners are sensitive to their needs and appreciate the limitations of the different approaches to treatment (11,13).

C. Acculturation

Acculturation is defined as the ability to deal effectively with a new culture, and may have both a positive and negative impact on mental health in Hispanics (11,14).

Though acculturation is difficult to quantify objectively, the ability to speak English is often used as a proxy measure for acculturation (15), and language difficulties may contribute to psychological stress. Less acculturated Hispanics may experience more stress when having to deal with American society, and may be limited in terms of ability to find gainful employment and advance socioeconomically. These individuals may become more vulnerable to mental illness, and may have greater difficulties with access to care. Acculturation, on the other hand, may also present a conflict of values, and more acculturated Hispanics may feel alienated from their "mother culture." This is especially true for offspring of immigrants, who often feel "stuck" between two cultures (11,14). The few research studies in this area suggest better outcomes for those who manage to integrate both sets of values (14).

D. Interpersonal Factors in the Treatment Setting

Clinicians who work with Hispanics need to be aware of several interpersonal issues that may emerge during their clinical work (11). For example, *respeto* (respect) is the expectation that respect be conveyed between the clinician and the patient, typically by the proper use of titles (*Señor, Señora,* Doctor, etc.) and the formal form of addressing a person (*usted,* as opposed to *tu*). Nonetheless, Hispanics also prefer to relate to their treaters as people rather than as representatives of an institution. *Personalismo* (personalism), therefore, is the expectation that the clinician behave in a more familiar manner with the patient and their family, once trust (*confianza*) has been established. Other manifestations of *personalismo* may include the patient's desire to sit or stand more closely to the doctor than would an Anglo-American patient (16).

Personalismo can at times be troublesome, particularly in the mental health field, because psychiatrists and psychologists are often trained not to disclose personal details—such as marital status, religious beliefs, and so forth—to patients. Other difficulties for the treater include the dilemma of whether to accept gifts from the patient (3). It is customary among many Hispanics to give occasional gifts to their treaters, as a sign of gratitude and respect. To decline a gift or other familiar gesture from the patient may be viewed by the patient as a personal rejection and/or lack of respect for his or her culture. This can strain the treatment alliance (3). Clinicians need to be comfortable when dealing with these gestures of gratitude from patients, and may consider relaxing boundaries in such cases, in order to protect the treatment alliance.

E. Time

It is often said that for Hispanics, "time walks rather than flies." Patients often arrive late (or too early) for appointments (3). Clinicians may perceive lateness as resistance to treatment, and early arrivals may be viewed as a sign of dependency. This phenomenon may, however, represent a differing view of time among Hispanics, focussing more on events than on time itself. Clinicians may develop different strategies for managing this situation. For example, some clinics may function on a walk-in basis, arranging for clinician availability between a given number of hours (e.g. flexible availability from 2–5 p.m.). Alternatively, individual clinicians may observe a patient's arrival pattern (late or early), and adjust their schedule appropriately, (e.g. instructing a patient to arrive at 2 p.m., and expecting to meet with him or her at 2:30 p.m.).

F. Fatalism

Hispanics often use the phrases "*si Dios quiere*" ("the Lord willing"), and "*que sera sera*" ("whatever will be will be") (10,11). They represent a belief that whatever will happen is predetermined and/or in the hands of a higher entity, usually the Christian God. In some extreme cases, it may encourage relinquishing of responsibility, and can present a problem in psychotherapy, in cases where the therapist may be working to empower the patient to take charge of his or her life. Emphasizing that "God helps those who help themselves" is a useful strategy that can encourage patients to be more proactive in their treatment and general life circumstances (16). This is especially important when medications are prescribed, and the clinician may have concerns about adherence. Clinicians may also have to be prepared to answer questions about their own religious and spiritual beliefs, in cases where the patient may be seeking similarity with their treater.

G. Gender Roles

The Hispanic culture tends to assign specific roles to men and women, and clinicians should be well acquainted with these. For example, *machismo* is a concept generally misunderstood by Anglo-Americans as the need for a man to signal sexual availability, or to behave in a raucous manner (e.g., drinking heavily or starting fights) (11). To Hispanics, in fact, it is the expectation that a man be a strong, loving provider for his family, and that he protect their welfare and their honor. The father is also expected to provide discipline among his children (17). For Hispanic men, therefore, it can be difficult to accept the need for mental health treatment, as they may interpret it as a sign of weakness, or may fear being perceived as weak by their peers or by their family.

The role of the Hispanic mother, on the other hand, is idealized and equated with self-denial. *Marianismo* is the belief that the woman is spiritually superior to the man, and must defer her own physical and emotional needs for those of the family, particularly her children (11). This is important to appreciate when working with Hispanic women, because depression may result when emotional needs go unmet (18). Hispanic women may be more likely than their male counterparts to seek help from a psychiatrist (3). They may also be more forthcoming about distress (3), because they are not bound by the same code of strength as men are.

H. The Family

Among Hispanics, the family is considered the primary source of support. *Familismo* is the term for this phenomenon (11), which emphasizes collective family goals, rather than individual goals. The psychiatrist must consider the benefits of involvement of the patient's family members as part of the treatment team. Hispanic patients will often see their doctor while accompanied by one or several family members, including nonbiological "relatives" such as godparents. Patients may be reticent to accept a certain treatment if one or all of their family members are opposed to it. The psychiatrist must then work to ensure family consensus before a treatment plan can be agreed upon. The clinician needs to watch out for disagreement on the part of family members, because this can often undermine treatment. An understanding of the authority structure in the family can be helpful, because the approval of the "patriarch" (usually the father) will facilitate treatment. Extending an invitation to the family members to attend the patient's appointment may help to solidify the treater's alliance with the patient and his or her family.

I. Economics and Education

In general, the Hispanic-American population is characterized by limited income and education, as well as difficulties with access to medical care (3). About 26% of Hispanic Americans live in poverty, and less than 50% have completed high school (3). As mentioned before, many Hispanics are limited by the fact that they speak Spanish only. Even Hispanics who have fairly good access to care may not be able to take full advantage of treatment. For example, some patients may have difficulty understanding the rationale or schedule for certain treatments. This may result in nonadherence and poor follow-up (19). The psychiatrist must have a good understanding of the patient's level of education and economic situation, in order to determine how feasible a particular treatment may be, and what resources may be available to maximize the effectiveness of the treatment plan.

III. DIAGNOSTIC ISSUES IN HISPANIC PATIENTS

A. Underreporting of Symptoms

The rate of psychiatric disorders such as depression may be higher in Hispanics than in the general population (15). Unfortunately, depression often goes undiagnosed, especially in primary care settings. Underreporting of symptoms, as well as limited physician education about psychiatric illness, may contribute to this problem in general (20).

Hispanics may be particularly reluctant to discuss mental illness and may express mental anguish differently compared to individuals from other cultures (21). As mentioned earlier, somatization, the manifestation of emotional distress in the form of physical symptoms, is frequently seen, particularly in women. This is thought by some to result from the suppression of emotional needs, which may make one vulnerable to illness. Somatic symptoms commonly seen include fatigue, headache, backache, stomach upset, insomnia, and loss of appetite (15).

Hispanics in general may rely more on primary care physicians for their emotional care (3,19,22–25), in part because of the tendency toward somatic symptoms, and in part because of the greater acceptability of a general physician as opposed to a psychiatrist. In many instances, patients may exhibit outright denial of a problem. This is especially true among Hispanic men, who may view themselves as weak if they acknowledge emotional pain (4).

B. Diagnosis and the Category Fallacy

Misdiagnoses are common in Hispanic populations, in part because of language barriers, but also because it can be difficult to apply diagnostic categories across different cultures (26–28). Symptoms that may be considered pathologic in one culture may be acceptable and normal in another (29). In addition, different beliefs and customs may be subject to misinterpretation. Overdiagnosis may occur if the clinician is not familiar with cultural beliefs responsible for a patient's symptoms. Conversely, underdiagnosis may occur when the clinician mistakenly considers pathologic symptoms as culturally acceptable behaviors or experiences. This dilemma led to the development of the term "category fallacy," which is defined as the application of a nosological category to members of a culture without first establishing its validity in that culture (30).

C. Psychiatric Illness and Culture-Bound Syndromes

When diagnosing psychiatric disorders in Hispanics, it is important to begin by assessing for the classic symptoms and signs of illness, as defined by the *Diagnostic and Statistical Manual of Mental Disorders, Fourth Edition* (DSM-IV) (31). Careful history of alcohol and drug use should be obtained, because these problems may be more frequent in Hispanics compared to other ethnic groups (4), and may contribute to symptoms of mood, thought, and anxiety disorders.

Other types of symptomatology may also be present, some of which may constitute unique syndromes unto themselves. These are often referred to as "culture-bound syndromes" (32). Culture-bound syndromes consist of atypical collections of symptoms that do not fit into the usual DSM-IV categories, and are specific to a particular society or cultural area (31–33). We will review a few representative "Hispanic-specific" syndromes.

1. *Ataque de Nervios* (Attack of Nerves)

This syndrome, also referred to as *ataque,* is similar to a panic attack, but often exhibits more violent behavior, and may occur without intense fear. *Ataque* is a culturally sanctioned phenomenon, and is often precipitated by an upsetting event such as a threat of harm, a family conflict, or the death of a relative. *Ataques* are often seen at a family member's funeral or at the scene of an accident (33–36).

The presentation of *ataque* may include uncontrollable shouting, trembling, palpitations, a sensation of heat in the chest rising to the head, fainting, and seizurelike episodes. These events often mobilize the family to support the individual with the attack, and recovery tends to be fast, with limited recollection of the event. Two thirds of individuals with *ataque* may have comorbid depressive or anxiety disorders. This syndrome, like most Hispanic-specific syndromes, may be seen in women more often than in men. Frequent and/or very intense attacks may require symptomatic treatment, usually with benzodiazepines, and sometimes with low-dose neuroleptics, but there is no firm consensus regarding optimal treatment approaches (18).

2. *Nervios* (Nerves)

This syndrome is analogous to generalized anxiety disorder in that it constitutes a baseline anxiety state rather than an episodic one like panic disorder or *ataque*. It usually involves emotional upset, somatic distress, feelings of isolation, restlessness, affective instability, and a sense of loss of control (37). External stressors that may contribute to *nervios* include trauma, the loss of a loved one, socioeconomic difficulties, or the loneliness resulting from being in an unfamiliar culture or place. Treatment approaches tend to vary from family to family, and may include herbal teas (sometimes prescribed by *curanderos,* or folk healers), supportive interactions, or anxiolytic medications, as well as individual psychotherapy (18,37).

3. *Susto* (Fright)

This condition is based on the notion that a sudden fright or trauma may cause the soul or spirit to exit the body, thus leaving the individual vulnerable to many ills. Presenting symptoms may include anxiety, irritability, anorexia, insomnia, trembling, sweating, tachycardia, diarrhea, depression, and vomiting (18). Spiritists (*espiritistas*) may be especially helpful in the treatment of this condition, because their therapeutic rituals often seek to expel evil spirits (9). Pharmacological treatment is usually recommended in cases where an underlying anxiety, depressive, or post-traumatic stress disorder is present (18).

4. Atypical Psychotic Symptoms

Psychotic symptoms described by Hispanic patients often differ from those seen in other populations, and may include auditory and visual hallucinations in the presence of otherwise unremarkable mental status examination findings (38). Hallucinations often reported by Hispanics include the sound of someone knocking at the door, the telephone or doorbell ringing, and children calling the patient's name. Visual hallucinations may include shadows, spots, or balls flying across the visual field, faces of adults or children on the wall, and visions of a dead spouse or relative.

These hallucinations are seldom a part of the chief complaint, and may go unnoticed by the clinician. Practitioners who observe these symptoms may feel uncertain of whether to treat their patients with neuroleptics. Failure to treat may result in a more serious decompensation, but overdiagnosis of psychotic disorders may cause unnecessary stigmatization, and antipsychotic medications may result in a variety of unpleasant adverse effects. These atypical psychotic symptoms are frequently discussed among psychiatrists who treat Hispanic patients, but the phenomenon is not well understood, and may represent a cultural entity without a psychopathologic significance (39).

Clinical Vignette #1

JT was a 19-year-old single Puerto Rican woman, who was brought to the inpatient unit with bizarre affect, disorganized behavior, poor self-care, and poverty of speech. She had no significant past psychiatric or medical history. JT was started on olanzapine (5 mg/day), but she continued to behave strangely. She would often stand in the unit's lounge area, making bizarre gestures with her hands and smiling inappropriately at the staff and other patients. She would speak a little bit with her treating physician (who spoke Spanish), but disclosed almost no useful information about her mental state, other than reporting occasional black "spots" flying across her field of vision. A few days after her admission, JT's family, including her father, mother, and two brothers, came to visit, and a family meeting was held with the treatment team. During the meeting, the patient was able to engage with the family and her treaters. She disclosed that before admission, she was date-raped by a boyfriend with whom she had been meeting in secret because her father had disapproved of him. JT's mother gave the patient some consolatory words, and asked her to apologize to her father for disobeying him. JT apologized, and the father accepted her apology. The patient's symptoms resolved shortly thereafter, and she was discharged to outpatient care a few days later. She was able to taper off her olanzapine with no recurrence of her symptoms.

IV. PHARMACOLOGICAL APPROACHES TO TREATMENT

A. Ethnopsychopharmacology

There is a very limited body of knowledge about comparative psychotropic medication trials involving Hispanics (18), and there is no consensus on the optimal treatment approach to psychiatric disorders in the Hispanic population (3,40). Nonetheless, this modest body of evidence has spurred a growing interest in ethnopsychopharmacology, particularly with regard to the cytochrome P-450 (CYP-450) drug-metabolizing enzymes and their polymorphisms, some of which may be more prevalent in Hispanics and other ethnic minorities (40,41).

The lack of a Hispanic-specific response pattern to psychotropic medications may be explained in part by the fact that Hispanics have a varied and mixed heritage, including Asian/Mongoloid, white/Spaniard, and black/African contributions (40). This mixed heritage has had a substantial impact on the genetics of the CYP-450 enzymes. Particular interest has focused on the 2D6, 2C19, 1A2, and 3A4 subtypes, which metabolize psychotropic drugs (40). The 2D6 and 2C19 subtypes exhibit genetic polymorphisms, which can result in varied efficacy (42). The 1A2 and 3A4 subtypes have shown limited evidence for polymorphisms, but may nonetheless account for ethnic-based variation in sensitivity to psychotropic drugs (43).

The CYP-450 2D6 variants are among the better-studied polymorphisms, especially in Hispanics. This enzyme family metabolizes a wide variety of psychotropics, including tricyclic antidepressants (TCAs), selective serotonin reuptake inhibitors (SSRIs), serotonergic-noradrenergic reuptake inhibitors, and antipsychotics. A small percentage of Spaniards and Mexican Americans have been found to be rapid metabolizers of certain antidepressants such as fluoxetine, paroxetine, and tricyclics. This may be due to multiple copies of the CYP-450 2D6 enzyme (44,45), and these individuals may require higher medication doses in order to obtain a clinical effect. Other individuals have been described as poor metabolizers because they usually lack a functional form of the enzyme. Approximately 2% to 10% of various Hispanic groups qualify as poor metabolizers, and may be more sensitive to side effects (40).

Specific mutations may affect metabolic status. For example, superextensive metabolizers, individuals with increased enzyme activity, have a 2D6-L mutation and multiple copies of the enzyme. This pattern has been observed in 7% of Spaniards (40,44). Slow metabolizers, individuals who metabolize drugs somewhat faster than poor metabolizers, are thought to result from a 2D6-J mutation. This mutation is present in 47% to 70% of Asians, 23% of whites, and 11.6% of Spaniards (40). Slow metabolism may also result from a 2D6-Z mutation, which occurs in 40% of African blacks and 15% to 26% of African Americans, and may therefore be found in Hispanics with African heritage (40). Finally, intermediate patterns of metabolism may be observed in Hispanics with combinations of mutations resulting from mixed heritage (40).

Dietary practices, as well as the use of caffeine and tobacco, which may be higher in Hispanic populations (18), may affect the metabolism of psychotropics. For example, a high-protein diet may increase drug metabolism (46). Cyclic aromatic hydrocarbons, which are present in smokers and in people who eat grilled meats, may increase activity of CYP-450 1A2 (40). Indoles, which are found in cabbage and brussel sprouts, may also increase CYP-450 1A2 activity (46). Grapefruit, as well as the flavonoids in corn, may decrease metabolic activity of CYP-450 3A4 (40). The aforementioned foods are all staples of the diet of many Hispanics, and may therefore have an impact on how these individuals metabolize psychotropics.

Along these lines, drug–drug interactions must also be taken into account, because polypharmacy is commonly used among Hispanics. For example, SSRIs may increase TCA levels via competition for CYP-450 2D6 and this combination may have a greater impact in Hispanic patients. Similarly, extensive metabolizers may sometimes convert to poor metabolizers, as a result of competitive inhibition between different psychotropics that are used in combination (40).

Regarding medication choice, there is some evidence that Hispanics may respond to TCAs at doses lower than those needed in Caucasians (47). However, we also tend to see higher rates of side effects and discontinuation in Hispanics. Because TCAs are metabolized by 2D6 and 2C19, we would expect genetic control and slow metabolism to account for greater sensitivity to side effects, but the evidence for this is limited (40). Finally, some studies have suggested that Hispanics may tolerate SSRIs better than Caucasians do (48), but again, the evidence is too scant to recommend a particular agent as a specific first line treatment for Hispanic patients.

When choosing a treatment approach, it is preferable to focus on the target symptoms, rather than trying to "settle" on a diagnosis in cases where the clinical picture may be complicated by comorbidity or by the presence of a culture-bound syndrome. For example, if the patient presents with depressive symptoms as the main complaint, it may be best to initiate treatment with an antidepressant. If mild and atypical psychotic symptoms are present, it may be reasonable to defer neuroleptics, unless the patient is very troubled by the symptoms. Anxiolytics can be a useful adjunct in cases where significant stress and anxiety are present.

Finally, many Hispanics tend to view medication as something to be taken on an as-needed basis, as with a "prn" anxiolytic (11,18). This stems in part from a belief that "too much" medication may be harmful, and perhaps also from limited education about mental illness and the ways in which psychotropics function. Psychiatrists must emphasize to patients the importance of taking their medication on a daily basis, regardless of whether or not they are feeling well (19). This is especially the case with antidepressants, which require standing doses to be effective. As mentioned earlier, negotiation with the patient and family about the treatment may be necessary in order to ensure optimal adherence.

Clinical Vignette #2

RV was a 30-year-old married woman from Spain, who presented to a new psychiatrist for treatment of chronic depression. The patient had tried several SSRIs and other newer antidepressants in the past, with little success. The psychiatrist suggested a tricyclic antidepressant, and started RV on imipramine (25 mg/day). After 3 weeks, the patient returned, saying she was feeling better, but was having severe constipation and daily headaches from the medication. The psychiatrist obtained a serum level of imipramine and found that RV's levels were much higher than expected, based on her dose. He concluded that RV was probably a slow metabolizer. He decreased the dose of imipramine to 10 mg/day, and the patient reported no further side effects. Her depression continued to abate and she achieved remission a few weeks later.

B. Natural Remedies

A psychiatrist who works with Hispanics should be familiar with some of the natural or alternative remedies that are often used by Hispanics (11), as well as by the general population (49). It is important for physicians to routinely ask about use of such remedies. Many patients will neglect to mention herbal remedies, sometimes because they think that "Western-trained" physicians do not believe in such treatments, or because the patients may not consider over-the-counter remedies as true medications (49). Some popular herbal remedies used by Hispanics include valerian, kava, St. John's wort, and maca. Although the effectiveness and safety data for these treatments are limited, they may serve as a viable option for individuals with mild-to-moderate illness who have a strong interest in natural treatments, or in individuals who have been refractory to US Food and Drug Administration (FDA)-approved psychotropics and/or are very sensitive to side effects (49).

Valerian (*Valeriana officinalis*) is a sedative and mild hypnotic that decreases sleep latency and improves sleep quality (50,51). It is popular among Hispanics, and some have studied it specifically in this population (52). It does not appear to cause dependence or daytime drowsiness, though there is evidence of benzodiazepinelike activity (53). It is not thought to be ideal for acute treatment of insomnia, but rather it promotes natural sleep after several weeks of use. The suggested dosage of valerian is 450 to 600 mg daily 2 hours before bedtime (50,51).

There are relatively few published well-designed, adequately powered research studies at this time (54) and many of these studies have produced contradictory results. Valerian has been compared against oxazepam (55) and against kava (56). In both instances, valerian appears to have comparable efficacy to the other medications. Toxic reactions with valerian are rare, and may include blurry vision, dystonias, and hepatotoxicity (50). Mexican or Indian valerian may have a carcinogenic risk, and therefore is not recommended (50).

Kava (*Piper methysticum*) originated in the Polynesian Islands, and is believed to have a calming, relaxing effect (50,51). Its active components consist of central muscle relaxants and anticonvulsants, and may interact with the GABA receptor to reduce the excitability of the limbic system (50,51). So far, kava has shown no evidence of dependence or withdrawal. Kava is available in various preparations (tablets, tincture, and "tea bag"). Its suggested dosages are 60 to 120 mg/day. Common side effects may include gastrointestinal upset, allergic skin reactions, headaches, and dizziness (50). Toxic reactions may occur with high doses or with prolonged use. These may include ataxia, hair loss, visual problems, respiratory problems, and a transient yellowing of the skin (kava dermopathy). For this reason, it is generally not advisable to use kava for more than 3 months (50).

Recently, over 70 cases of severe kava-related liver toxicity (including hepatitis, cirrhosis, and liver failure requiring liver transplant) have been reported in Canada and parts of Europe, though a direct relationship between kava and liver disease was not clear in all cases, and some individuals had taken excessive doses. Several European countries have banned kava products from the market, and the FDA is currently investigating kava to determine whether similar restrictions are necessary in the United States (57). The sudden emergence of kava-related toxicity may reflect increasing use of kava, as well as a lack of physician supervision. At this time, extreme caution is advised for individuals who are considering use of kava. Individuals with a history of liver disease or alcohol use, or those who take medications that are potentially hepatotoxic, should not use kava, and those who choose to use kava should consult with a physician.

St. John's wort (SJW; *Hypericum perforatum*) is believed to be effective for mild-to-moderate depression (50,58–60), though recent large-scale studies comparing SJW against placebo and SSRI (61–63) have raised questions about the efficacy of SJW. It has various presumed active components, including polycyclic phenols, hypericin, pseudohypericin, and hyperforin. Its mechanism of action is unclear, and may involve interaction with the hypothalamus-pituitary-adrenal axis to decrease cortisol secretion. It has some minimal monoamine oxidase inhibitor activity, and therefore should not be combined with SSRIs because the combination may cause serotonin syndrome (64).

The suggested dosage of SJW is between 900 and 1,800 mg/day (often divided into a thrice-daily dosage). Most preparations are standardized to hyperforin or hypericin, which are thought to play an active role in the antidepressant effect. Adverse effects may include dry mouth, dizziness, constipation, and phototoxicity (50). SJW has been associated with cycling to mania in persons with bipolar disorder, and therefore should be used with care in such patients (65,66). Use of SJW has been shown to decrease serum levels of some protease inhibitors in HIV-positive patients, and therefore should not be recommended for these individuals (67). Likewise, cyclosporin levels may be decreased by SJW, and in some cases has resulted in transplant rejection (64,68). Finally, women who use oral contraceptives must also be careful because SJW may decrease hormone levels (64,68) and result in unwanted pregnancies.

Maca (*Lepidium meyenii*) is a Peruvian root vegetable (69,70) that has been used as a food since before the time of the Incas (69), and is thought to act as a fertility and sexual enhancer. The maca root contains essential substances, such as amino acids, proteins, complex carbohydrates, minerals, vitamins, and fatty acids. It also contains *p*-methoxybenzyl isothiocyanate, which may function as an aphrodisiac, and glucosinolates, which may enhance fertility (71–76). Maca may also alleviate menstrual irregularities and female hormonal imbalances, as seen in menopause and chronic fatigue syndrome (69,77).

The maca tuber is usually stored and later cooked or prepared as a sweet drink called *maca chicha* (71–73). Maca is also consumed as *mazzamora,* a porridgelike dish with up to 60 g of the root per serving. In traditional Peruvian medicine, maca powder is delivered at doses of 5 to 20 g in tablets or capsules, stirred into water or juice, or sprinkled over food. In the United States, maca is sold in capsule form, with most preparations containing about 500 mg in each capsule. Typical dosages range from 3 to 6 g/day, but there is no consensus on the ideal therapeutic dose of maca.

Despite its popularity, there is no systematic human research on maca for sexual dysfunction, though some animal studies are encouraging (78,79). So far, maca has shown no toxicity in humans or animals. However, maca is not recommended for men with elevated prostate-specific antigen or history of prostate cancer, or for women with a history of breast or other hormonal cancers (80).

Clinical Vignette #3

CR was a 35-year-old single Mexican-American man with a long history of mild but persistent major depression. He presented to a new outpatient psychopharmacologist with a chief complaint of depression and classic neurovegetative symptoms. The patient reported that he was taking no medications at the time. The psychiatrist started CR on 20 mg of fluoxetine, and increased the dosage to 40 mg/day after 4 weeks. A few days later, the patient called the doctor, complaining of fever, sweating, and palpitations. The psychiatrist asked CR if he had taken any other substances. The patient disclosed that he had been taking SJW for several weeks, but had not realized that the over-the-counter drug was considered a "true" medication, so he had not mentioned it before. The psychiatrist instructed the patient to go to his nearest emergency room. CR was successfully treated for serotonin syndrome, which had resulted from the interaction between fluoxetine and SJW.

V. NONPHARMACOLOGIC APPROACHES TO TREATMENT

A. Psychotherapy

Supportive therapy can be a useful part of the treatment program, especially if the patient is exposed to situational stressors (11,37). A therapist may help the patient to develop better coping mechanisms for dealing with the general difficulties of life. Enlisting alternative treaters of the patient's choice may also be of value, both from a clinical standpoint as well as for solidification of the treatment alliance by showing respect for other treatment approaches the patient's cultural beliefs (11). Above all, the clinician should encourage the patient to feel comfortable discussing treatment and concerns. Some examples of alternative treaters, also referred to as folk healers, are discussed below.

B. *Espiritistas, Curanderos,* and the Church

Espiritismo (spiritism) involves a combination of Catholic and African mystical beliefs about witchcraft, magic, and the use of herbs and potions that target the influence of spirits (9,11). A session with an *espiritista* is similar in many ways to a psychotherapy session. Generally the *espiritista* diagnoses a specific problem, aligns him or herself with the patient, and tries to identify ego strengths and access good protective spirits, offering concrete solutions in the process. *Curanderos* may use specific medicines or recipes of their own preparation to combat the patient's symptoms. Hispanics may also rely heavily on their Church or priest (usually Roman Catholic) for support during difficult times (10,11).

VI. CONCLUSION

Mental health professionals who work with Hispanic patients may face a series of challenges and obstacles to effective treatment. A good diagnostic assessment requires an awareness of culture-bound syndromes and atypical symptoms, so that the clinician may recommend appropriate treatment. Furthermore, the clinician must appreciate cultural differences regarding mental illness, the role of medications, and the role of "non-Western" healers in the management of Hispanics. These differences must be carefully discussed and negotiated with the patient when working out a treatment plan.

Research on culture-bound syndromes and ethnopsychopharmacology will eventually yield a better understanding of ways in which to maximize treatment effectiveness and outcomes. However, there are not yet enough systematic data to allow for differential recommendations of specific treatments for Hispanic patients, as compared to other ethnic groups. For now, flexibility in the approach to treatment may be the clinician's best tool. In that spirit, we recommend the "LEARN" mnemonic (81), which reminds clinicians to: *listen* with sympathy, *explain* their perception of the problem, *acknowledge* differences and similarities between their views and those of their patient, *recommend* a treatment, and *negotiate* agreement on the treatment plan. This approach should work well for clinicians who treat Hispanic patients.

REFERENCES

1. US Census Bureau. *The Hispanic population in the United States: population characteristics.* Washington, DC: US Census Bureau, March 2001.
2. US Census Bureau. *Profiles of general demographic characteristics: 2000 census of population and housing.* Washington, DC: US Census Bureau, May 2001.
3. Ruiz P. Assessing, diagnosing, and treating culturally diverse individuals: a Hispanic perspective. *Psychiatr Q* 1995;66:329–341.
4. Caudle P. Providing culturally sensitive health care to Hispanic clients. *Nurs Pract* 1993;18:40–51.
5. Rogler LH. Hispanic Perspectives. In: Mezzich J, Kleinman A, Fabrega H, et al., eds. *Culture and psychiatric diagnosis: a DSM-IV perspective.* Washington, DC: American Psychiatric Press, 1996: 39–41.
6. Kline F, Acosta FX, Austin W, et al. The misunderstood Spanish-speaking patient. *Am J Psychiatry* 1980;137:1530–1533.
7. Gomez R, Ruiz P, Rumraut RD. Hispanic patients: a linguo-cultural minority. *Hispanic J Behav Sci* 1985;7:177–186.
8. Vasquez C. The problem with interpreters: communicating with Spanish-speaking patients. *Hosp Commun Psychiatry* 1991;42:163–165.
9. Bird HR, Canino I. The sociopsychiatry of espiritismo. *J Am Acad Child Psychiatry* 1981;20: 725–740.
10. Guarnaccia PJ, Parra P, Deschamps A, et al. Si Dios quiere: Hispanic families' experiences of caring for a seriously mentally ill family member. *Cult Med Psychiatry* 1992;16:187–215.
11. Comas-Diaz L. Culturally relevant issues and treatment implications for Hispanics. In: Koslow DR, Salett EP, eds. *Crossing cultures in mental health.* Washington DC: SIETAR International, 1989: 31–48.
12. Kline LY. Some factors in the psychiatric treatment of Spanish-Americans. *Am J Psychiatry* 1969; 125:88–95.
13. Greenblatt M, Norman M. Hispanic mental health and use of mental health services: a critical review of the literature. *Am J Social Psychiatry* 1982;11:25–31.
14. Rogler LH, Cortes DE, Malgady RG. Acculturation and mental health status among Hispanics. *Am Psychol* 1991;46:585–597.
15. Lagomasino I, McColl R, Mulroy R, et al. Prevalence and symptoms of depression among primary care patients of different ethnic groups. Presented at the Academy of Psychosomatic Medicine Annual Meeting, November 14–17, 1996, San Antonio, TX.

16. Herrerias C. Guidelines for working with Hispanics. Presented at NIDA National Conference on Drug Abuse Research and Practice, January 14, 1991, Washington, DC.
17. Bird HR, Canino G. The Puerto Rican family: cultural factors and family intervention strategies. *J Am Acad Psychoanal* 1982;10:257–268.
18. Jacobsen FM, Comas-Diaz L. Psychopharmacologic treatment of Latinas. *Essent Psychopharmacol* 1999;3:29–42.
19. Ruiz P, Venegas-Samuels K, Alarcon RD. The economics of pain. Mental health care costs among minorities. *Psychiatr Clin North Am* 1995;18:659–670.
20. Mischoulon D, McColl R, Howarth S, et al. Management of major depression in the primary care setting. *Psychother Psychosom* 2001;70:103–107.
21. Dassori A, Miller A, Saldana D. Schizophrenia among Hispanics: epidemiology, phenomenology, course, and outcome. *Schizophr Bull* 1995;21: 303–312.
22. Hough RL, Landsverk JA, Karno M, et al. Utilization of health and mental health services by Los Angeles Mexican Americans and non-Hispanic whites. *Arch Gen Psychiatry* 1987;44:702–709.
23. Leaf PJ, Bruce ML, Tischler GL, et al. The relationship between demographic factors and attitudes toward mental health services. *J Commun Psychol* 1987;15:275–284.
24. Leaf PJ, Bruce ML, Tischler GL, et al. Factors affecting the utilization of specialty and general medical mental health services. *Med Care* 1988;26:9–26.
25. Briones DF, Heller PL, Chalfant HP, et al. Socioeconomic status, ethnicity, psychological distress, and readiness to utilize a mental health facility. *Am J Psychiatry* 1990;147:1333–1340.
26. Rogler LH. The role of culture in mental health diagnosis: the need for programmatic research. *J Nerv Ment Dis* 1992;180:745–747.
27. Littlewood R. Cultural comments on culture-bound syndromes: I. In: Mezzich J, Kleinman A, Fabrega H, et al., eds. *Culture and psychiatric diagnosis: a DSM-IV perspective.* Washington, DC: American Psychiatric Press, 1996:309–312.
28. Skilbeck WM, Acosta FX, Yamamoto J, et al. Self-reported psychiatric symptoms among black, Hispanic, and white outpatients. *J Clin Psychol* 1984;40:1184–1189.
29. Corin E. Cultural comments on organic and psychotic disorders: I. In: Mezzich J, Kleinman A, Fabrega H, et al., eds. *Culture and psychiatric diagnosis: a DSM-IV perspective.* Washington, DC: American Psychiatric Press, 1996:63–69.
30. Good B, Good MD. The cultural context of diagnosis and therapy: a view from medical anthropology. In: Miranda, M., and Kitano, L., eds, *Mental health research in minority communities: development of culturally sensitive training programs.* Rockville, MD: National Institute of Mental Health, 1985: 1–27.
31. American Psychiatric Association. *Diagnostic and statistical manual of mental disorders, fourth edition.* Washington, DC: APA, 1994.
32. Levine RE, Gaw AC. Culture bound syndromes. In: Alarcon R, ed. *Cultural psychiatry.* Philadelphia, PA: WB Saunders Company, 1995:523–526.
33. Guarnaccia PJ, Rubio-Stipec M, Canino G. Ataques de nervios in the Puerto Rican diagnostic interview schedule: the impact of cultural categories on psychiatric epidemiology. *Cult Med Psychiatry* 1989;13:275–295.
34. Guarnaccia P. Ataques de nervios in Puerto Rico: culture-bound syndrome or popular illness? *Med Anthropol* 1993;15:157–170.
35. Liebowitz MR, Salman E, Jusino CM, et al. Ataque de nervios and panic disorder. *Am J Psychiatry* 1994;151:871–875.
36. Oquendo MA. Differential diagnosis of ataque de nervios. *Am J Orthopsychiatry* 1996;65:60–64.
37. Dresp CSW. Nervios as a culture-bound syndrome among Puerto Rican women. *Smith Coll Stud Soc Work* 1985;Mar:115–135.
38. Mischoulon D, Lagomasino I, Harmon C. Psychotic depression in a Hispanic population: diagnostic dilemmas and implications for treatment. Presented at the annual meeting of the American Psychosomatic Society, Clearwater, FL, March 12, 1998. Also presented at the American Psychiatric Association Annual Meeting, Toronto, Ontario, June 1, 1998.
39. Al-Issa I. The illusion of reality or the reality of illusion: hallucinations and culture. *Br J Psychiatry* 1995;166:368–373.
40. Mendoza R, Smith MW. The Hispanic response to psychotropic medications. In: Ruiz P, ed. *Ethnicity and psychopharmacology.* Washington, DC: American Psychiatric Press, 2000:55–89.
41. Lin K-M, Smith MW. Psychopharmacology in the context of culture and ethnicity. In: Ruiz P, ed. *Ethnicity and psychopharmacology.* Washington, DC: American Psychiatric Press, 2000:1–36.

42. Gonzalez FJ, Nebert DW. Evolution of the P450 gene superfamily: animal-plant "warfare," molecular drive and human genetic differences in drug oxidation. *Trends Genet* 1990;6:182–186.
43. Smith M, Mendoza R. Ethnicity and pharmacogenetics. *Mt Sinai J Med* 1996;63:285–290.
44. Agundez JA, Ledesma MC, Ladero JM, et al. Prevalence of CYP2D6 gene duplication and its repercussion on the oxidative phenotype in a white population. *Clin Pharmacol Ther* 1995;57: 265–269.
45. Lam WYF, Castro DT, Dunn JF. Drug metabolizing capacity in Mexican Americans. *Clin Pharmacol Ther* 1991;49:159–163.
46. Anderson KE, McCleery RB, Vesell ES, et al. Diet and cimetidine induce comparable changes in theophylline metabolism in normal subjects. *Hepatology* 1991;13:941–6.
47. Marcos LR, Cancro R. Pharmacotherapy of Hispanic depressed patients: clinical observations. *Am J Psychiatry* 1982;26:505–512.
48. Alonso M, Val E, Rapaport MH. An open-label study of SSRI treatment in depressed Hispanic and non-Hispanic women. *J Clin Psychiatry* 1997;58:31.
49. Mischoulon D, Rosenbaum JF. The use of natural medications in psychiatry: a commentary. *Harv Rev Psychiatry* 1999;6:279–283.
50. Schulz V, Hansel R, Tyler VE. *Rational phytotherapy: a physicians' guide to herbal medicine.* 4th ed. Berlin: Springer, 2001.
51. Mischoulon D. The herbal anxiolytics kava and valerian for anxiety and insomnia. *Psychiatr Ann* 2002;32:55–60.
52. Dominguez RA, Bravo-Valverde RL, Kaplowitz BR, et al. Valerian as a hypnotic for Hispanic patients. *Cult Divers Ethnic Minor Psychol* 2000;6:84–92.
53. Marder M, Viola H, Wasowski C, et al. 6-methylapigenin and hesperidin: new valeriana flavonoids with activity on the CNS. *Pharmacol Biochem Behav* 2003;75:537–545.
54. Stevinson C, Ernst E. Valerian for insomnia: a systematic review of randomized clinical trials. *Sleep Med* 2000;1:91–99.
55. Ziegler G, Ploch M, Miettinen-Baumann A, et al. Efficacy and tolerability of valerian extract LI 156 compared with oxazepam in the treatment of non-organic insomnia: a randomized, double-blind, comparative clinical study. *Eur J Med Res* 2002;7:480–486.
56. Wheatley D. Stress-induced insomnia treated with kava and valerian: singly and in combination. *Hum Psychopharmacol* 2001;16:353–356.
57. Packer-Tursman J. Anxiety over kava. *Washington Post,* Tuesday, Jan. 22, 2002:HE01.
58. Schrader E. Equivalence of St John's wort extract (Ze 117) and fluoxetine: a randomized, controlled study in mild-moderate depression. *Int Clin Psychopharmacol* 2000;15:61–68.
59. Brenner R, Azbel V, Madhusoodanan S, et al. Comparison of an extract of hypericum (LI 160) and sertraline in the treatment of depression: a double-blind, randomized pilot study. *Clin Ther* 2000; 22:411–419
60. Linde K, Ramirez G, Mulrow CD. St. John's wort for depression—an overview and meta-analysis of randomized clinical trials. *BMJ* 1996;313:253–258.
61. Shelton RC, Keller MB, Gelenberg A, et al. Effectiveness of St John's wort in major depression: a randomized controlled trial. *JAMA* 2001;285:1978–1986.
62. Hypericum Depression Trial Study Group. Effect of Hypericum perforatum (St John's wort) in major depressive disorder: a randomized controlled trial. *JAMA* 2002;287:1807–1814.
63. Lecrubier Y, Clerc G, Didi R, et al. Efficacy of St. John's wort extract WS 5570 in major depression: a double-blind, placebo-controlled trial. *Am J Psychiatry* 2002;159:1361–1366.
64. Fugh-Berman A. Herb-drug interactions. *Lancet* 2000;355:134–138.
65. Moses EL, Mallinger AG. St. John's Wort: three cases of possible mania induction. J *Clin Psychopharmacol* 2000;20:115–117.
66. Nierenberg AA, Burt T, Matthews J, et al. Mania associated with St. John's wort. *Biol Psychiatry* 1999;46:1707–1708.
67. Piscitelli SC, Burstein AH, Chaitt D, et al. Indinavir concentrations and St John's wort. *Lancet* 2000; 355:547–548
68. Baede-van Dijk PA, van Galen E, Lekkerkerker JF. [Drug interactions of Hypericum perforatum (St. John's wort) are potentially hazardous.] *Ned Tijdschr Geneeskd* 2000;144:811–812.
69. Rea J. Raices andinas: maca. In: Bermejo H, Leon, JE, eds. *Cultivos marginados, otra perspectiva de 1492.* Rome: The Botanic Garden of Cordoba, 1992:163–166.
70. King S. Ancient buried treasure of the Andes. *Garden* 1986;Nov/Dec.
71. Report of an Ad Hoc Panel of the Advisory Committee on Technical Innovation, Board on Science

and Technology for International Development. *Lost Crops of the Incas: Little Known Plants of the Andes with Promise for Worldwide Cultivation.* National Research Council, 1989.
72. Johns T. The anu and the maca. *J Ethnobiol* 1981;1:208–212
73. Quiros C, Epperson A, Hu J, et al. Physiological studies and determination of chromosome number in maca, *Lepidium meyenii. Econ Bot* 1996;50:216–223.
74. Leon J. The "maca" (*Lepidium meyenii*) a little known food plant of Peru. *Econ Bot* 1964;18:122–127.
75. Chacon RC. Estudio fitoquimico de *Lepidium meyenii* [dissertation]. Universidad Nacional, Mayo de San Marcos, Peru, 1961.
76. Dini A, Migliuolo G, Rastrelli L, et al. Chemical composition of *Lepidium meyenii. Food Chem* 1994;49:347–349.
77. Steinberg P. *Phil Steinberg's Cat's Claw News* 1995; July/August:1(2).
78. Cicero AF, Bandieri E, Arletti R. *Lepidium meyenii Walp.* improves sexual behaviour in male rats independently from its action on spontaneous locomotor activity. *J Ethnopharmacol* 2001;75: 225–229.
79. Zheng BL, He K, Kim CH, et al. Effect of a lipidic extract from *lepidium meyenii* on sexual behavior in mice and rats. *Urology* 2000;55:598–602.
80. Mischoulon D. Polypharmacy and side effects management with natural psychotropic medications. In: Mischoulon D, Rosenbaum J, eds. *Natural medications for psychiatric disorders: considering the alternatives.* Philadelphia: Lippincott Williams & Wilkins, 2002:207–215.
81. Berlin EA, Fowkes WC. A teaching framework for cross-cultural health care. *West J Med* 1983; 139:934–938.

6

Postpartum Mood Disturbance in Cross-Cultural Perspective

*Anna M. Georgiopoulos, †Amy B. Saltzman, and
*Anne E. Becker

*Department of Psychiatry, Massachusetts General Hospital,
Boston, Massachusetts 02114; and †Department of Anthropology, Princeton University,
Princeton, New Jersey 08544

I. INTRODUCTION

Postpartum mental illness is prevalent and associated with serious risks to mother and baby (1–4). Although its distribution appears to be global, important differences in incidence and clinical presentation across culturally diverse populations pose diagnostic and therapeutic challenges. Notwithstanding that childbirth is a biologically well-defined event, sociocultural variation in the way the postpartum is defined, structured, experienced, and supported is substantial. In this chapter, we review cross-cultural population and ethnographic data on postnatal depression relevant to etiologic understandings and potential preventive and therapeutic interventions.

Within Western psychiatric nosology, postpartum mood disturbance is conventionally classified into postpartum blues, postpartum depression (minor or major), and postpartum psychosis. Depressive symptoms are common in women of childbearing age, often beginning during pregnancy or in the first months postpartum (5). Most studies have defined postpartum depression as an episode of depression starting within the first 3 months after delivery, with symptoms similar to depressive episodes occurring at other times (6,7). More recently, use of the *Diagnostic and Statistical Manual of Mental Disorders, Fourth Edition* (DSM-IV) Postpartum Onset Specifier with a Major Depressive, Mixed, or Manic Episode is restricted to symptoms beginning within 4 weeks postpartum (8). Although affective lability that does not impair functioning may be quite common soon after childbirth, symptoms of puerperal affective psychosis also most often begin precipitously within the first 2 to 14 days postpartum; in many cases, these episodes appear similar to a bipolar manic or mixed state (5,9). Perhaps because of its relative rarity, occurring in less than 1% of childbearing women (9,10), postpartum affective psychosis has received less attention in recent literature than postpartum depression. Kendell and colleagues' (10) classic study in Edinburgh indicated that the incidence of psychiatric disorder, particularly psychotic illness, was substantially elevated for postpartum women, with a rate of psychiatric hospitalization nearly quadruple baseline in the first 3 months after delivery and staying elevated for 2 years thereafter. Other population-based work in Western cultures has not found major differences in the rates of major depression in postpartum women and age-matched controls (10% to 15%), and this epidemiologic issue remains controversial (5). Nonetheless, depression often emerges for the first time in the postpartum period. In one illustration of this, in a prospective study of 119 primiparas, more than 50% of the women with ongoing psychiatric problems at 4 years postpartum had never needed professional help for emotional problems before the onset of postpartum depression (11).

Postpartum mood disturbance appears to have a multifactorial etiology with familial (6), hormonal (12–20), psychological (21–23), and sociocultural contributions to risk. Interventions have been typically therapeutic rather than preventive. The development of successful primary and secondary prevention interventions for women with postpartum depression will depend on the further clarification of modifiable risk factors. Three bodies of literature suggest that an exploration of how social factors could be addressed to protect women from postpartum depression might be a productive first step toward a strategy to modify risk. First, strong evidence associates social support with attenuation in risk for postpartum mood symptoms across diverse contexts (24–27). Second, ethnographic data have documented striking cross-cultural diversity in how much support and rest is formally sanctioned for postpartum women (28,29). Finally, cross-cultural epidemiologic data suggest some variation in the incidence of postpartum illness across populations. Limited data further suggest that traditional supports may protect women's mental health in the postpartum.

The impressive cultural diversity in emotions, traditions, and practices surrounding pregnancy, childbirth, and the postpartum also have important implications for medically optimal and culturally sensitive delivery of health care in international settings and multiethnic populations. As mentioned earlier, risk for postpartum depression may be increased or attenuated by the routine absence or availability of specific supports to new mothers (25). Inasmuch as local, culture-specific explanatory models (30) differ, patterns of help-seeking and treatment adherence are likely to vary as well. Moreover, distress in postpartum women may present in various ways in different contexts depending on whether a psychological or somatic idiom is most culturally salient (31). Hence, not only is help-seeking behavior likely to differ markedly across cultures, but phenomenologic manifestations of postpartum distress will vary as well. For these reasons, clinicians will benefit from being informed of and attuned to culturally particular idioms of distress (32) in order to identify patients who require intervention. They will also need to be skilled in negotiating a shared perspective that allows a solid therapeutic alliance. In addition, because many women with illness may not actually be able to seek help for themselves, outreach to postpartum women attending maternal and child health clinics for infant care may be necessary to identify and treat women at risk.

II. CROSS-CULTURAL EPIDEMIOLOGY OF POSTPARTUM DEPRESSION

Although worldwide estimates of postpartum depression do appear to fall within a fairly consistent range of 8% to 14%, notable outliers have been observed. Much of the compelling evidence that sociocultural factors may moderate risk for postpartum illness stems from studies that suggest variability in the incidence of postpartum depression in non-Western populations. However, the cross-cultural comparison of the prevalence and etiology of postpartum illness has been complicated by evolving diagnostic criteria, phenomenologic variation, and numerous methodologic limitations in assessment. As a result, study findings have been inconclusive in establishing the scope of variation in prevalence across populations.

Ethnographic data have suggested that both postpartum traditions and postpartum illness may be culturally specific (33). Although some anthropologists have even suggested that postpartum depression does not exist in some societies (28), most investigations of postpartum illness have reported some evidence of it across diverse social contexts. However, population studies do suggest some variability in incidence (see Table 6-1). For example, a low prevalence of postpartum depression has been reported in some Asian populations. A study of 200 women in Singapore found that only 1% scored higher than 12 on a modified 16-item Edinburgh Postnatal Depression Scale (EPDS) at 3 months postpartum (34). Similarly, in a study of Malaysian women (of Indian, Malay, and Chinese ethnicity), only 3.9% of 154 assessed with the EPDS at 6 weeks postpartum scored higher than 12 (35). However, elsewhere in Asia, among a population of 781 Chinese women in Hong Kong, a prevalence of 6.1% for major depression and 5.1% for minor depression was reported at 3 months postpartum (36). In addition, a study of 88 postpartum women in Japan reported 8% cumulative incidence of major depression and 9% cumulative incidence of minor depression at 3 months (37), and a study of Japanese women living in London revealed similar results, with 12% meeting criteria for major or minor depression at 3 months (38). In contrast to earlier work in Nepal (28), postpartum depressive symptoms were common in a recent study of 100 women in Kathmandu at 2 or 3 months postpartum, with 12% scoring greater than 12 on the EPDS. However, there were no significant differences in EPDS scores when compared with control group women who were not puerperal (39).

In a prospective study in the United Arab Emirates, 15.8% of 95 women delivering at a hospital in Dubai were identified as having "psychiatric morbidity" at 6 to 10 weeks postpartum based on the Present State Examination (PSE) (40). Among 257 women in Manisa, Turkey, 14% had likely postpartum depression, with scores greater than 12 on a Turkish version of the EPDS, measured before 6 months postpartum (41). A prospective study of 327 Jewish women in Jerusalem showed that 11%

TABLE 6-1. *Selected Studies of Postpartum Mood Disturbance Outside of North America and Europe*

Author(s)	Year	Study population	Sample size	Timing of postpartum assessment	Assessment(s) used	Findings
Yamashita et al. (37)	2000	Kyushu, Japan: married Japanese	88	3 weeks 3 months	SADS/RDC: Japanese translation	6% major depression, 8% minor depression at 3 weeks 8% (cumulative incidence) major depression at 3 months 9% (cumulative incidence) minor depression at 3 months
Yoshida et al. (38)	1997	Greater London: Japanese	98	3 months postpartum	SADS/RDC: Japanese translation	6% major depression 6% minor depression
Lee et al. (36)	2001	Hong Kong; Chinese	959 (781)	1 month (3 months)	GHQ-12: Chinese version SCID-NP for DSM-III-R for GHQ $>$ 4 and 10% of those with GHQ $<$ 5	5.5% prevalence major depression at 1 month 4.7% minor depression at 1 month 6.1% major depression at 3 months 5.1% minor depression at 3 months
Kok et al. (34)	1994	Singapore: uncomplicated delivery	200	Day 5, 3 and 6 months postpartum	Modified 16-item EPDS	At 3 months, 0.5% scored $>$ 15, 0.5% scored 13–15 At 5 months, 0.5% scored $>$ 15, 1% scored 13–15
Kit et al. (35)	1997	Seremban, Malaysia	154	6 weeks	Modified 16-item EPDS: Malay translation (cut-off $\geq$ 13)	3.9% point prevalence overall Ethnicity-specific point prevalence: 8.5% among Indians, 3% among Malays, 0% among Chinese
Patel et al. (60)	2002	Goa, India	252 235	6–8 weeks 6 months	EPDS: Konkani translation (cut-off $\geq$ 12)	23% at 6–8 weeks 22% at 6 months
Regmi et al. (39)	2002	Kathmandu, Nepal	100	2–3 months postpartum	EPDS (cut off $>$ 12)	12%
Ghubash and Abou-Saleh (40)	1997	Dubai, United Arab Emirates	94 90	Day 2 postpartum Day 7 postpartum	SRQ (cut-off $\geq$ 6) EPDS (cut-off $\geq$ 12) PSE	24.5% prevalence "psychiatry morbidity" on SRQ, on day 2 17.8% prevalence "psychiatry morbidity" on EPDS, day 7

			95	6–10 weeks		15.8% "psychiatry morbidity" by PSE at 6–10 weeks
			95	28–32 weeks		4.2% "psychiatry morbidity" by PSE at 28–32 weeks
Danaci et al. (41)	2002	Manisa, Turkey	257	Up to 6 months	EPDS (cut-off ≥ 13)	14% prevalence
Dankner et al. (42)	2000	Jerusalem, Israel	327	6–10 weeks	EPDS: Hebrew (cut-off ≥ 9)	11% prevalence
Jadresic et al. (45)	1995	Chile: middle class	108	2–3 months	Standardized interview with Psychiatric Assessment Schedule (based on PSE) using RDC criteria	10% prevalence of major or minor depression by RDC criteria (11/108)
Cooper et al. (44)	1999	Peri-urban Capetown, South Africa	147	2 months	SCID	34.7% point prevalence of major depression 18% had postpartum onset; 17% had antenatal onset
Uwakwe (43)	2003	Nigeria: Igbo-speaking, tertiary care hospital	225	1–8 weeks	Structured clinical interview adapted from the CIDI and affective module of ICD-10 SCL	10.7% prevalence of depression
Cox (70)	1983	Uganda: Ganda women	183	3 months	Luganda modification of Goldberg's SPI; ICD-8 criteria	10% prevalence of depressive illness by SPI

CIDI, Composite International Diagnostic Interview; EPDS, Edinburgh Postnatal Depression Scale; GHQ, General Health Questionnaire; ICD-10 SCL, ICD-10 Symptom Check List; PSE, Present State Exam; RDC, Research Diagnostic Criteria; SADS, Schedule for Affective Disorders and Schizophrenia; SCID-NP, Structured Clinical Interview for DSM (nonpatient version); SPI, Standardized Psychiatric Interview; SRQ, Self Report Questionnaire.

scored 9 or above on the EPDS at 6 to 10 weeks postpartum; in this study, there was a higher prevalence of postpartum depression in those women born outside of Israel (42).

In a Nigerian study of 225 Igbo-speaking women at a semiurban tertiary care hospital assessed with the ICD-10 Symptom Check List and structured interview between 1 and 8 weeks postpartum, a 10.7% prevalence of depression was reported. By contrast, in a 5-year period before this study, only two referrals for postpartum mental illness had been made to mental health clinicians at this hospital, where over 1,000 deliveries occur every year (43). This disparity in incidence is puzzling, and further research will clarify whether it reflects poor access to psychiatric care (43), lack of salience of postpartum illness in this population, or changes in help-seeking patterns. An usually high point prevalence of major depression at 2 months postpartum was reported in a population of 147 women in a periurban settlement outside of Cape Town, South Africa, living under extremely socially adverse conditions (i.e., predominantly living in shacks without electricity or running water in overcrowded conditions). Using the major depression section of the Structured Clinical Interview for DSM-IV (SCID) at 2 months postpartum, Cooper and colleagues (44) reported that 34.7% of the sample met criteria for major depression; 18% had postpartum onset of the depression, whereas 17% had had antenatal onset. Finally, in Chile, 10% of a sample of 108 middle class women interviewed at 2 or 3 months postpartum were found to have major or minor depression using Research Diagnostic Criteria (RDC) (45).

Ideally, comparative studies would use consistent means of assessing and classifying postpartum illness across different populations. Such ideal studies in non-Western societies would also begin with ethnographic data to identify whether local categories of postpartum disorders exist, and if they do, how phenomenologic presentations and help-seeking may compare with Western nosologic categories. Because such integrated studies are rare, systematic bias introduced by misclassification is likely to make prevalence data difficult to interpret.

Even within culturally similar Western populations, the prevalence of postpartum illness can vary substantially, depending on study population, assessments, definition of duration of the postpartum, and diagnostic criteria used. For example, in prospective studies, postpartum depression varied from a point prevalence of 3.5% in a middle class, fairly well-educated, primarily white population in Iowa at 8 weeks postpartum (46), to a point prevalence of 23.4% in one study of largely impoverished, racially diverse, urban women in the midwestern United States at 7 to 9 weeks postpartum (47). Despite the apparently large between-population differences, classification was made with the Hamilton Rating Scale for Depression in the former study and with a version of the Schedule for Affective Disorders and Schizophrenia (SADS) adapted by O'Hara for use with pregnant and postpartum women using RDC in the latter. A cohort of 104 primarily African American (93%) urban adolescent mothers in the United States evidenced an even higher prevalence of depressive symptoms at 2 months postpartum (36%) and 4 months postpartum (32%) on the Center for Epidemiological Studies of Depression—Children's Scale (48). By contrast, a study of urban US adolescent mothers (69.0% black, 20.9% Hispanic, and 10.1% white) using the Beck Depression Inventory (BDI) with a cut score of more than 20 yielded a much lower prevalence of depression at 5 weeks postpartum, with 7.0% becoming depressed postpartum and an additional 3.1% becoming depressed during pregnancy and remaining so after delivery (49). There were no significant differences by race (49), and results were more similar to those found in the study of a more affluent, and predominantly white, population cited earlier that also used the BDI (46), suggesting that the instrument chosen may have influenced the results, attenuating possible between-population differences. By comparison, a less specifically characterized South London population was found to have a 12% prevalence of affective disorder at 6 weeks postpartum; assessment in this study was by a different form of semistructured interview (50). Finally, in Portugal, a study using a semistructured interview (SADS) found that 24.5% of 54 primiparas met criteria for major depression, minor depression, or intermittent depressive disorder during the first 3 months postpartum (51).

A variety of additional methodological limitations have impacted epidemiological studies of postpartum depression. These have seriously undermined meaningful comparison of prevalence among studies. As noted previously, studies use a wide variety of measurement tools, including structured and nonstructured clinical interviews and self-report scales such as the EPDS, which was designed specifically for use in postpartum women, and the BDI. Often, instruments designed as screening tools are used to measure the prevalence of postpartum depression, and studies may be designed without the ability to distinguish minor and major depression. Many depression scales evaluate study subjects by a checklist of symptoms and classify them with a numerical score. Thus, the same individual could be classified as having probable depression using one tool, but as not depressed when assessed at the same point in time with a different instrument. In one Australian study of four self-report scales in 260 postpartum women, agreement between instruments in identifying the 25 women who were "most depressed" was low, averaging 40% (52).

Even in studies in which the same scale is used, there can be a lack of consensus as to which cut scores correspond to clinically significant postpartum illness (53); different cut-off scores may have been selected by researchers for use in different populations, complicating comparison across studies. For instance, a population-based study of one county in the midwestern United States found that the percentage of women screening positive for postpartum illness ranged from 11.4% to 19.8% depending on the EPDS cut-score used (54). In a related study in this population, the incidence of postpartum depression diagnosed in the community in the course of usual medical care in the first year postpartum increased from 3.7% to 10.7% following the introduction of EPDS screening (55). Although often used to define "caseness" in clinical research (and perhaps by busy clinicians in some primary care settings), the EPDS and similar tools have been developed as screening instruments; even when women identified as having a "positive" screen are similar to the populations in which these instruments have been validated, these patients require further clinical assessment to confirm a diagnosis of postpartum depression (56,57). In some cases where the specificity and positive predictive value of screening tools have been found to be relatively low in a particular population, a two-stage screening process has been suggested (58). Studies validating these instruments against the "gold standard" of structured psychiatric interview are important in determining the specificity and sensitivity of these tools, and should be repeated when research instruments are translated or used in populations quite different than those for which they were originally designed.

In addition, measurements of postpartum depression are affected by the timing of assessment relative to childbirth. Inconsistencies in timing will affect cumulative incidence rates and case definition. For example, in one study of a Swedish population using the EPDS with a cut-off score greater than 9, there was an 18% prevalence of postpartum depression when measured in the maternity ward (likely including cases of transient baby blues), whereas the prevalence decreased to 13% both at 6 to 8 weeks and at 6 months postpartum (59). In a Swedish community sample, the point prevalence of women with EPDS scores greater than 11 decreased from 12.5% at 8 weeks to 8.3% at 12 weeks postpartum, with only 4.5% screening positive at both measurements (58). In addition, many studies do not assess antenatal depression in their study population; thus postpartum onset is unconfirmed. For example, Patel and colleagues would have obtained very different results in their determination of the incidence of postpartum depression in Goa, India, if they had not accounted for the high numbers in their sample with antenatal depression. Although they found that 23% of mothers were depressed 6 to 8 weeks after delivery, only 13 of the 252 mothers assessed (5%) had developed their depression in the postpartum period (60).

The inconsistent validation of assessment measures across culturally and linguistically diverse populations also limits interpretation of findings. Translation and back-translation, while a necessary first step, are not sufficient to guarantee conceptual equivalence or clarity across culturally different populations. Despite some investigators utilizing more than one means of assessment as a cross-validation technique, correlated measurement errors could potentially render this strategy insufficient in obtaining valid estimates of true incidence. Some tools used in research on postpartum depression have not been specifically validated—even in the West—in populations of postpartum women, in which perinatal somatic changes can complicate assessment for postpartum depression (61). For example, the BDI was compared to the EPDS against a criterion standard of psychiatric interview using *Diagnostic and Statistical Manual of Mental Disorders, Third Edition* (DSM-III) criteria for major depression in a group of postpartum women in South Wales (many of whom were thyroid antibody positive); the EPDS performed far better, with sensitivity of 95% and specificity of 93% at a cut point greater than 12, compared to the 68% sensitivity and 88% specificity found with BDI scores greater than 10. This difference was attributed to a relative overemphasis on items asking about energy level, sleep and appetite in the BDI (53). Even so, when the EPDS was validated in a large British community sample (N = 702) of primiparous women at 6 weeks postpartum against the criterion standard of assessment with the Standardized Psychiatric Interview (SPI) modified to fit the RDC, results were somewhat less reassuring, with a sensitivity of 67.7%, specificity of 95.7%, and positive predictive value of 66.7% at the same cut point used by Harris and colleagues (62). In the case of the EPDS, which was designed for use in postpartum women, some cross-cultural validation studies have now been conducted, for example in Chile (45), Portugal (51), Sweden (63), Norway (64), the United Arab Emirates (65), Nigeria (43), China (66), Nepal (39), Spain (67), and Australia (68). These studies utilize varying standards for validation (39,43,45,51,63–68). Not surprisingly, although these studies were each felt to lend support to use of the EPDS as adapted for their respective populations, they yielded varying sensitivities and specificities for detection of postpartum depression in each population group and at each cut point assessed. For example, in a Chilean validation study in women 2 or 3 months postpartum against standardized interview based on the PSE/RDC, the best cut point on the EPDS was determined to be a score greater than 9, yielding a sensitivity of 100%, specificity of 80%, and positive predictive value of 37%; using the cut point of scores greater than 12 in this population resulted in a sensitivity of only 55%, with a specificity of 94% and positive predictive value of 50% (45). Similarly, in the Chinese validation study, scores greater than 9 on the EPDS were recommended as optimal for screening use, with a sensitivity of 82%, specificity of 86% and positive predictive value of 44% (66). In Spain, the best EPDS cut point was found to be a score greater than 10, with a sensitivity of 79%, specificity of 95.5%, and positive predictive value of 63.2% for combined major and minor depression (67). Of note, few validation studies of the EPDS have been carried out in the United States. In an unpublished validation study by Swain and colleagues (69), conducted at the University of Iowa, of nearly 200 married US women near 6 weeks postpartum, the EPDS yielded a 90.5% sensitivity for major and minor depression, with a specificity of 86.1% and positive predictive value of 79.2%, when measured against the RDC assessed by a semistructured interview adapted from the SADS.

Finally, meaningful descriptive statistical comparisons among results based on small sample sizes are limited. Though a few studies evaluated hundreds of mothers, many only evaluated samples of approximately100 people (see Tables 6-1- and 6-2). Small differences in the number of subjects classified as cases can contribute to large variations in percentage when they are calculated in samples of that size. Moreover, limited statistical power in small studies may bias toward null results in looking for associations between social support and disease. In addition, studies may not adequately adjust for factors influencing their data such as the mother's antenatal mental health status.

A handful of cross-cultural comparative studies have used consistent methodology in comparisons of two populations. These few studies show a very similar prevalence of postpartum depression in Western and non-Western populations. For example, using the SPI and ICD-8 criteria to diagnose depression in a home interview, Cox and colleagues found similar point prevalences of postpartum depression in 183 Ganda women in Uganda seen near 3 months postpartum (10%) (70) and 105 mothers in Scotland assessed 3 to 5 months after delivery (13%) (71) in a direct comparison of the two study populations. In a study comparing Taiwanese and British women

TABLE 6-2. *Selected Studies Investigating the Association between Social Support and Postpartum Depression or Distress*

Author(s)	Year	Study population	Sample size	Timing of assessment(s)	Assessment(s) used	Selected outcomes related to social support
O'Hara (21)	1986	Iowa City, Iowa: 98% white	99	Second trimester, approximately 9 weeks postpartum	SADS-RDC, PLES, CSI, SSI Peripartum Stress Scale, PSSQ, DAS	Postpartum depression significantly associated with more life events since delivery, childcare-related stressful events, inadequate instrumental and emotional support from spouse, dissatisfaction with frequency of supportive behaviors from spouse/parents/parents-in-law, lower marital satisfaction
Gjerdingen and Chaloner (22)	1994	St. Paul, Minnesota: primiparous, married, ethnically diverse	436	1, 2, 3, 6, 9, and 12 months postpartum	Mental Health Inventory from RAND Health Insurance Experiment, checklists on physical health and obstetric complications, work and baby, social support questions, Work Activity Scale, Recreational Activity Scale	Mother's better mental health significantly associated with emotional support from spouses/others, number of support persons, satisfaction with husband's help in household, income; inversely associated with infant illness
Sèguin et al. (23)	1999	Montreal: nulliparous, diverse SES	116	Week 30 of pregnancy, 3 and 9 weeks postpartum	BDI: French translation, Life Conditions Questionnaire adapted from Makosky, Kanner's Hassle Scale (adapted), DAS (French), ASSIS (adapted)	Fewer people to provide social support, frequent conflict with social network prospectively significantly associated with higher BDI score at 9 weeks postpartum
Logsdon et al. (106)	1994	United States: primiparous, married	105	1 month before delivery, 6 weeks postpartum	Postpartum Support Questionnaire CES-D	Lack of postpartum closeness to husband and difference between expected and received support (in areas perceived to be important when assessed prenatally) significantly associated with postpartum depression

Neter et al. (27)	1995	United States: ethnically diverse, low-income	108	Multiple prenatal visits, 4–8 weeks postpartum	CES-D; unique measures of satisfaction with social support, life events inventory adapted from Los Angeles Epidemiological Catchment Area Study, PSS, STAI	Higher levels of depressed mood significantly associated with less satisfaction with prenatal support and life events distress
Barnet et al. (48)	1996	United States: Low income, urban adolescents, primiparous, 93% black	125	Third trimester, 2 and 4 months postpartum	CES-D Children's Scale (cut-off > 20) ASSIS Coddington's Life Events Scale	Lack of emotional or material support from adolescent's mother or baby's father, conflict with baby's father, high (vs. low) levels of stress all significantly associated with CES-D > 20 at 4 months
Romito et al.) (101)	1999	France and Italy: first or second baby	629 French 724 Italian	Several days, 5 months, and 12 months postpartum	GHQ-12 as measure of "psychological distress"	Postpartum psychological distress significantly associated with lack of confidante, financial worries, poor relationship with partner (at birth and especially at 12 months postpartum), infant illness
Paykel et al.) (99)	1980	London, England: white	120	Approximately 5–8 weeks postpartum	Clinical Interview for Depression with Raskin Three Area Depression Scale rating (cut off > 6), Interview for Recent Life Events, unique interview measures of social variables	Postpartum depression significantly associated with number of undesirable life events in past 11 months, less communication with and help from husband, inadequacy of confidante, and housing problems
Brugha et al. (100)	1998	Leicestershire, United Kingdom: nulliparous	427	Antenatal care visit, 12 weeks postpartum	GHQ-30 (modified 28-item version), IMSR, LTE, EPQ-N	Higher scores (i.e., indicative of depression) significantly associated with living without a partner, unemployment, and perceived lack of support

(*continues*)

TABLE 6-2. *(Continued)*

Author(s)	Year	Study population	Sample size	Timing of assessment(s)	Assessment(s) used	Selected outcomes related to social support
Escribá et al. (102)	1999	Valencia, Spain	498	1 year postpartum	GHQ-12 (cut off > 3; Spanish version) plus unique measures of symptoms and medical care consumption to determine "psychological distress," unique measures of social variables	Psychological distress significantly associated with living without partner; financial problems; fair/poor marital relationship after 12 months; arguments about domestic chores/childcare, infant illness
Augusto et al. (103)	1996	Urban Portugal	352	2–5 months postpartum	EPDS Zung self-rating depression scale, social and demographic factor checklist	Higher EPDS scores significantly associated with lower occupational status, educational level, income, quality of housing, and residential area
Danaci et al. (41)	2002	Manisa, Turkey	257	Up to 6 months postpartum	EPDS demographic information questionnaire	Significantly higher EPDS scores were associated with history of migration, living in a squatter area, infant health problem, moderate or bad relationship with husband, mother-in-law, or father-in-law
Dankner et al. (42)	2000	Jerusalem, Israel	327	6–10 weeks postpartum	EPDS (cut-off ≥ 9), sociodemographic questionnaire	EPDS ≥ 9 significantly correlated with being an immigrant, secular religious practices
Ghubash and Abou-Saleh (40)	1997	Dubai, United Arab Emirates: affluent population	95	6–10 weeks postpartum	PSE (Level 5) Assessment of life events and marital relationship with nonstandardized/unvalidated measures	Depression significantly associated with previous divorce, marital problems before or after delivery, primiparity, unwanted pregnancy, infant's illness, life event during past year
Cooper et al. (44)	1999	Periurban Capetown, South Africa	147	2 months	SCID Interview assessing sociodemographic information	Postpartum major depression was significantly inversely related to both "regular emotional support" and "reliable practical support" from the partner

Tamaki et al. (105)	1997	Suzuka, Mie Prefecture, Japan	627	Antenatal; 1, 3, and 4 months postpartum	EPDS (cut-off ≥ 9) STAI Unique life-events questionnaire	EPDS scores ≥ 9 significantly associated with primiparity at 1 month postpartum, with adverse life events in previous 12 months at 3 and 4 months, and with worries about baby care at 1, 3, and 4 months
Hung and Chung (104)	2001	Kaohsiung City, Taiwan	526	1, 3, and 5 weeks postpartum	HPSS: includes subscales of maternal role attainment, lack of social support, body changes, SSS, CHQ-12 (cut off > 2 to define "minor psychiatric morbidity")	"Minor psychiatric morbidity" significantly associated with lack of social support
Lee et al.	2004	Hong Kong	959	Third trimester, Immediately after delivery, 3 months	EPDS, IMS, SRRS Medical Outcome Study Social Support Survey Semistructured interview	Marital dissatisfaction, inadequate social support, life events in pregnancy, poor mother-in-law relationship, and absence of *peiyue* were significantly associated with probable postpartum depression (in univariate analyses)

Abbreviations as in Table 6-1, also ASSIS, Barrera's Arizona Social Support Interview Schedule; BDI, Beck Depression Inventory; CES-D, Center for Epidemiological Studies-Depression; CHQ-12, 12-item Chinese Health Questionnaire; CSI, Childcare Stress Inventory; DAS, Dyadic Adjustment Scale; EPQ-N, Eysenck Personality Questionnaire Neuroticism Subscale; IMS, Index of Marital Satisfaction; IMSR, Interview Measure of Social Relationships; HPSS, 66-item Hung Postpartum Stress Scale; LTE, List of Threatening Experiences; PLES, Pilkonis Life Events Schedule; PSS, Perceived Stress Scale; PSSQ, Postpartum Social Support Questionnaire; SPI, Standardized Psychiatric Interview; SRRS, Social Adjustment Rating Scale; SSI, Social Support Interview; SSS, Smilkstein's Social Support Scale; STAI, State Anxiety Scale from State-Trait Anxiety Inventory.

with the EPDS (using a cut score of greater than 12) at 3 months postpartum, a very similar prevalence of depression (18% in Keelung,Taiwan and 19% in Sheffield, United Kingdom) was found (72). However, sampling differences for the two study populations (in the former case at public health stations and in the latter, from among patients of community midwife teams) may have introduced some bias into the results. Only 62% of the 50 UK mothers studied were married, compared to 92% of the 101 Taiwanese mothers, and there were significant differences in educational level, with 66% of British women and 34% of Taiwanese women having higher education. The British women were more likely to attend parenting classes, but also more likely to have had a shorter hospital stay. In addition, the Chinese-language version of the EPDS was specifically prepared by the investigators for this study and was not systematically validated prior to use; the cut point was selected based on validations of the English version (72). This suggests the possibility of a higher rate of false negatives in the Chinese women than in the English-speaking women, given that a previous validation study in a different Chinese-speaking population showed the optimal EPDS cut point to be scores greater than 9 (66).

III. CROSS-CULTURAL DIFFERENCES IN POSTPARTUM DISTRESS AND EXPERIENCE

Whereas cross-cultural epidemiologic data for the incidence of postpartum depression remain inconclusive, ethnographic data provide strong evidence of variability in the presentation and incidence of postpartum illness. Substantial variability in the presentation of major depression is reflected in the DSM–IV diagnostic criteria that allow for different combinations of neurovegetative symptoms to constitute a major depressive episode. Moreover, the signal of an emerging clinically significant postpartum depression might be partially obscured against the background noise of the fairly common sleep, energy, and appetite changes in the postpartum related to recovery from childbirth, breastfeeding, and infant care. Cross-cultural differences in attention to emotional states and formulation of postpartum distress may further substantially influence symptom reporting and help-seeking behavior. Finally, application of Western psychiatric nosologic categories to non-Western contexts must proceed with informed caution as this risks a "category fallacy" (73) (i.e., that symptoms are not recognized or experienced as the same illness elsewhere). In such situations, patterns of symptom expression could easily be misinterpreted clinically (74).

Reactions to childbirth can differ in individual women, but also by culture. Hrdy (75) notes that, unlike in other mammals, in humans, there are no "fixed action patterns" surrounding the birthing period, with the clearest universal customs involving some way of cleaning and inspecting the baby soon after birth. In some cultures, as in much of the United States, mothers are usually expected to express joy immediately following delivery. However, women from other cultures, such as the Machiguenga in South America, Mayan-speaking women in the Yucatan, and even affluent British mothers, often appear indifferent after giving birth (75).

Even for women who may not have postpartum depression, maternal feelings following delivery remain far more complex than is often publicly stated among American mothers. This may suggest cultural-specific pressures for a self-presentation that is less conflicted or stressed than experienced. Some nonmedical writers have begun to address these issues (76–79), as have a few more systematic research studies. Levitzky and Cooper (80) studied 23 well-educated, married mothers with colicky infants living in New York City who had been referred for the study by the physicians treating the infants' colic. Most of the women (70%) had aggressive fantasies toward their infants, and six women (26%) admitted to thoughts of killing the baby. They reported that 91% of mothers felt their relationship with their husbands had been adversely affected. They also noted that women in the study complained that people in their support system generally focused on the well-being of the baby, rarely asking mothers how they were feeling, despite their distress.

Oates and colleagues (81) recently performed a qualitative study including mothers of babies 5 to 7 months old, relatives, and health care workers from France, Ireland, Italy, Portugal, Austria, Switzerland, Sweden, the United Kingdom, the United States, Uganda, and Japan. Informants from all cultures studied identified some form of "morbid unhappiness" as frequently occurring in their society after childbirth. In all cases, the symptoms described dovetailed with the Western concept of depression. However, these feelings were explicitly conceptualized as postpartum depression in only some of the populations. The Portuguese, Swiss, Ugandans, and Asians living in the United Kingdom did not formulate these symptoms in this way. Informants from all cultures endorsed the ability of psychosocial factors such as poor social support to cause this postpartum distress and talking to others (whether informally or in the course of psychotherapy) as potentially ameliorative. Some of the study populations also posited an etiologic role for hormones (although the Japanese, Ugandans, and Asians living in the United Kingdom did not), but the United States was the only study population that indicated an explanatory model that antidepressant treatment might be therapeutic. Interestingly, some specific stressors appeared nearly universal, with all study populations but the Swedes bringing forth concerns about relationships with the mother-in-law. Others appeared more culture specific, with Ugandans, for example, noting that family delay in naming the baby commonly contributes to unhappiness postpartum, and others citing inability to engage in traditional perinatal practices as distressing.

Important phenomenologic variation has been noted across different populations even when diagnoses of postpartum depression have been made in a similar systematic manner. For example, although rates of postpartum depression were quite similar in the aforementioned comparison of postpartum women in Scotland and Uganda, Scottish women reported relatively more self-blame and guilt (70,71). By the same token, some symptoms commonly experienced among postpartum mothers in non-Western cultures would be unfamiliar to and unanticipated by Western-trained psychiatrists. Thus, assessment tools developed for Western populations may entirely miss important markers of postpartum distress, and research protocols designed for use in the West, if not adapted for use elsewhere, could ignore demographic and social categories affecting symptom presentation. For example, a prospective study of 400 Nigerian Yoruba mothers identified both insomnia and feeling "heat-in-the-head" as the most common symptoms of postpartum distress. Although certain symptom constellations (worry, guilt, and "heat-in-the-head") were more likely to occur in younger than older women, others (anorexia, worry, and palpitations) were more likely to occur in women living in polygamous instead of monogamous marriages, a demographic variable not typically assessed in the West (82).

Thus, whereas uniform diagnostic criteria are essential to conduct systematic epidemiologic and clinical research on postpartum depression, these criteria may be too limiting in clinical practice in multicultural and international settings. Clinicians caring for pregnant and postpartum women should be aware of the varieties of manifestations of distress that can occur before, during, and after childbirth. For example, a prospective study investigating postpartum illness among ethnic Fijian women identified a culturally unique presentation of postpartum illness, called *na tadoka ni vasucu.* The cumulative incidence of this syndrome was 9% among a sample of 82 ethnic Fijian mothers followed up for 2 to 5 months postpartum. Whereas many of the women experiencing this syndrome also reported mood symptoms in the postpartum, this illness was locally formulated as primarily somatic (i.e., consisting of flulike symptoms and nonspecific aches). Moreover, it was quite transient and clinically benign, usually remitting in days (24). Although ethnic Fijians recognize a form of postpartum psychosis (*cavuka*), they do not recognize illnesses that would correspond to either maternity blues or postpartum depression in their local nosology.

Other culturally specific postpartum syndromes have been identified, including *Amakiro* among Baganda mothers in Uganda. *Amakiro* is regarded as a serious mental illness that usually affects postpartum women but could also begin during pregnancy. Symptoms of *Amakiro* include the mother's wish not to feed her baby and possibly the desire to eat it; it is considered potentially fatal to mother or child. The most common perceived causes of *Amakiro* cited by a study sample of 28 Ugandan informants were the promiscuity of the mother or father during pregnancy, as well as the failure to use preventive herbal baths (83).

Ethnographic data have also identified cross-cultural differences in practices in defining and structuring the postpartum period. Consideration of the unique social structuring of the postpartum period in a particular population may suggest locally practical interventions for postpartum distress. Moreover, postpartum practices that appear to be protective against mood disturbance might inform prevention strategies in other populations as well (25).

IV. POSTPARTUM TRADITIONS IN CROSS-CULTURAL CONTEXT

There is great cultural diversity in postpartum practices—many of which formally or informally demarcate the puerperium as a unique time for special supports for women. Postpartum traditions have both practical and symbolic significance and reflect cultural values placed on children and motherhood as well as the social status of women. In many societies, a woman's status is critically tied to her fertility and ability to bear children. Childbirth thus marks a major social-role transition in many areas of the world. Approximately half of societies expect a full return to work within 2 weeks of giving birth (29). However, some societies have quite formal and highly elaborate traditions that allow women to rest after giving birth, support the maternal–infant dyad, and recognize the milestone. The range of formal support varies from an extended period of up to 12 months and assignment of a caregiver to look after the mother (for example, in Fiji) to virtually no formal social support except for medical care (for example, a widespread practice in many communities in the United States). Intermediate postpartum traditions include a 7-day period of mandated rest and seclusion among the Kokwet in Kenya (84) to month-long rest periods among the Chinese (85), Japanese (86), and Hmong (87).

In addition to seclusion and rest, many traditions prohibit specific activities and foods for the protection of the mother or the healthfulness of the breastmilk. For example, the Chinese practice *zuo yue zi,* what they call "doing the month," for 30 days after childbirth. They are specifically prohibited from any activity, including walking, exposing themselves to the sun, or leaving their home (85). They must practice abstinence from sexual activity and must avoid getting wet. Thus they avoid bathing, washing their hair, and contact with cold water. Some Chinese traditions emphasize that postpartum women must be kept warm and dry during this period and must be protected from the wind for fear of developing "wind illness" (88). Ethnographic data suggest that women perceive wind's effect on the postpartum body as predisposing to future asthma, aches, pains, and arthritis (85). During this period, new mothers in China are supported by a specially designated caretaker, usually their mothers-in-law, in a tradition locally called *peiyue* (25,88–90).

Postpartum traditions in several other East and Southeast Asian populations are comparable to those of the Chinese. For example, in Japan, postpartum women typically spend a month at their parents' home (86). Likewise, new Indian mothers are confined for up to 40 days in order to protect themselves from evil spirits and from illness (89). Thai practices include a similar period of seclusion that is also called "doing the month." Those 30 days include confinement to the home, seclusion, significant help with household work, and sexual abstinence. New mothers are restricted to eating only plain foods such as rice and soup, as well as white foods and boiling water, thought to stimulate breast milk. They practice *Yue Fai,* or "lying by the fire," in which mothers either lie close to a fire or place a fire-heated stone on their abdomens to respond to the locally held perception that "childbirth leaves the mother cold and wet" (91).

Vietnamese puerperal practices bear some resemblance to those of the Chinese, Hmong, Indian, and Thai populations. A Vietnamese tradition of "roasting of the mother" involves warming her with a charcoal fire in a clay stove near her bed for the month-long postpartum period and feeding her spicy foods. She is also advised to avoid water and use an herbal alcohol solution for cleaning herself and her baby in order to keep herself warm (92). Malaysian mothers follow a similar month-long course, called *pantang larang,* involving confinement, sexual abstinence, restriction to "hot" foods, and traditional massage that helps rejuvenate the mother after pregnancy and birth (35).

In Melanesia, ethnic Fijian women have extraordinarily strong social support in the postpartum. Women are relieved of their domestic responsibilities for 2 or 3 months and are given respite from agricultural work for up to 12 months after the birth (24).Women are encouraged to rest (lie down) in the immediate postpartum and avoid sun exposure, sexual activity, and combing their hair. They are prohibited from eating specific foods that are thought to pose a risk to the baby; other foods are encouraged to enhance the quality and supply of breast milk. The community brings supplies for the baby in a ceremony called the *roqoroqo* and cooks for the mother's household for weeks to months (*kabekabe*). In contrast to a rather low social status before giving birth, new mothers are protected, nurtured, and admired.

Palestinian Bedouin women in the Negev enjoy a celebratory meal with their family and their community that includes an animal sacrifice. They receive support with household chores from nearby relatives. Thus, they can stay secluded for the 40 days of the puerperium in order to avoid *kabsa,* or perceived contamination by menstruating women, that is believed to threaten the baby's well-being or interfere with the mother's fertility. Similar to practices in East Asia, they attempt to maintain an appropriate balance of hot and cold humours through specific dietary proscriptions (93).

The *cuarentena* of Zapotec Indian and other Latin American populations also lasts about 40 days and is reported to include seclusion and dietary restriction (85). Traditional Guatemalan midwives who care for the indigenous Mayan population in Guatemala emphasize the importance of (re)warming the mother, and new mothers are often bathed in hot water both to stimulate milk flow and to cleanse their bodies (94).

Though the specifics of postpartum practices vary considerably across cultures, (e.g., prohibitions against bathing in China vs. encouragement of baths with warm water in Guatemala), overarching similarities can be observed. Most generally, formal provisions to allow rest and promote support during a period when the mother and baby may be perceived as vulnerable appear to be globally widespread. In many societies, there is detailed attention to restoring balance to the postpartum body through regulation of temperature through foods and exposures (89,95). In some cases, seclusion is emphasized, and in others, specific practices are meant to neutralize perceived threats to the mother and baby (whether of medical or spiritual nature) (28,95).

Postpartum traditions in the United States have undergone wide variation over the past century in response to a changing social status of women and health care economics. In the first half of the 20th century and before, women in the United States and other Western cultures spent a significant amount of time resting at home after giving birth (96), with plenty of family and friends caring for the mother and her new baby. This practice of "confinement" or "lying in" structured the postpartum period for American women at least to some extent, resembling the culturally sanctioned or mandated rest period traditional in some populations described earlier.

However, during World War II, economic and political pressures, shortened hospital stays, and urbanization resulting in fewer family members living under one roof ushered in the now more common practice of an almost immediate return to daily life—with the added responsibility of a new child (97). By the 1990s, advocates worried about poor parenting education, inadequate social and informational support for new parents, and postpartum depression were lobbying for legislation to ban increasingly short hospital stays. The Newborns' and Mothers' Health Protection Act of 1996 was passed at the beginning of 1998 to protect new mothers and their babies (96). At the same time, European countries were increasing their maternity leave entitlements substantially between 1969 and 1994, to an average of 26 weeks of job-protected time off, mostly at full pay; although longer paid maternity leaves clearly reduce early childhood mortality, the United States has not followed suit, mandating only 12 weeks' unpaid leave through the Family and Medical Leave Act (98).

In other societies, traditions promote affiliation of new mothers with experienced mothers. It might be interesting to observe how baby showers, mothers' groups, lactation consultants, postpartum *doulas,* and baby "nurses" address these needs in some US populations. By contrast to the emphasis on social support for role transition elsewhere, among upper middle class US women there is a cultural premium on minimizing "disruption" by the baby, with an emphasis on portability of the baby and rapid restoration of the mother's body. This is also evident in the special interest expressed about how the baby is sleeping (i.e., read as how disruptive is the baby?), whereas elsewhere there is relatively greater interest in how the baby is feeding. Trends in maternity clothes illustrate this as well, as within two decades, they evolved from disguising the pregnancy to disregarding it in favor of paralleling fashions for nonpregnant women.

V. THE RELATION OF SOCIAL SUPPORT TO POSTPARTUM HEALTH

Cross-cultural illustrations of the diversity of postpartum support suggest that a woman's experience may differ substantially depending on what formal support, protection, and recognition is available for postpartum women and how well a she might perceive these traditions to be implemented in her own case. That is, women might be particularly vulnerable when support is withdrawn or if their expectations exceed the practical support that is available. Although there has been relatively little investigation into how the level of culturally sanctioned social support might impact the risk of postpartum illness within a population, solid empirical evidence suggests that poor social support is associated with postpartum depression. Puerperal maternal distress has also been specifically linked to dissatisfaction with relationships, adverse health/life experiences, and economic stressors.

Numerous studies have investigated the impact of social support on postpartum mood disturbance. In a seminal study among postpartum women in London, Paykel and colleagues (99) found that relatively poor social support was significantly associated with postpartum depression. In another landmark study of 99 postpartum women in the midwestern United States, O'Hara (21) similarly found that postpartum depression was significantly associated with a number of prospectively assessed social stressors as well as relatively poor social support. Another study of 436 primiparous, married, socioeconomically diverse midwestern women similarly found that the mother's favorable mental health is significantly associated with emotional support of spouses or other members of the mother's social network, number of support persons, satisfaction with husband's help with household duties, and income (22). Several additional studies demonstrated a comparable inverse association between social support and postpartum depression even among more ethnically and socioeconomically diverse North American women (see Table 6-2). For example, a prospective study of socioeconomically diverse, primiparous women in Montreal found that less social support as well as conflictual relationships within a woman's social network measured at 3 weeks postpartum were significantly associated with higher BDI scores at 9 weeks postpartum (23). Moreover, a prospective study of a primarily Latina population of 108 mothers in the United States at 4 to 8 weeks postpartum found that lower satisfaction with prenatal support and life events distress were associated with increased levels of depressed mood in the postpartum (27). As described earlier, a study of 125 adolescent mothers in the United States found that depression at 4 months postpartum was significantly associated with lack of emotional or material support from the adolescent's mother or the infant's father, conflict with infant's father, and high levels of stress (48).

In the United Kingdom and Western Europe, a comparable inverse association between social support and postpartum depression has been reported in a number of studies. Among a sample of 427 mothers in Leicestershire, United Kingdom, living without a partner, unemployment, and perceived lack of support were significant predictors of high General Health Questionnaire (GHQ-30) scores in the postpartum (100). In a sample of 724 Italian and 629 French postpartum women, GHQ scores above 5 were significantly associated with a lack of confidante, financial worries, poor relationship with partner, and infant illness (101). Moreover, a study conducted in Valencia, Spain, found that psychological distress at 1 year postpartum was significantly associated with living without a partner, poor marital relationship after 12 months, arguments about the division of household chores and childcare, financial problems, and infant illness (102). Finally, a study conducted in urban Portugal reported that lower occupational status, educational level, income, as well as quality of housing and residential area were significantly associated with higher EPDS scores in a sample of 352 women at 2 to 5 months postpartum (103).

The association between inadequate social support and postpartum mood disturbance has also been noted in the Middle East. For example, in a sample of 257 Turkish postpartum women, a history of migration, living in a squatter area, baby health problems, as well as moderate or bad relationships with a husband, mother-in-law, or father-in-law were associated with significantly higher EPDS scores as compared with postpartum women without these social stressors (41). In addition, in the United Arab Emirates, a study of 95 women in Dubai at 6 to 10 weeks postpartum found that depression was significantly associated with previous divorce, marital problems before or after delivery, primiparity, unwanted pregnancy, poor infant health, or life events during the past year (40). Another study conducted in Jerusalem found that a score of 9 or above on the EPDS was significantly associated with immigrant status among 327 Jewish women at 6 to 10 weeks postpartum (42). Moreover, in a sample of 147 women living under socially adverse conditions in periurban Capetown, emotional and practical support from a partner was significantly inversely associated with SCID-diagnosed major depression at 2 months postpartum (44).

In Asia, in a sample of 526 postpartum Taiwanese women, "minor psychiatric morbidity" was significantly associated with lack of family and social support (104). In addition, marital dissatisfaction, inadequate social support, life events in pregnancy, poor mother-in-law relationship, and absence of *peiyue* were significantly associated with probable postpartum depression in univariate analyses in a large sample of Hong Kong women (90). Finally, EPDS scores greater than 8 and State-Trait Anxiety Inventory (STAI) Trait and State scores greater than 44 were significantly more likely among postpartum women who experienced stressful life events in a sample of 627 Japanese women in Japan (105).

Although some of the aforementioned studies report the association of a prospective assessment of social support with subsequent postpartum depression, direction of causality cannot be established in other studies. That is, it is quite conceivable that postpartum illness could undermine social support systems. We are also aware that negative studies may be less likely to be reported and published. Moreover, these studies have used disparate measures for assessing both social support and postpartum mood disturbance. Finally, the ways in which the adequacy of social support could impact on depression are probably complex. For example, in a sample of 105 married, primiparous US women, postpartum depression was prospectively significantly associated with a discrepancy between the amount of support expected or desired and the amount actually received (according to areas identified as being important during the prenatal assessment) (106). However, the consistency of the inverse relationship between social support and postpartum mood disturbance across diverse social contexts is striking and has great potential relevance to preventive interventions.

Thus, there is substantial evidence that postpartum depression is associated with the perceived availability and quality of social support. To the extent that culture-specific postpartum traditions might ensure adequate social support in the postpartum, it will be imperative to investigate whether these practices might be protective at a population level. For example, the low prevalence of postpartum depression (only 3.9%) in a Malaysian sample was observed in a social context in which a majority of women followed traditional postpartum practice of *pantang larang* and the vast majority followed a postpartum diet. However, the association between adherence to traditional practices and protection from postpartum depression in this population has not been examined (35). In addition, formalized substantive support for ethnic Fijian women in the postpartum in the Fiji appears to possibly attenuate postpartum illness. That is, women who report poorer social support are at higher risk for an episode of the postpartum (largely somatic) illness, *natadoka ni vasucu,* but presentation of symptoms rapidly mobilizes social support and symptoms resolve quickly (24,25). Similarly, in a prospective study of Hong Kong Chinese, women who did not practice *peiyue* (having a designated caregiver) were significantly more likely to have an episode of postpartum depression compared with women who did practice it (90). Further evidence that culture and social structure can play a protective role is provided by a study of Jewish women in Jerusalem. Among a sample of 327 secular, traditional, religious, and orthodox women, secular practice was associated with a significantly increased odds of postpartum depression. The study investigators hypothesized that clear delineation of social structure and social roles reduces a woman's risk for developing postpartum illness either by eliminating stressors or by enhancing coping mechanisms (42). Perhaps traditional, non-Western social structures (most likely in the form of social support), preserved despite immigration, confer some protection for new mothers against postpartum mood disturbance; however, more evidence is needed to support this hypothesis. The strong empirical evidence that social support moderates the risk of postpartum illness suggests the need for potential prevention strategies, either by reinforcing and sustaining traditions that provide support or by adapting traditions for other social contexts.

VI. CULTURALLY RELEVANT INTERVENTIONS FOR POSTPARTUM DEPRESSION

Conflict, migration, urbanization, modernization, and Westernization are contributing to rapid social, economic, and political change around the world. This change will undoubtedly threaten to undermine the social support networks that may protect women from postpartum illness. In light of these global changes, several essential questions arise. Can traditional social support systems be maintained or reinforced (or transplanted, in the case of immigration) despite social disruption? How can health policy makers and clinicians working within immigrant and refugee populations support traditions that protect the health of mothers and infants in the postpartum? Minimally, clinicians can inquire about traditional practices around the time of childbirth and role expectations for extended families in order to reinforce support mechanisms that may be available but not yet fully engaged (107). Finally, can protective traditions be revived or adapted as a prevention strategy for postpartum depression in populations in which postpartum women are at high risk for poor social support?

However, social mechanisms are often complicated and subtle, and it is important that even powerful and established support structures be considered with a critical eye. For example, the Japanese postpartum tradition *Satogaeri bunben*—in which women return to live with their parents from late in the third trimester of pregnancy to approximately 2 months postpartum, in order to rest and receive care—has been a presumed protective factor partially responsible for low rates of postpartum depression in Japanese women (108). Although disadvantages of the practice include a period of spousal separation, discontinuity in obstetric care, and potentially difficult relationships with the pregnant woman's family of origin (108), Oates and colleagues

(81) found that Japanese women did consider the inability to participate in *Satogaeri bunben* as likely to be distressing. Yoshida's group (108) combined a validation study of the EPDS as a screening tool for postpartum depression in Japanese women living in England and Japan with a qualitative study of *Satogaeri bunben.* Using the SADS/RDC, postpartum depression was found in 12% of the Japanese women living in England and in 17% of those living in Japan, incidences comparable to those in Western samples. They found, however, that sensitivity (82%) and specificity (95%) in identifying depression were optimized by a lower EPDS cut-off (greater than 8) than is typically used in Western subjects, and that even then the EPDS remained inadequately sensitive to identify depression in the subgroup of Japanese women living abroad. In addition, they found that adherence to *Satogaeri bunben* had no association with the presence or absence of postpartum depression. By using this combination of culturally sensitive quantitative and qualitative research methods, this group was able to question the assumptions that postpartum depression is particularly rare in Japanese women (rather, adjustment in research instruments may be required to adequately detect postpartum depression in this population) and that traditional practices are necessarily purely protective.

Cultural differences between patients and physicians can critically influence how medical care is offered and received, with potentially devastating effects on the outcome of care (109). These factors can become especially important in the case of postpartum mental illness. In the cross-cultural qualitative study of postpartum depression by Oates and colleagues (81), it was noted, for example, that whereas Asian mothers living in the United Kingdom expressed explicit concerns about interference from extended family, health care providers appeared to incorrectly assume that these extended family relationships would serve as a buffering force for this group of women. It is easy to see how this kind of misunderstanding could lead to offering unhelpful or even counterproductive interventions.

Tseng (110) discusses the concept of "culturally relevant psychotherapy," which can be used in working with any patient. In this model, clinicians incorporate patient-specific cultural meanings of life stories, stressors, and coping strategies as well as the cultural mediation of psychopathology into their formulations. Clinicians must come to understand how these cultural issues affect what patients expect and need from treatment, and be ready to modify therapeutic goals and technique appropriately.

This kind of "culturally relevant" approach is especially crucial around the time of childbirth, given the unique meanings and stresses of the transition to motherhood. Saintfort and Stern (111) describe a case of a Somali woman who presented at term with preeclampsia and no history of prenatal care. Postpartum, she developed complex neuropsychiatric symptoms, including psychotic and affective components, requiring rehospitalization on a neurology service. She and her family shared the belief that she was the victim of an evil spirit with whom her mother had made a contract in order to prevent the patient's death during a childhood illness. By the terms of this contract, the patient was to have made an offering to the spirit when she grew up and had a child of her own; she and her baby were now at risk because she had not done so. Although her family recognized the presence of "madness" in the patient that extended beyond their shared belief system, they remained unsupportive of treatment recommendations. Crucial to management of the case was the treatment team's decision to allow her family to take her home for several hours against medical advice for a culturally sanctioned healing ritual.

Some intervention studies have attempted to more systematically engage social support factors in order to prevent distress after childbirth. For example, prenatal and postpartum home visits by trained peers were associated with reduced psychological distress compared with that experienced by women without these visits (112). Another study found that straightforward prenatal instructions designed to enhance spousal support and ensure that a new mother receive help and rest were associated with significantly less postpartum distress compared with receiving no such instruction (113). However, a randomized controlled trial offering counseling to Hong Kong Chinese women with "suboptimal" childbirth outcomes did not have a significant effect in reducing postpartum depression (114). Finally, a pilot study assessed the effects of a community-based program to provide postpartum mothers with emotional support, practical infant care advice, and coaching on responsiveness to their infant in a population of women in periurban South Africa. Although no significant difference in prevalence of major depression was found between the intervention and control groups at 6 months postpartum, significant improvements in maternal–infant engagement were noted (115). It remains to be seen if such psychosocial interventions can have specific effects on preventing postpartum depression and improving family functioning in high-risk samples, and if they can be adapted to other settings in culturally appropriate ways.

Based on their review of randomized, controlled trials of efforts to prevent postpartum depression, Ogrodniczuk and Piper (116) suggest that continuity of care by midwives and brief psychotherapy for high-risk women may be useful strategies. They note that prevention research using biologically based interventions has been minimal to date, and randomized, controlled prevention studies that specifically address poor social support to reduce the incidence of postpartum depression have not yet been conducted. Although such research is conceivably straightforward to design, the interventions might prove to be highly culture-specific. Thus, future research will benefit from a thoughtful integration of ethnographic and epidemiologic approaches (81). Although still at an early stage, efforts have begun to establish research instruments and methods that will facilitate systematic cross-cultural studies on the causes and consequences of postpartum depression and culturally relevant interventions (117).

VIII. CONCLUSIONS

Childbirth is widely viewed as an event of enormous importance for women and their families—a time of physical, psychological, and social change as well as, potentially, stress. There is growing recognition that the postpartum period can be a time of distress as well as happiness, and that even normative experiences can differ substantially across and within cultures. Attempts to address this issue have ranged from first-person accounts that complicate the popular understanding of what it means to become a mother, to anthropological studies of traditional practices and culture-specific experiences of distress in the puerperium, to efforts by psychiatric researchers to define and understand pathological syndromes occurring in the perinatal period. The medical literature reveals burgeoning research that attempts to identify and characterize the syndrome of postpartum depression across ethnically diverse populations. Substantial efforts have been made to identify both biological and social factors that moderate the risk of postpartum depression. Although we have reported on some of the methodological challenges in the cross-cultural study of postpartum illness, we also feel that such research will make essential contributions to the development of effective therapeutic and preventive strategies for postpartum mood disturbance.

Whereas postpartum distress may not be universally experienced or recognized as a mental illness, it appears that postpartum illness consistent with the biomedical nosologic category of postpartum depression is globally widespread. It is also evident that there is substantial cross-cultural variability in postpartum practices that support mothers. Moreover, empirical data strongly suggest that poor social support is associated with increased risk of postpartum illness. Finally, some data suggest the possibility that postpartum traditions that enhance social support may protect women from postpartum illness. Thus, in clinical encounters with individual patients, it is essential to be curious about a woman's expectations and experiences in the perinatal period and the ways in which these may be influenced by cultural factors. This information and sensitivity may suggest means of mobilizing the kinds of support networks—traditional, untraditional, or developed through health care or social service systems—that she may find useful, as well as to recommend more specific treatments that may be indicated. Future research that thoughtfully integrates epidemiologic, anthropologic, and psychiatric perspectives will be invaluable in identifying psychosocial therapies and preventive and social policy interventions for postpartum depression.

REFERENCES

1. Grace SL, Evindar A, Stewart DE. The effect of postpartum depression on child cognitive development and behavior: a review and critical analysis of the literature. *Arch Womens Ment Health* 2003; 6:263–274.
2. Hay DF, Pawlby S, Sharp D, et al. Intellectual problems shown by 11-year-old children whose mothers had postnatal depression. *J Child Pscyhiatry* 2001;42:871–889.
3. Caplan HL, Cogill SR, Alexandra H, et al. Maternal depression and the emotional development of the child. *Br J Psychiatry* 1989;154:818–822.
4. Cohen LS, Altshuler LL. Pharmacologic management of psychiatric illness during pregnancy and the postpartum period. *Psychiatr Clin N Am Annu Drug Ther* 1997;4:21–60.
5. Nonacs R, Cohen LS. Postpartum mood disorders: diagnosis and treatment guidelines. *J Clin Psychiatry* 1998;59(Suppl 2):34–40.
6. Wisner KL, Parry BL, Piontek CM. Postpartum depression. *N Engl J Med* 2002;347:194–199.
7. Steiner M, Tam WYK. Postpartum depression in relation to other psychiatric disorders. In: Miller LJ, ed. *Postpartum mood disorders.* Washington, DC: American Psychiatric Press, 1999:47–63.

8. American Psychiatric Association. *Diagnostic and Statistical Manual of Mental Disorders, Fourth Edition, text revision.* Washington, DC: American Psychiatric Association, 2000.
9. Attia E, Downey J, Oberman M. Postpartum psychoses. In: Miller LJ, ed. *Postpartum mood disorders.* Washington, DC: American Psychiatric Press, 1999:99–117.
10. Kendell RE, Chalmers JC, Platz C. Epidemiology of puerperal psychoses. *Br J Psychiatry* 1987; 150:662–673.
11. Kumar R, Robson KM. A prospective study of emotional disorders in childbearing women. *Br J Psychiatry* 1984;144:35–47.
12. Halbreich U, Endicott J. Possible involvement of endorphin withdrawal or imbalance in specific premenstrual syndromes and postpartum depression. *Med Hypoth* 1981;7:1045–1051.
13. Wieck A. Endocrine aspects of postnatal mental disorders. *Baillieres Clin Obstet Gynaecol* 1989; 3:857–877.
14. Smith R, Cubis J, Brinsmead M, et al. Mood changes, obstetric experience and alterations in plasma cortisol, beta-endorphin and corticotrophin releasing hormone during pregnancy and the puerperium. *J Psychosom Res* 1990;34:53–69.
15. Henrick V, Altshuler LL, Suri R. Hormonal changes in the postpartum and implications for postpartum depression. *Psychosomatics* 1998;39:93–101.
16. Henrick V, Altshuler LL. Biological determinants of postpartum depression. In: Miller LJ, ed. *Postpartum mood disorders.* Washington, DC: American Psychiatric Press, 1999:65–82.
17. O'Hara MW, Schlechte JA, Lewis DA, et al. A controlled prospective study of postpartum mood disorders: psychological, environmental, and hormonal factors. *J Abnorm Psychol* 1991;100:63–73.
18. O'Hara MW. *Postpartum depression: causes and consequences.* New York: Springer-Verlag, 1995.
19. Parry BL. Postpartum depression in relation to other reproductive cycle mood changes. In: Miller LJ, ed. *Postpartum mood disorders.* Washington, DC: American Psychiatric Press, 1999:21–45.
20. Bloch M, Schmidt PJ, Danaceau M, et al. Effects of gonadal steroids in women with a history of postpartum depression. *Am J Psychiatry* 2000;157:924–930.
21. O'Hara MW. Social support, life events, and depression during pregnancy and the puerperium. *Arch Gen Psychiatry* 1986;43:569–573.
22. Gjerdingen DK, Chaloner KM. The relationship of women's postpartum mental health to employment, childbirth, and social support. *J Fam Pract* 1994;38:465–472.
23. Sèguin L, Potvin L, St-Denis M, et al. Socio-environmental factors and postnatal depressive symptomatology: a longitudinal study. *Womens Health* 1999;29:57–72.
24. Becker AE. Postpartum illness in Fiji: a sociosomatic perspective. *Psychosom Med* 1998;60: 431–438.
25. Becker AE, Lee DTS. Indigenous models for attenuation of postpartum depression: case studies from Fiji and Hong Kong. In: Cohen A, Kleinman A, Saraceno B, eds. *The world mental health casebook.* New York: Kluwer/Academic Publishers, 2002.
26. Beck CT. A meta-analysis of predictors of postpartum depression. *Nurs Res* 1996;45:297–303.
27. Neter E, Collins NL, Lobel M, et al. Psychosocial predictors of postpartum depressed mood in socioeconomically disadvantaged women. *Womens Health* 1995;1:51–75.
28. Stern G, Kruckman L. Multi-disciplinary perspectives on post-partum depression: an anthropological critique. *Soc Sci Med* 1983;17:1027–1041.
29. Jiminez MH, Newton N. Activity and work during pregnancy and the postpartum period: a cross-cultural study of 202 societies. *Am J Obstet Gynecol* 1979;135:171–176.
30. Kleinman A. *Patients and healers in the context of culture: an exploration of the borderland between anthropology, medicine, and psychiatry.* Berkeley: University of California Press, 1980.
31. Kirmayer LJ, Young A. Culture and somatization: clinical, epidemiological, and ethnographic perspectives. *Psychosom Med* 1998;60:420–30.
32. Nichter M. Idioms of distress: alternatives in the expression of psychosocial distress: a case study from South India. *Cult Med Psychiatry* 1981;5:379–408.
33. Kumar R. Postnatal mental illness: a transcultural perspective. *Soc Psychiatry Psychiatr Epidemiol* 1994;29:250–264.
34. Kok LP, Chan PSL, Ratnam SS. Postnatal depression in Singapore women. *Singapore Med J* 1994; 35:33–35.
35. Kit LK, Janet G, Jegasothy R. Incidence of postnatal depression in Malaysian women. *J Obstet Gynaecol Res* 1997;23:85–89.
36. Lee DTS, Yip ASK, Chiu HFK, et al. A psychiatric epidemiological study of postpartum Chinese women. *Am J Psychiatry* 2001;158:220–226.

37. Yamashita H, Yoshida K, Nakano H, et al. Postnatal depression in Japanese women: detecting the early onset of postnatal depression by closely monitoring the postpartum mood. *J Affect Disord* 2000;58:145–154.
38. Yoshida K, Marks MN, Kibe N, et al. Postnatal depression in Japanese women who have given birth in England. *J Affect Disord* 1997;43:63–77.
39. Regmi S, Sligl W, Carter D, et al. A controlled study of postpartum depression among Nepalese women: validation of the Edinburgh Postnatal Depression Scale in Kathmandu. *Trop Med Int Health* 2002;7:378–382.
40. Ghubash R, Abou-Saleh MT. Postpartum psychiatric illness in Arab culture: prevalence and psychosocial correlates. *Br J Psychiatry* 1997;171:65–68.
41. Danaci AE, Dinc G, Deveci A, et al. Postnatal depression in Turkey: epidemiological and cultural aspects. *Soc Psychiatry Psychiatr Epidemiol* 2002;37:125–129.
42. Dankner R, Goldberg RP, Fisch RZ, et al. Cultural elements of postpartum depression: a study of 327 Jewish Jerusalem women. *J Reprod Med* 2000;45:97–104.
43. Uwakwe R. Affective (depressive) morbidity in puerperal Nigerian women: validation of the Edinburgh postnatal depression scale. *Acta Psychiatr Scand* 2003;107:251–259.
44. Cooper PJ, Tomlinson M, Swartz L, et al. Post-partum depression and the mother-infant relationship in a South African periurban settlement. *Br J Psychiatry* 1999;175:554–558.
45. Jadresic E, Araya R, Jara C. Validation of the Edinburgh Postnatal Depression Scale (EPDS) in Chilean postpartum women. *J Psychosom Obstet Gynecol* 1995;16:187–191.
46. Cutrona CE. Causal attributions and perinatal depression. *J Abnorm Psychol* 1983;92:161–172.
47. Hobfoll SE, Ritter C, Lavin J, et al. Depression prevalence and incidence among inner-city pregnant and postpartum women. *J Consult Clin Psychol* 1995;63:445–453.
48. Barnet B, Joffe A, Duggan AK, et al. Depressive symptoms, stress, and social support in pregnant and postpartum adolescents. *Arch Pediatr Adolesc Med* 1996;150:64–69.
49. Steer RA, Scholl TO, Beck AT. Revised Beck Depression Inventory scores of inner-city adolescents: pre-and postpartum. *Psychol Rep* 1990;66:315–320.
50. Watson JP, Elliot SA, Rugg AJ, et al. Psychiatric disorder in pregnancy and the first postnatal year. *Br J Psychiatry* 1984;144:453–462.
51. Areias MEG, Kumar R, Barros H, et al. Comparative incidence of depression in women and men, during pregnancy and after childbirth: validation of the Edinburgh Postnatal Depression Scale in Portuguese mothers. *Br J Psychiatry* 1996;169:30–35.
52. Condon JT, Corkindale CJ. The assessment of depression in the postnatal period: a comparison of four self-report questionnaires. *Aust N Z J Psychiatry* 1997;31:353–359.
53. Harris B, Huckle P, Thomas R, et al. The use of rating scales to identify post-natal depression. *Br J Psychiatry* 1989;154:813–817.
54. Georgiopoulos AM, Bryan TL, Yawn BP, et al. Population-based screening for postpartum depression. *Obstet Gynecol* 1999; 93:653–657.
55. Georgiopoulos AM, Bryan TL, Wollan P, et al. Routine screening for postpartum depression. *J Fam Pract* 2001;50:117–122.
56. Cox J. Origins and development of the 10-item Edinburgh Postnatal Depression Scale. In: Cox J, Holden J, eds. *Perinatal psychiatry: use and misuse of the Edinburgh Postnatal Depression Scale.* London: Royal College of Psychiatrists (Gaskell), 1994:115–124.
57. Holden J. Using the Edinburgh Postnatal Depression Scale in clinical practice. In: Cox J, Holden J, eds. *Perinatal psychiatry: use and misuse of the Edinburgh Postnatal Depression Scale.* London: Royal College of Psychiatrists (Gaskell), 1994:125–144.
58. Wickberg B, Huang CP. Screening for postnatal depression in a population-based Swedish sample. *Acta Psychiatr Scand* 1997;95:62–66.
59. Josefsson A, Berg G, Nordin C, et al. Prevalence of depressive symptoms in late pregnancy and postpartum. *Acta Obstet Gynecol Scand* 2001;80:251–255.
60. Patel V, Rodrigues M, DeSouza N. Gender, poverty, and postnatal depression: a study of mothers in Goa, India. *Am J Psychiatry* 2002;159:43–47.
61. O'Hara MW. Postpartum depression: identification and measurement in a cross-cultural context. In: Cox J, Holden J, eds. *Perinatal psychiatry: use and misuse of the Edinburgh Postnatal Depression Scale.* London: Royal College of Psychiatrists (Gaskell), 1994:145–168.
62. Murray L, Carothers AD. The validation of the Edinburgh Post-natal Depression Scale on a community sample. *Br J Psychiatry* 1990;157:288–290.

63. Wickberg B, Huang CP. The Edinburgh Postnatal Depression Scale: validation on a Swedish community sample. *Acta Psychiatr Scand* 1996;94:181–184.
64. Berle JO, Aarre TF, Mykletun A, et al. Screening for postnatal depression: validation of the Norwegian version of the Edinburgh Postnatal Depression Scale, and assessment of risk factors for postnatal depression. *J Affect Disord* 2003;76:151–156.
65. Ghubash R, Abou-Saleh MT, Daradkeh TK. The validity of the Arabic Edinburgh Postnatal Depression Scale. *Soc Psychiatry Psychiatr Epidemiol* 1997;32:474–476.
66. Lee DTS, Yip SK, Chiu HFK, et al. Detecting postnatal depression in Chinese women: validation of the Chinese version of the Edinburgh Postnatal Depression Scale. *Br J Psychiatry* 1998;172: 433–437.
67. Garcia-Esteve L, Ascaso C, Ojuel J. Validation of the Edinburgh Postnatal Depression Scale (EPDS) in Spanish mothers. *J Affect Disord* 2003;75:71–76.
68. Boyce P, Stubbs J, Todd A. The Edinburgh Postnatal Depression Scale: validation for an Australian Sample. *Aust N Z J Psychiatry* 1993;27:472–476.
69. Swain AM, Stuart S, O'Hara MW. Validation of the Edinburgh Postnatal Depression Scale with an American community sample. Unpublished data, 1996.
70. Cox JL. Postnatal depression: a comparison of African and Scottish women. *Soc Psychiatry* 1983; 18:25–28.
71. Cox JL, Connor Y, Kendell RE. Prospective study of the psychiatric disorders of childbirth. *Br J Psychiatry* 1982;140:111–117.
72. Huang Y, Mathers N. Postnatal depression–biological or cultural? A comparative study of postnatal women in the UK and Taiwan. *J Adv Nurs* 2001;33:279–287.
73. Kleinman A. Depression, somatization and the new cross-cultural psychiatry. *Soc Sci Med* 1977; 11:3–10.
74. Green AR, Betancourt JR, Carrillo JE. The relation between somatic symptoms and depression. *New Engl J Med* 2000;342:658–659.
75. Hrdy SB. *Mother Nature: a history of mothers, infants, and natural selection.* New York: Pantheon Books, 1999.
76. Neisslein J. Happy, happy, joy, joy. *Brain Child* 2004;5:5.
77. Buchanan AJ. *Mother shock: loving every (other) minute of it.* New York: Seal Press, 2003.
78. Lamott A. *Operating instructions: a journal of my son's first year.* New York: Ballantine Books, 1993.
79. Slater L. When love doesn't come easily. *Self* 2004;26:182–191.
80. Levitzky S, Cooper R. Infant colic syndrome—maternal fantasies of aggression and infanticide. *Clin Pediatr* 2000;39:395–400.
81. Oates MR, Cox JL, Neema S, et al. Postnatal depression across countries and cultures: a qualitative study. *Br J Psychiatry* Suppl 2004;184:s10–s16.
82. Jinadu MK, Daramola SM. Emotional changes in pregnancy and early peruperium among the Yoruba women of Nigeria. *Int J Soc Psychiatry* 1990;36:93–98.
83. Cox JL. Childbirth as a life event: sociocultural aspects of postnatal depression. *Acta Psychiatr Scand Suppl* 1988;78:75–83.
84. Harkness S. The cultural mediation of postpartum depression. *Med Anthropol Q* 1987;1:194–209.
85. Pillsbury BLK. "Doing the month": confinement and convalescence of Chinese women after childbirth. *Soc Sci Med* 1978;12:11–22.
86. Shimizu YM, Kaplan BJ. Postpartum depression in the United States and Japan. J *Cross Cult Psychol* 1987;18:15–30.
87. Stewart S, Jambunathan J. Hmong women and postpartum depression. *Health Care Women Int* 1996;17:319–330.
88. Matthey S, Panasetis P, Barnett B. Adherence to cultural practices following childbirth in migrant Chinese women and relation to postpartum mood. *Health Care Women Int* 2002;23:567–576.
89. Kim-Godwin, YS. Postpartum beliefs and practices among non-western cultures. *Am J Matern Child Med* 2003;28:74–78.
90. Lee DT, Yip AS, Leung TY, et al. Ethnoepidemiology of postnatal depression. Prospective multivariate study of sociocultural risk factors in a Chinese population in Hong Kong. *Br J Psychiatry* 2004; 184(Suppl):34–40.
91. Kaewsarn P, Moyle W, Creedy D. Traditional postpartum practices among Thai women. *J Adv Nurs* 2003;41:358–366.

92. Bodo K, Gibson N. Childbirth customs in Vietnamese traditions. *Can Fam Physician* 1999;45: 690–697.
93. Hundt GL, Phil M, Beckerleg S, et al. Women's health custom made: building on the 40 days postpartum for Arab women. *Health Care Women Int* 2000;21:529–542.
94. Lang JB, Elkin ED. A study of the beliefs and birthing practices of traditional midwives in rural Guatemala. *J Nurs Midwifery* 1997;42:25–31.
95. Davis RE. The postpartum experience for southeast Asian women in the United States. *Am J Matern Child Med* 2001;26:208–213.
96. Martell LK, Zwelling E. The hospital and the postpartum experience: a historical analysis. *J Obstet Gynecol Neonat Nurs* 2000;29:65–72.
97. Temkin E. Driving through: postpartum care during World War II. *Am J Public Health* 1999;89: 587–595.
98. Ruhm CJ. Parental leave and child health. *J Health Econ* 2000;19:931–960.
99. Paykel ES, Emms EM, Fletcher J, et al. Life events and social support in puerperal depression. *Br J Psychiatry* 1980;136:339–346.
100. Brugha TS, Sharp HM, Cooper SA, et al. The Leicester 500 project: social support and the development of postnatal depressive symptoms, a prospective cohort study. *Psychol Med* 1998;28:63–79.
101. Romito P, Saurel-Cubizolles MJ, Lelong N. What makes new mothers unhappy: psychological distress one year after birth in Italy and France. *Soc Sci Med* 1999;49:1651–1661.
102. Escribà V, Más R, Romito P, et al. Psychological distress of new Spanish mothers. *Eur J Public Health* 1999;9:294–299.
103. Augusto A, Kumar R, Calhieros JM, et al. Post-natal depression in an urban area of Portugal: comparison of childbearing women and matched controls. *Psychol Med* 1996;26:135–141.
104. Hung CH, Chung HH. The effects of postpartum stress and social support on postpartum women's health status. *J Adv Nurs* 2001;36:676–684.
105. Tamaki R, Murata M, Okano T. Risk factors for postpartum depression in Japan. *Psychiatr Clin Neurosci* 1997;51:93–98.
106. Logsdon MC, McBride AB, Birkimer JC. Social support and postpartum depression. *Res Nurs Health* 1994;17:449–457.
107. Wile J, Arechiga M. Sociocultural aspects of postpartum depression. In: Miller LJ, ed. *Postpartum mood disorders.* Washington, DC: American Psychiatric Press, 1999:83–98.
108. Yoshida K, Yamashita H, Ueda M, et al. Postnatal depression in Japanese mothers and the reconsideration of 'Satogaeri bunben.' *Pediatr Int* 2001;43:189–193.
109. Fadiman A. *The spirit catches you and you fall down: a Hmong child, her American doctors, and the collision of two cultures.* New York: Farrar, Straus and Giroux, 1997.
110. Tseng W. Culture and psychotherapy: an overview. In: Tseng W, Streltzer J, eds. *Culture and psychotherapy: a guide to clinical practice.* Washington, DC: American Psychiatric Press, 2001: 3–12.
111. Saintfort R, Stern TA. Cross-cultural and neuropsychiatric aspects of a postpartum delusional state. *Harv Rev Psychiatry* 2000;8:141–147.
112. Marcenko MO, Spence M. Home visitation services for at-risk pregnant and postpartum women: A randomized trial. *Am J Orthopsychiatry* 1994;64:468–478.
113. Gordon RE, Gordon KK. Social factors in the prevention of postpartum emotional problems. *Obstet Gynecol* 1960;15:433–438.
114. Tam WH, Lee DT, Chiu HF, et al. A randomised controlled trial of educational counselling on the management of women who have suffered suboptimal outcomes in pregnancy. *Br J Obstet Gynaecol* 2003;110:853—859
115. Cooper PJ, Landman M, Tomlinson M, et al. Impact of a mother-infant intervention in an indigent peri-urban South African context: a pilot study. *Br J Psychiatry* 2002; 180:76–81.
116. Ogrodniczuk JS, Piper WE. Preventing postnatal depression: a review of research findings. *Harv Rev Psychiatry* 2003;11:291–307.
117. Asten P, Marks MN, Oates MR, et al. Aims, measures, study sites and participant samples of the Transcultural Study of Postnatal Depression. *Br J Psychiatry* 2004;46:s3–s9.

7

Bipolar Disorder in African Americans

William B. Lawson

Department of Psychiatry, Howard University Hospital, Washington, DC 20060

I. INTRODUCTION

Bipolar affective disorder is a serious but treatable mental disorder that is often either misdiagnosed or underrecognized (1,2). As a consequence, treatment is often inappropriate or simply not provided (3). African Americans, like most ethnic minorities, experience disparities in general health and mental health care (4). Misdiagnosis is more common and treatment is less likely to be accessible. Contrary to recent findings, bipolar disorder was once thought to be rare in African Americans and appropriate treatment was just as uncommon (5). This chapter presents a review of recent findings about the diagnosis and treatment of bipolar disorder in African Americans, providing illustrative vignettes.

II. DIAGNOSIS AND MISDIAGNOSIS

Diagnosing Bipolar Disorder: The Premed Student

A 22-year-old African American premed student was admitted to an acute care community psychiatric facility with a working diagnosis of schizophrenia. He was a student at a top-ten private university, one of only a handful of African American students. He would go into the undergraduate women's dormitory claiming he was the world's greatest lover and "feel up" female students. He often would go to the cafeteria and simply take food without paying. He was generally euthymic or irritable and never expressed hallucinations. He once received a psychological evaluation in which he stated that he sometimes would just "lay in the cut" (in Chicago and other inner city neighborhoods, this is a term that also means "taking it easy"). The psychologist noted this statement as an example of a thought disorder. He had only one prior admission during the past 2 years. He had been on a first-generation antipsychotic, fluphenazine, and later fluphenazine decanoate alone. The school had earlier delayed taking action because he made excellent grades. On the acute unit, bipolar disorder was quickly diagnosed. He was started on lithium and later was admitted to medical school on lithium monotherapy. He had not had any hospitalizations over the intervening 5 years.

Discussion: This vignette describes a common experience—persistent misdiagnosis despite clear symptoms of bipolar disorder, a tendency to interpret nonpathological symptoms as psychosis, and improved responsiveness as measured by fewer relapses and a better outcome when appropriate treatment is given.

Bipolar disorder is frequently misdiagnosed. On initial presentation, patients are often first diagnosed with major depression, as much as 50% of the time (1,6). African Americans with bipolar disorder are often diagnosed with schizophrenia despite clear-cut bipolar symptoms. Schizophrenia was previously thought to occur up to ten times more commonly in African Americans and bipolar disorder rarely if ever (5). Large multisite studies using reliable structured assessment tools have consistently found that ethnic differences in the prevalence of bipolar disorder tend to be small or nonexistent (7,8).

III. REASONS FOR MISDIAGNOSIS

A. Clinician-Related Reasons for Misdiagnosis

Overall, the factors leading to misdiagnosis can be divided into clinician-related variables and patient variables. Variables resulting from the behavior of the provider include:

1. *Failure to apply diagnostic criteria.* A consistent finding is the disconnect between clinical diagnosis and the diagnoses derived from structured interviews. The third and fourth editions of the *Diagnostic and Statistical Manual of Mental Disorders* (DSM) were designed to be criteria driven to improve reliability and validity. However, misdiagnosis for bipolar disorder continues to persist regardless of ethnicity (9).
2. *Failure to elicit symptoms.* A recent study suggests that information variance (i.e., the quality or type of history and symptoms used) rather than criterion variance (i.e., disagreement about the diagnostic criteria used) accounted for most diagnostic disagreement around race (10). Providers may spend less time with African American patients or simply fail to ask about affective symptoms and overemphasize psychotic symptoms.
3. *Failure to understand ethnic differences in expression.* African Americans may have different idioms of distress. Irritability may be expressed more often than euphoria in mania. Protective wariness and cultural distrust are common. These nonpathological expressions may be interpreted as psychotic symptoms (5,9).
4. *Overt or covert stereotyping.* African Americans were once thought to have little intrapsychic life. Bipolar disorder was thought to be virtually nonexesistent (5). An extensive literature has labeled African Americans as psychotic and rarely depressed. African American males are often portrayed as violent in the media (5,11). Social distance—because the provider is often of a different race, income

level, and professional status than the patient—probably contributes to a persistence of these and other stereotypes. Recent studies with investigators trained to use diagnostic criteria have shown that clinicians readily recognize psychotic symptoms in African Americans but often miss affective symptoms (11).

5. *Selection bias.* Information about African Americans comes from clinic population or prevalence studies, yet these samples are often biased because they probably do not represent the larger population of African Americans. The National Comorbidity Study, purportedly the best epidemiological study to date, has a number of inherent problems with assuming the assessing instruments are reasonably valid and reliable for African American populations, a question that is still under considerable debate (8). First, the study did not oversample African Americans. Reliability may be questionable for smaller subsets, including such relatively uncommon illnesses as bipolar disorder, even though reliability of the overall sample may be quite good. Secondly, African Americans may be less likely to be included in clinical trials. Finally, the sample did not include incarcerated or hospitalized individuals, yet African Americans are far more likely to be in those settings.

B. Patient-Related Reasons for Misdiagnosis: The Ex-Inmate

A 46-year-old African American single man had been released from prison (for drug dealing) with a follow-up appointment for outpatient psychiatric care. He had had over ten psychiatric admissions for "schizophrenia" until his most recent admission for bipolar disorder. He had 20 arrests and ten incarcerations, usually for cocaine abuse. He had never received substance abuse treatment or psychiatric care during his incarcerations, except for the most recent one. He would present with irritability and grandiosity, seek prostitutes, and ultimately use cocaine heavily. After his release, he was maintained on divalproex, lithium, and quetiapine, and participated in Narcotics Anonymous. He improved sufficiently to work full-time, get an apartment, and regularly take his wheelchair-bound, elderly mother to church. He did well for over 2 years; then, he started skipping his medication and his appointments with his parole officer, where drug screens were done. He was evicted from his apartment for wild parties and cocaine use, threatened his mother, and was subsequently arrested. He remains in custody while prosecutors are seeking a lengthy sentence for cocaine possession.

Discussion: This vignette demonstrates the problem of misdiagnosis and comorbid drug use that led to a diversion to the criminal justice system. This patient's course might have been different if he had gotten his initial treatment services for his bipolar disorder and substance abuse in a noncorrectional setting.

1. Real differences in symptom expression

Cultural and ethnic differences in idioms of distress and willingness to seek treatment can also contribute to diagnostic error. Misdiagnosis also may reflect "true" differences in symptom presentation for a given disorder. African Americans appear to be more likely to present with psychotic symptoms. Clinicians will often attend more to the psychotic symptoms and ignore affective symptoms, leading to a misdiagnosis of schizophrenia (11). These symptom differences may reflect a different presentation of the disorder, but they also may represent ethnic differences in willingness to verbalize certain types of symptoms. They may also represent a misinterpretation of ethnic differences in expression. African Americans, for example, often show a protective wariness around providers of a different ethnicity, which has been referred to as a healthy paranoia. However, this is often misinterpreted as schizophrenia (5). Moreover, as the vignette of the premedical student shows, unfamiliar idioms may be interpreted as a thought disorder.

2. *Treatment delay or refusal, especially with mental health professionals.* African Americans with mental disorders often refuse to seek treatment from mental health professionals or delay doing so (3,4). Distressed individuals may not have adequate or up-to-date knowledge about the mental health system. They often fear hospitalization or involuntary commitment (3,12). Treatment or help is more likely to be sought apart from mental health professionals. These sources of help include primary care providers, family members, and the faith community (13). Unfortunately, they are often unfamiliar with the management of bipolar disorder.
3. *Settings with limited mental health services.* Many bipolar patients may be followed up in primary care clinics, which can be excellent for general medical questions and very adequate for managing depression. However, the management of bipolar disorder is often beyond the capacity of these clinics (14). Additionally, with deinstitutionalization and limited community resources, many of the mentally end up on the streets or in jail. Up to 50% of jail inmates may be mentally ill, yet fewer than a third of surveyed jails offer any mental health services or training to staff (15,16). Bipolar patients, with dramatic symptoms that include irritability, probably face a high risk of arrest. The problem is especially acute for African Americans, who disproportionately receive mental health services in primary care settings and constitute up to 50% of the prison population (1).
4. *The problem of comorbidity.* Substance abuse is common in bipolar disorder. Alcohol and substance abuse may occur in over half of patients with bipolar disorder (17). Substance abuse may contribute to misdiagnosis in African Americans (18). These disorders may further confuse the diagnostic picture because substance abuse often mimics psychopathology and may alter symptom presentation.

III. TREATMENT: HOW MISDIAGNOSIS IMPACTS PHARMACOTHERAPY

A. Overuse of Antipsychotics: The Singer

A 43-year-old, tall, muscular African American man is brought into the emergency room of a Veterans Administration hospital for what was thought to be a psychotic episode. He was found shouting and singing in front of a fast food restaurant at 1 a.m. Records from previous emergency room visits show that he always had an admitting diagnosis of paranoid schizophrenia. He was brought into the hospital in four-point leather restraints. His restraints were removed and he sat quietly, even though he had no additional medication given. He had been treated with depot fluphenazine but had missed several appointments. A review of his inpatient record revealed a different story. He would, after some coaxing, express the belief that he was the Son of God. His affect on those admissions was elevated with rapid speech and complaints of "thoughts like race horses." At other times, he was despondent with slowed speech, lowered eyes, and deep shame over his actions. He had a history of six suicide attempts, including sticking his head in a gas oven and barely escaping with his life after being discovered. He was invariably discharged on lithium but returned on a first generation antipsychotic alone. The psychiatrists at his outpatient agency were finally called to share their thoughts about his diagnosis. They were convinced and remained convinced that he had schizophrenia, despite a recitation of his symptoms, which they generally endorsed as well. They saw no reason for him to receive lithium and did not understand why the depot medication was stopped. They admitted that he was generally compliant with lithium but gave him the depot shots anyway. They also noted that whenever he was interviewed he was not willing to provide much information at all, and considered this behavior reflective of paranoia. A year later, after two more admissions, he eventually attempted to gas himself in an oven and suffered severe anoxic damage. He was referred to nursing home care.

Discussion: This case illustrates that misdiagnosis often persists despite evidence to the contrary. Misdiagnosis affects treatment, encouraging excessive use of conventional antipsychotics and depot medication at the expense of antimanic medication.

African Americans are more likely to receive antipsychotics in the treatment of mania (18,19). This use of antipsychotics may be a consequence of misdiagnosis, with patients often overdiagnosed with schizophrenia and thus treated for schizophrenia rather than bipolar disorder. Consequently, African Americans are likely to receive antipsychotics rather than antimanic agents (18–21).

Antipsychotic agents are often used to treat acute mania. First generation agents such as neuroleptics are effective in treating acute mania but there is some question about their efficacy in preventing relapse (22). Moreover, African Americans given antipsychotics are far more likely to receive first generation than atypical or second-generation agents (23,24). Second-generation agents have fewer extrapyramidal side effects and a probable lower tardive dyskinesia risk. The tendency of first-generation agents to produce extrapyramidal symptoms may be problematic, especially for African Americans. African Americans may be more likely to develop tardive dyskinesia with the use of first-generation antipsychotics (25–27). Thus, African Americans with bipolar disorder may, because of misdiagnosis, receive conventional antipsychotics, which may be less tolerable for African Americans, rather than more appropriate antimanic or even second-generation antipsychotic agents. African Americans are more likely to receive depot or long-acting injectable medication (28,29). It is likely that the increased use of depot injections may reflect poor compliance as a result of excessive use of agents with poorly tolerated side effects.

B. Effects of Misdiagnosis on Antidepressant Use

Antidepressant medications are often used in the treatment of bipolar disorder. Depressive symptoms can occur in bipolar I, and must occur in bipolar II disorder. Moreover, many bipolar patients demand antidepressant treatment because they often perceive euthymia as depression. Most guidelines now recommend sparing use of antidepressants in the treatment of bipolar depression because they are often associated with the induction of often-treatment-resistant rapid cycling (30). Tricyclic antidepressants in particular have been associated with "switching" into manic states (31).

Many bipolar patients, however, are treated with antidepressants because they are initially misdiagnosed as having unipolar depression (1). The problem is particularly acute in the primary care setting, where clinicians may be quite good at recognizing and treating depression but have limited knowledge and skills in recognizing bipolar disorder (14).

Several points are especially relevant to African Americans. As noted earlier, African Americans are more likely to seek mental health treatment in the primary care setting (13). In addition, African Americans are more likely to receive tricyclic antidepressants rather than newer antidepressants such as selective serotonin reuptake inhibitors. As previously noted, the tricyclic antidepressants may be the worse offenders in inducing manic states in bipolar depression.

C. Improving Access To and Use of Antimanic Agents

Standard antimanic agents such as lithium and divalproex remain the treatments of choice for bipolar disorder (22). They are often able to treat both mania and depression, and can be used effectively for acute and maintenance treatment. The excessive use of other medications, such as conventional antipsychotics and antidepressants, instead of antimanic agents probably contributes to poorer outcomes for African American bipolar patients (34). Many second-generation antipsychotics appear to have properties that would qualify them as antimanic agents (22). However, as noted earlier, African Americans are more likely to receive first-generation agents.

Recent evidence suggests that African Americans may be less likely to tolerate lithium. African Americans receiving lithium tend to have a higher red blood cell to plasma ratio. This higher ratio has been associated with more evidence of lithium-related side effects (35,36). Recent findings suggest that lithium may be more effective in preventing suicide (37). The clinician treating African American patients will have to decide how to balance the relatively uncommon but lethal risk of suicide against the less lethal but more common risk of medication side effects.

IV. CONCLUSION

African Americans with bipolar disorder face a greater burden of illness (34). The problem of misdiagnosis continues to be an important issue despite the widespread use of the DSM-IV. More needs to be done to determine the reasons for this misdiagnosis and possible protective actions. Misdiagnosis affects pharmacotherapy, with African Americans often not receiving optimal treatment; instead they are often prescribed older medications with lesser efficacy and more side effects.

Tremendous strides have been made in the psychological, sociocultural, and biological understanding of bipolar disorder. However, a number of steps must still be taken to promote optimal care. We need to:

- Improve our knowledge about how to address ethnic and racial disparities.
- Plan more studies to determine why misdiagnosis continues to occur.
- Conduct more research in primary care settings and jails, where African Americans often receive their care.
- Design more research on the idioms of distress in the African American community to better understand them and to train providers in understanding them.
- Complete more research on the relative tolerability of the psychotropic medications that manage this disorder in African Americans.
- Better educate mental health providers about the diagnosis and treatment of African Americans.
- Do more to educate professionals outside the mental health field as well, because African Americans are often in their care. Similarly, patients and their families must be informed about this disorder.

Addressing these issues in African Americans will benefit more than this single ethnic group. Addressing such issues will lead to a paradigm that will better account for ethnic differences and disparities that are becoming increasingly relevant as our country becomes more culturally diverse.

REFERENCES

1. Ghaemi SN, Boiman EE, Goodwin FK. Diagnosing bipolar disorder and the effects of antidepressants: a naturalistic study. *J Clin Psychiatry* 2000;61:804–808.
2. Strakowski SM, Lonczak HS, Sax K, et al. The effects of race on diagnosis and disposition from a psychiatric emergency service. *J Clin Psychiatry* 1995;56:101–107.
3. Wells KB, Miranda J, Bauer MS, et al. Overcoming barriers to reducing the burden of affective disorders. *Biol Psychiatry* 2002;52:655–675.
4. US Department of Health and Human Services. *Mental health: culture, race, and ethnicity. A supplement to mental health: a report of the Surgeon General.* Rockville, MD: US Department of Health and Human Services, Substance Abuse and Mental Health Services Administration, Center for Mental Health Services, National Institutes of Health, National Institute of Mental Health, 2001.
5. Jones BE, Gray BA. Problems in diagnosing schizophrenia and affective disorders among blacks. *Hosp Community Psychiatry* 1986;37:61–65.
6. Mukherjee S, Shukla S, Woodle J, et al. Misdiagnosis of schizophrenia in bipolar patients: a multiethnic comparison. *Am J Psychiatry* 1983;140:1571–1574.
7. Robins LN, Locke B, Regier DA. An overview of psychiatric disorders in America. In: Robins LN, Regier DA, eds. *Psychiatric disorders in America. The Epidemiologic Catchment Area Study.* New York: The Free Press, 1991:328–366.
8. Kessler RC, McGonogle KA, Zhao S, et al. Lifetime and 12 month prevalence of DSM III-R psychiatric disorders in the United States. *Arch Gen Psychiatry* 1994;51:8–19.
9. Adebimpe VR. Race, racism, and epidemiological surveys. *Hosp Community Psychiatry* 1994;45: 27–31.
10. Strakowski SM, Hawkins JM, Keck PE Jr, et al. The effects of race and information variance on disagreement between psychiatric emergency service and research diagnoses in first-episode psychosis. *J Clin Psychiatry* 1997;58:457–463.
11. Arnold LM, Keck PE Jr, Collins J, et al. Ethnicity and first-rank symptoms in patients with psychosis. *Schizophr Res* 2004;67:207–212.

12. Sussman LK, Robins LN, Earls F. Treatment seeking for depression by black and white Americans. *Soc Sci Med* 1987;24:187–196.
13. Neighbors HW. The distribution of psychiatric morbidity in black Americans: a review and suggestion for research. *Community Ment Health J* 1984;20:169–181.
14. Manning JS, Haykal RF, Akiskal HS. The role of bipolarity in depression in the family practice setting. *Psychiatr Clin North Am* 1999;22:689–703.
15. Teplin LA. The prevalence of severe mental disorder among male urban jail detainees: comparison with the Epidemiologic Catchment Area Program. *Am J Public Health* 1990;80:663–669.
16. Teplin LA. Detecting disorder: the treatment of mental illness among jail detainees. *J Consult Clin Psychol* 1990; 58:233–236.
17. Regier DA, Farmer ME, Rae DS, et al. Comorbidity of mental disorders with alcohol and other drug abuse: results from the Epidemiological Catchment Area (ECA) Study. *JAMA* 1990;264:2511–2518.
18. Chung H, Mahler JC, Kakuna T. Racial differences in the treatment of psychiatric inpatients. *Psychiatr Serv* 1995;46:586–591.
19. Arnold LM, Strakowski SM, Schwiers ML, et al. Sex, ethnicity, and antipsychotic medication use in patients with psychosis. *Schizophr Res* 2004;66:169–175.
20. Bell CC, Mehta H. The misdiagnosis of black patients with manic-depressive illness. *J Natl Med Assoc* 1980;72:141–145.
21. Bell CC, Mehta H. Misdiagnosis of black patients with manic-depressive illness: Second in a series. *J Natl Med Assoc* 1981;73:101–107.
22. Sachs GS. Decision tree for the treatment of bipolar disorder. *J Clin Psychiatry* 2003;64(Suppl 8): 35–40.
23. Copeland LA, Zeber JE, Valenstein M, et al. Racial disparity in the use of atypical antipsychotic medications among veterans. *Am J Psychiatry* 2003;160:1817–1822.
24. Opolka JL, Rascati KL, Brown CM, et al. Ethnic differences in use of antipsychotic medication among Texas Medicaid clients with schizophrenia. *J Clin Psychiatry* 2003;64:635–639.
25. Morgenstern H, Glazer WM. Identifying risk factors for tardive dyskinesia among chronic outpatients maintained on neuroleptic medications: results of the Yale tardive dyskinesia study. *Arch Gen Psychiatry* 1993;50:723–733.
26. Glazer WM, Morgenstern H, Doucette J. Race and tardive dyskinesia among outpatients at a CMHC. *Hosp Community Psychiatry* 1994;45:38–42.
27. Lindamer L, Lacro JP, Jeste DV. Relationship of ethnicity to the effects of antipsychotic medication. I. In: Herrera JM, Lawson WB, Sramek, JJ, eds. *Cross cultural psychiatry*. Chichester: Wiley, 1999.
28. Price N, Glazer W, Morgenstern, H. Demographic predictors of the use of injectable versus oral antipsychotic medications in outpatients. *Am J Psychiatry* 1985;142:1491–1492.
29. Segal SP, Bola J, Watson M. Race, quality of care, and antipsychotic prescribing practices in psychiatric emergency services. *Psychiatr Serv* 1996;47:282–286.
30. Ghaemi SN, Hsu DJ, Soldani F, et al. Antidepressants in bipolar disorder: the case for caution. *Bipolar Disord* 2003;5:421–433.
31. Bottlender R, Rudolf D, Strauss A, et al. Mood-stabilisers reduce the risk of developing antidepressant-induced maniform states in acute treatment of bipolar I depressed patients. *J Affect Disord* 2001; 63:79–83.
32. Blazer DG, Hybels CF, Simonsick EM, et al. Marked differences in antidepressant use by race in an elderly community sample: 1986–1996. *Am J Psychiatry* 2000;157:1089–1094.
33. Melfi CA, Croghan TW, Hanna MP, et al. Racial variation in antidepressant treatment in a medicaid population. *J Clin Psychiatry* 2000;61:16–21.
34. Miranda J, Lawson W, Escobar J. NIMH Affective Disorders Workgroup. Ethnic minorities. *Ment Health Serv Res* 2002;4:231–237.
35. Okpaku S, Frazer A, Mendels J. A pilot study of racial differences in erythrocyte lithium transport. *Am J Psychiatry* 1980;137:120–121.
36. Strickland TL, Lin K-M, Fu P, et al. Comparison of lithium ratio between African-American and Caucasian bipolar patients. *Biol Psychiatry* 1995;37:325–330.
37. Goodwin FK, Fireman B, Simon GE, et al: Suicide risk in bipolar disorder during treatment with lithium and divalproex. *JAMA* 2003;290:1467–1473.

SECTION II

Psychotherapy in Cross-Cultural Context

8

Psychoanalytic Therapy with Asians and Asian Americans

Alan Roland

National Psychological Association for Psychoanalysis, New York, New York 10014

I. INTRODUCTION

Over 25 years ago, as a third-generation Jewish American psychoanalyst, I embarked on a clinical psychoanalytic journey to India and Japan to ascertain the psychological effects of modernization and Westernization, and the extent to which their psychology is significantly different from the ethnically diverse Euro-Americans I have worked with in New York City. Both India and Japan have longstanding psychoanalytic traditions, the former dating back to 1922 when India became a member of the International Psychoanalytic Association, the latter to the 1930s. Seeing patients there in short-term psychoanalytic therapy and supervising Indian and Japanese psychoanalytic therapists was necessary but not sufficient for understanding the subtleties of their psyche and ways of relating. I also needed the perceptive contributions of not only indigenous psychoanalysts and others in the mental health professions but also anthropologists, writers, historians, and philosophers. I came to understand that culture and social change are not simply "out there" but influence the deepest layers of our psyche. Upon returning home, I began to work psychoanalytically with a number of Asian Americans, the majority being Indian but also with Japanese, Chinese, and Koreans. I would like to share some of the insights and experiences of my therapeutic work with these Asian and Asian American patients.

II. THE NORMALITY/PSYCHOPATHOLOGY CONTINUUM

I shall start with the most difficult part of doing psychoanalytic therapy with someone from an Asian culture, especially if the therapist is from a Euro-American background. When we work with patients in psychoanalytic therapy, we are always making implicit judgments as to what is more or less normal in their relationships and work, including the relationship with the therapist, and what seems skewed or in some way psychopathological. When these patients are more or less from our own culture, we unreflectedly judge on implicit understandings of what goes or doesn't go in our culture, or what is generally considered normal or psychopathological. It is not that psychoanalytic therapy is a well-laid-out roadmap. Far from it. It is full of ambiguities and a great deal of uncertainty, often for extended periods. However, in working with someone from a radically different culture, such as those from an Asian background, a Euro-American therapist can feel not only uncertain but at sea. This is because there is a different normality/psychopathology continuum from the one we are used to, influenced by radically different cultural patterns than our own; indeed, the norms of development, structuralization, and functioning can differ from what we have been taught in our training. Plainly put, psychoanalytic norms are often more Western-centric and less universal than most therapists realize.

A simple example of this is different forms of child rearing. Asian children often sleep next to their parents for several years, or with each other, or an aunt or uncle, but rarely alone. To have your own bed and bedroom, as is the ideal for middle class America, is often considered dire punishment. The emphasis is far more on symbiotic modes of dependency and interdependence, with considerable nonverbal communication, than the Euro-American stress on developing autonomy, independence, and verbal communication. Asian child-rearing results in quite different ego boundaries where outer boundaries are more permeable with semimerger relationships but there is a formation of a highly private self, much more private and secretive than is usually the case for Westerners. A great deal of individuality is maintained in this private self. Thus, typical Indian or Japanese mother–toddler relationships can easily be misinterpreted as psychopathological if viewed from the norms of separation-individuation in American psychoanalysis.

As difficult as this other continuum may sometimes be to learn, even more difficult is to locate a patient's psychopathology on this different continuum. And then to ascertain the idiosyncratic, disturbed family relationships that have given rise to the patient's emotional problems. Understanding the unconscious factors is always a challenge in psychoanalytic therapy, but this is doubly difficult when working with someone from a radically different culture than oneself. I still struggle with this.

Thus, cultural patterns deeply embedded in the psyche interact with internalized idiosyncratic, problematic familial relationships from childhood, as well as with the unique temperament and proclivities of the patient. Moreover, these cultural patterns vary from one Asian culture to another, and to some extent within each society. By taking into account the deeply embedded cultural patterns, a psychoanalytic therapist can be more effective, while paradoxically, psychoanalytic therapy can help elucidate the inner world of Asians and Asian Americans. It is in effect a depth ethnography. Although psychoanalysis developed within the modern Western culture of individualism, it has, as mentioned earlier, been in India and Japan for many decades, and is now being taught in China and Korea as a result of certain modernizing, individualizing social changes. Emotional problems and stress do tend to be universal, although the content may vary from one culture to another.

To illustrate the difficulties a psychoanalytic therapist can have in sorting out embedded cultural patterns from internalized, problematic familial relationships, I shall give a couple of case examples. Some years ago, I saw a Japanese man in psychoanalysis because of problems he was having in a doctoral counseling psychology program in New York City. His well-off family was subsidizing him in his graduate work, living expenses, and psychoanalysis. We agreed on a fee, my minimum fee at the time. Over a year later, he was granted an assistantship by the university, from which he earned a significant amount of money. As is customary after a year or two, especially when a patient's income increases, I asked for a small fee increase. He became indignant, telling me that he thought I knew about Japanese culture and the *amae* (dependency) relationship, that because he was dependent on me, I shouldn't raise the fee. This was even more important because his mother was not a nurturing person. Further, that once a fee is set in Japan, it lasts a lifetime. However, should I insist on raising the fee, he would have to go along with it, as one must always obey what a superior wants. As he expressed it, "it can't be helped."

Thus, he unreflectedly structured the therapy relationship as both a dependency relationship in which the therapist is nurturing, and a hierarchical relationship in which he as the subordinate has to obey the superior. This is totally consonant with Japanese relationships. I found myself in the position of being highly uncertain whether the resistance to the fee raise was due to normal Japanese cultural expectations or to unconscious factors of which we were both unaware, or even to a combination of the two. Further, if I decided to raise the fee, he would have paid it, but would then have kept all feelings to himself in a very private self, also characteristic of Japanese.

I therefore decided not to raise the fee at the time, but instead to keep a very close watch as to what money meant to him. It was only after well more than a year later that it became apparent that money was a central dynamic in his family, especially with his mother, who bought off people right and left, including him. Instead of being emotionally nurturing, she would give him money to buy things. With this in mind, I told him that I thought it was very important that there be a fee raise, even if it was just 25 cents, for its symbolic meaning. It was a turning point in the therapy because the rage he had toward his mother began to be directed toward me in the transference. We could further analyze all kinds of defenses he had to contain his rage, including being very obsessive-compulsive. This resulted in significant change.

Another example is that of a highly cultured Indian woman in her 40s, who had had a disturbed relationship with her mother, who had been living in New Delhi after a great deal of closeness throughout their lives. At varied points in the therapy, Mrs. K would come late to sessions or pay her monthly fee late, or sometimes she would miss a session, expecting not to be held responsible for it. She would graciously excuse herself, citing one reason or another, from work at her publishing firm to her daughter's illness. I sensed that I couldn't easily investigate what was becoming an ongoing pattern because she would experience it as an affront, and might even discontinue therapy. She would on occasion come into my consulting room if I were in the restroom or if she had arrived earlier. I would ordinarily investigate the meanings of this with a Euro-American patient, but it was not so unusual with other Indian patients. It was part of the intimacy dimension of the hierarchical relationship. Again, I couldn't easily delve into it.

Nevertheless, I began to feel intruded upon, that my boundaries were being subtly breached. Although I am very much attuned to unconsciously induced countertransference reactions, I reflected that I have often felt swallowed up in India, as people will ask a great deal of you, much more than in America or Japan. By asking, they try to convert an outsider relationship (insider and outsider relationships are extremely important in all of the Asian cultures) into a more intimate one of the extended family where asking and giving is commonplace. Asking is a subtle form of giving: it establishes the other as the superior and enhances the esteem of the superior whose ego-ideal is to be nurturing. It is a psychology foreign to Euro-Americans and is also present in Japan but only in their insider relationships. Thus, I asked myself whether my feelings of being intruded upon, of not having my usual boundaries, was a basic experience for an American working with an Indian. Or was there something else operating? I waited and listened to see if any light could be thrown on my reactions while attending to a few important issues that she was struggling with.

After close to 2 years, she mentioned for the first time that as a child she had had her own bedroom (something on the unusual side in India), and that her mother would periodically come into her bedroom after a fight with her father, spend the night, and confide in my patient what their problems were. By then I knew enough about Indian child-rearing and relationships to realize that this was out of the realm of the normal. To be raised in the parental bedroom was one thing, but to have her mother come to her bedroom to complain about her father was another. I then understood that my feelings of being intruded upon were related to this childhood experience with her mother, and that she had unconsciously induced in me her feelings as a child. As we worked on this, it became apparent that she had a great deal of difficulty dealing with anyone who would intrude on her, including her daughter. Thus, my experience in the therapy relationship was subtly related to this idiosyncratic, disturbed mother–daughter relationship rather than to more general boundary differences characteristic of Indians and Euro-Americans.

III. THE THERAPY RELATIONSHIP

In psychoanalytic therapy, we assume a Western contractual relationship in which the patient pays a fee for our time, during which we are expected to be of help in their resolving their emotional conflicts, relationships, and self feelings. Asian Americans structure the therapy relationship in significantly different ways. To understand how they do this, one must be aware of the three psychosocial dimensions of Asian hierarchical relationships, ones that vary from one Asian culture to another, as well as a dual self-structure that differs from the typical European American one. (See Roland 1988 [1] for a much fuller description of Asian hierarchical relationships.)

The first psychosocial dimension is that of the formal hierarchy based on age and gender, in which there are deeply internalized reciprocal expectations of both the superior and the subordinate. The subordinate is supposed to show deference, respect, and obedience to the superior, mainly keeping disagreements to oneself; whereas the superior is to be responsible and nurturing toward the subordinate, each maintaining and enhancing the esteem of the other. There is a dual self-structure in the subordinate who in social presentation will observe the social etiquette of these expectations, while keeping all kinds of feelings and fantasies in a private self (1,2). Thus, in the therapy relationship, Asian American patients will usually try to sense what the therapist expects of them while being polite and obedient. Indian immigrants, for instance, will often ask for a great deal of advice and guidance in handling their problems because they are used to this from family elders. I usually handle this by telling them that I am sure that they have already gotten a great deal of advice from family elders and others, but the problems still remain. They generally nod agreement to this. I then say that obviously there are deeper roots to their problems than they, others, or I am aware of, and that by working together and telling me whatever is on their mind, we can gradually learn what is causing their emotional problems.

The second psychosocial dimension is that of hierarchical intimacy relationships. In this dimension, there is an expectation for caring, empathy, and closeness in insider relationships and much less in outsider relationships. In the therapy relationship, the timing of this varies considerably from South Asian to East Asian. With Indians, Pakistanis, and Bangladeshis, if the patient senses that you are concerned and empathic, and that you will keep their communications confidential, they may open up very quickly as they immediately establish a familial insider relationship. With Japanese, however, it may take some time for the therapist to progress from an outsider relationship to an insider one. There is then an expectation for a close "we" relationship. For a Japanese man with a male therapist, once it becomes an insider relationship, the therapist is expected to become a mentor for life.

The third psychosocial dimension is that of hierarchy by personal qualities. I have found that persons from all different Asian backgrounds make quiet evaluations of the personal qualities of their superiors and others, reserving deeper respect and veneration for those with personal qualities they truly respect than simply for all superiors. Of course, the superior in the hierarchical relationship may indeed be a superior person, but by no means always. Younger brothers, sisters, wives, and servants may all have superior qualities. Thus, the therapist will always be deferred to but only some will be really respected.

Anger is another important element in psychoanalytic therapy with Asian Americans. All of them are usually easily able to express anger and sometimes rage in sessions about someone who has mistreated them or not fulfilled responsibilities toward them. However, it is extremely difficult for someone from any of the Asian countries to express any ambivalence, criticism, or anger directly to a superior, including the therapist. In my experience with both an Indian and a Japanese man in New York City, it took approximately 2 years of intensive analytic work on a three- to four-times-a-week basis for them to express even indirect criticism of me. This was followed by their coming in to the following session in an anxiety state. I had to interpret to them that their anxiety is related to their criticism of me. This enabled them to be even more directly critical of me after a few more sessions, followed by another anxiety state, and then by interpretations connecting the two. Eventually, they became involved in an ongoing negative transference and transference neurosis (3). This progression was confirmed by a noted Chinese American social scientist who had exactly the same experience in his analysis.

Another important issue in the therapy relationship with Asian Americans is communication. In psychoanalytic therapy with Euro-Americans, we expect the main communication to be verbal, with nonverbal communication often being dissociated. Asian communication, however, is often consciously nonverbal, where each is attuned to the other's moods, gestures, behavior, and such, and where the verbal communication can be indirect and ambiguous. In South Asians, the communication is often multileveled, with considerable verbal communication, evident facial and body gestures, moods and feelings, and behavior, all of which may or may not be congruent with each other. One has to be cognizant of all of these levels. Japanese, however, rely a great deal on empathic sensing of what the other is feeling, needing, or thinking with a relative minimum of verbal communication from a Western standpoint. There is a saying in Japanese that nothing important is ever to be communicated verbally. Here, it calls upon the therapist to use a great deal of intuition and empathy.

IV. THE BICULTURAL SELF

When we talk about psychoanalytic therapy with Asian Americans, we not only have to distinguish between persons coming from different Asian cultures but also between the immigrant generation, "1.5s" (those who were born and spent the first several years in their indigenous culture before coming to the United States and going through American schools), and the second generation who are born here. All of them have a bicultural self, often with considerable turmoil, as the value systems and makeup of the self are significantly different from that of Euro-Americans. In the immigrant generation, there is a need to combine a more individualized American self with their Asian familial self. In 1.5s and the second generation, although it can vary between them, they both have a strong internalized individualized self from American schooling and peer social life but also strong aspects of a familial self from their parents, which can also make for conflict and confusion. Thus, the Indian second generation often refers to itself as ABCD, American born, confused *desei* (Indian).

What are the major dimensions of the bicultural self, and what differences do they make in psychoanalytic therapy? The Asian self is much more of a "we-self" tied in to the family, community, or group in contrast to the North American self-motivating, self-assertive, and relatively self-contained "I-self." In the intimacy dimension of Asian hierarchical relationships, the we-self is deeply embedded in the dependencies and interdependencies, and reputation, of the family, with self experience fluctuating from one relationship to another in a highly contextual way. There is much more prolonged mothering, with the child often sleeping next to the mother or to other siblings or family members for years. In the Indian and Chinese extended family, there may be a great deal of multiple mothering. This contrasts with the emphasis on autonomy and independence in American individualism. Thus, the therapy relationship has a feel of greater closeness and empathic concern than is characteristic with most Euro-American patients.

Another major value clash and structuring of the self takes place in the formal dimension of Asian hierarchical relationships versus egalitarianism in American individualism. Asians have a dual self-structure where there is a presentation of self in the well spelled-out social etiquette of formal hierarchical relationships on one hand, and a highly private self that can keep all kinds of thoughts, feelings, and fantasies secret to oneself on the other hand. These may be revealed to certain persons but not to others, again depending on context. Secrets can be kept in psychoanalytic therapy for prolonged periods. One Indian woman saw her Indian therapist for a year and a half in twice-a-week psychoanalytic therapy, never revealing to him her two most salient inner struggles. The strictness of the social etiquette can vary according to the Asian culture, it being much more rigorous in Japan and Korea than, say, in India and Pakistan. Indians, for instance, may nod agreement with the wishes of the superior but then not carry them out. Japanese, however, would tend to carry out these wishes even if in disagreement. This dual self-structure contrasts sharply with the American ideal of authenticity, and being oneself as much as possible in different social relationships.

There is another important psychological dimension to Asian hierarchical relationships that varies considerably from Western ones. In the formal hierarchy, there are deeply internalized reciprocal attitudes in superior and subordinate, as mentioned earlier. The latter is to be loyal, respectful, and obedient to the former, whereas the superior is to be nurturant and responsible to the subordinate, each maintaining or enhancing the other's esteem. This contrasts considerably with American hierarchical relationships based on rights and obligations, where American superiors can often be directly critical and confrontive. Asians can often feel intensely slighted in American hierarchical relationships when the expected kind of caring and concern for self-esteem is not present in the superior. A simple example is a Pakistani professional who worked hard and competently in an American corporate firm and didn't get a raise after a year. He felt deeply slighted by his superior. He then learned he had to ask for the raise, which he did and then got, but was still disappointed that the superior had not given it without his asking.

There are other important dimensions to the Asian familial self that contrasts with the American individualized self, and which also enter into a bicultural self. One is self-esteem, or we-self esteem, often strongly tied in to family reputation, which is far more central to Asian psychology than American. There is an emphasis on enhancing or at minimum not undermining each other's self-esteem, where preserving the esteem of the other is usually more important than the truth of any given matter. (See Chapter 7, "The Influence of Culture on the Self and Self-object Relationships: An Asian-North American Comparison," in Roland 1996 [3].) Asians can experience direct criticism, the hallmark of American hierarchical relationships, as quite hurtful.

In one interesting case, an Indian patient who had a medical fellowship was being exploited by the head of her program. She was supposedly in the program two-thirds time because she had a young child. The director not only pushed her to work almost full-time, but also wanted her to repeat rotations she had already completed because he was short-handed. As an American, I felt anger at him for his exploitation and abrogation of the contractual agreement. She also was angry, but kept saying over and over again, "he doesn't respect me." The issue of esteem was much more central to her than the unfairness involved in the breaking of their contractual relationship.

In another relevant example, Yoshiko came to psychoanalytic therapy because of being extremely emotionally upset in her job. She had come from Japan to do graduate work in the United States and married an American. She then decided to work in an American corporation rather than a Japanese trading company here because she felt she had become too individualized to work as a woman in a Japanese company. However, working in an American company often left her feeling upset for days. The major problem was her relationship with her supervisor. The supervisor would confront her on the very occasional mistakes she would make, by report far fewer than those of the other American workers there. Yoshiko felt extremely disturbed by these direct criticisms, feeling the supervisor should have tactfully and indirectly called her attention to any mistakes she made, which she would then have striven to rectify. For the Americans at work, such critiques seemed to roll off of them like water off a duck's back. But for Yoshiko, it was a tremendous blow to her sense of esteem. I had first to call her attention to the very different hierarchical styles in the United States as contrasted to Japan, where direct criticism here is usually characteristic. It was only after we had sorted out the problematic cultural/psychological interface between Japanese and American work relationships that she was able to associate to a grandmother who was very strict with her. This internalized problematic past relationship greatly intensified her emotionally upset reaction to her supervisor. In general, I have found it is important to attend first to the value clash between cultures, which then enables the therapist to delve into contributing factors from idiosyncratic disturbed family relationships.

Conscience also varies greatly between Asian and Western cultures. Proper behavior is far more contextual in Asian societies than the tendency toward universal principles in the West. Both Indian and East Asian Confucian cultures emphasize a contextual or situational ethic. Indian *dharma* calls for moral behavior in which the time, the place, the nature of the relationship, and the natures of the persons involved are all taken into account. Thus, what is said to one person about a given matter might be quite different from what is said to another. Moreover, the ego ideal of doing everything as well as possible, or even perfectly, is typically much stronger in Japanese and Koreans than in South Asians.

Communication is another central dimension that differs tremendously between the Asian familial self and a Euro-American individualized self. As stated earlier, in all of the Asian cultures, there is far more emphasis on conscious nonverbal communication in contrast to North American culture, where verbal communication is central, and if nonverbal communication is present, it is usually dissociated. There is a great deal of sensing of nonverbal communication in all Asian cultures, but it seems particularly strong in Japanese and Korean cultures. Indian communication seems more multilayered with a great deal of verbal communication, which may be ambiguous, and then with gestures, behavior, and moods, all of which may or may not be congruous with each other. Ascertaining another's motives may be difficult even for Asians, and is particularly so for European Americans interacting with someone from an Asian culture. Asians on the whole tend to be more receptive than assertive in their communication, sensing the other while fully expecting the other to sense one's own needs and feelings without having to verbalize them.

This can make for significant conflict in intercultural marriages. I have found in working with Japanese women that they generally expect their American husbands to sense their needs and wishes without having to express them verbally, something the husbands are unable to do. As one Japanese American put it, "In American couples, if there is a complaint that one doesn't express feelings, it is inevitably the man. But in a couple with a Japanese woman and an American man, it is inevitably the woman who doesn't express her feelings and wishes. She expects her husband to sense them." I tend to tell my married Japanese women patients that the kind of sensing they expect from a husband is something that most American men are unable to do, and that they may have to think about expressing their wishes and needs more verbally for their husbands to understand what they are. Americans, however, tend to be far more verbally assertive, which Asian Americans gradually learn to do.

The Asian self is thus both more horizontal and vertical than the typical Euro-American self. It is horizontal in terms of the self's embeddedness in the extended family, community, and group. It is vertical, especially in Indians, where there is an assumption of past and future lives, and a sense of personal destiny tied in to past lives and the effects of the planets, with the use of astrology, palmistry, psychics, and such to fathom one's destiny. I have found with all of the Hindu patients I have worked with, most with advanced degrees, that the assumption of personal destiny is very strong, and that astrology, psychics, palmistry, and such have played a major influence in their life.

A simple example will suffice. A woman who was involved in a highly verbally abusive marriage over many years came for psychoanalytic therapy to see if she could get out of the marriage. At one point, she sent the exact time of birth of her husband and herself to a cousin in India to see what an astrologer would say. The astrologer knew nothing of what was going on. When he put together their horoscopes, he angrily asked who was responsible for arranging this marriage, stating that the two were totally unsuitable for each other, and her husband was a disturbed man. Further, she should leave her husband immediately because he had something growing behind his right eye, and that as he became increasingly disabled, it would be harder for her to leave. (They actually already knew he had a brain tumor behind the right eye.) This analysis of the astrologer in conjunction with the therapy gave her more conviction in leaving.

Then, there is a sense of a long spiritual evolution. Indians I have worked with all assume there is an inner spiritual reality, but that it takes effort to realize it, something that will take more than one life. Only a small number of the approximately 30 patients I have seen have been actively involved in one spiritual discipline or another, some through their art and others through meditation or prayer, to realize this inner spiritual self. Not to recognize this other inner level of reality in therapy can be alienating to many Indian patients.

An example is Shakuntala (I discuss this case at length in Chapter 5, "Urban Indian Women," in Roland 1988 [1]), who was a seriously practicing mystic with many spiritual experiences, perhaps the first case reported in the psychoanalytic literature. She never revealed to her psychoanalytic therapist in Bombay in 1.5 years of two-times-a-week therapy that one of her most intense inner struggles was whether she should give up the idea of an arranged marriage, or even her involvement with a married man at the time, to move to her aunt's *ashram* and eventually become a guru. Her aunt, a well-respected guru herself, had told Shakuntala that she was one of the very few who was capable of becoming a spiritual teacher and guide. Shakuntala had accurately sensed her therapist was not oriented in this direction, in keeping with the traditional Freudian viewpoint that spiritual experiences are either regressive or psychopathological, and so kept this inner struggle completely to herself.

Another factor in working with Asian Americans that is sometimes overlooked is that of past trauma from their country of origin. A Chinese American woman, originally from mainland China, whom I saw in couple's therapy with her Jewish American husband, was diagnosed by a few other psychoanalysts and psychiatrists as having severe borderline psychopathology because of her highly irrational rage and anxiety reactions to seemingly minor incidents. On more careful inquiry, it turned out that from age 7 to 17 she had lived in the middle of the Cultural Revolution. Across the street from her apartment building was a wealthy merchant's mansion. The Red Guards had killed him and taken over the mansion as a place for torturing people. She would hear screams of people being tortured day and night coming from the mansion. To a great extent, it was this early trauma that underlay many of her irrational reactions in the present, rather similar to those of Holocaust survivors. Without taking this trauma into account, it was impossible to appreciate her psychopathology.

V. CONCLUSION

This chapter is a result of psychoanalytic clinical work in India and Japan, and with Indians, Japanese, Chinese, and Koreans in New York City, as well as collaborations with indigenous analysts, mental health professionals, and others from a variety of disciplines. Without such collaboration, it would be extremely difficult for a Euro-American to understand the Asian psyche. It became evident that culture and social change influence the psyche on the deepest levels. The most difficult therapeutic issue for a Euro-American psychoanalytic therapist working with Asians and Asian Americans is first recognizing and learning a different normality/psychopathology continuum from what one is used to, and then to ascertaining where the psychopathology lies along this other continuum.

As we have seen, the therapeutic relationship itself is structured differently according to the three psychosocial dimensions of Asian hierarchical relationships: the formal hierarchy, hierarchical intimacy relationships, and hierarchy by personal qualities. Also important to the therapeutic relationship are a dual self-structure, modes of communication that emphasize the nonverbal, and the issue of anger and ambivalence. It is also important to understand the bicultural self of Asian Americans. Considerable conflict and anguish can be generated in the immigrant generation. In the second generation, confusion is common regarding substantial differences between Asian Americans and Euro-Americans in the self, hierarchical relationships, modes of communication, conscience, and the salience of self-esteem. Psychoanalytic therapy is certainly very possible and helpful with Asians and Asian Americans once the various enumerated factors are taken into account; and in fact, it can be an excellent mode of exploring their inner world in psychological depth.

REFERENCES

1. Roland A. *In search of self in India and Japan: toward a cross-cultural psychology.* Princeton: Princeton University Press, 1988.
2. Doi T. *The anatomy of self: the individual versus the society.* Tokyo: Kodansha International, 1986.
3. Roland A. *Cultural pluralism and psychoanalysis: the Asian and North American experience.* New York: Routledge, 1996.

9

Telling "Ten Percent of the Story"

Narrative and the Intergenerational Transmission of Trauma among Cambodian Refugees

*Audrey Rubin and †Lorna Rhodes

**Department of Child and Adolescent Psychiatry, Boston University School of Medicine, Boston, Massachusetts 02118; and †Department of Anthropology, University of Washington, Seattle, Washington 98195*

I. INTRODUCTION

Studies of traumatized populations from a variety of eras and world regions indicate that when survivors become parents, their past experiences can have a profound effect on their children. Reverberations have been described in family dynamics (1–6) and atmosphere (7), and in children's personality traits (4,6,8), self-image (2,3), world view (6,9,10), and rates of psychiatric symptoms and disorders (4–7). The earliest investigations, dating from the 1960s, involved offspring of survivors of the Holocaust, and were subject to a great deal of criticism because of numerous methodological weaknesses including lack of controls, blending of clinical and non-clinical subjects, and lack of appreciation for cultural context and meanings (11,12). Studies conducted during the past 20 years have examined the consequences of a broad range of societal and personal traumatic exposures, recognized more subtle outcomes, and better appreciated the great individual variability within each generation. The mechanisms by which parents' trauma is "transmitted" to their offspring

---

While conducting this study, Dr. Rubin was a fellow in the Robert Wood Johnson Clinical Scholars Program at the University of Washington, Seattle. The views expressed in this chapter do not necessarily reflect the views of the Robert Wood Johnson Foundation.

The authors would like to offer their thanks to Jeniffer Huong who provided expert interpretation as well as cultural consultation during many aspects of this project.

remains a matter of conjecture, and it is likely that multiple pathways overlap and operate simultaneously. A variety of models have been proposed, ranging from parental modeling of posttraumatic symptoms (9,13); to impaired parenting abilities consequent to trauma, manifested, for example, through insecure attachments (14,15); to psychodynamic views focusing on parents' tendency to project onto the children parts of themselves split off by trauma (1,5,15); to genetic/biological vulnerability to posttraumatic stress disorder (PTSD) (16,17). Another mechanism appears to be narrative, through the way in which parents share or withhold the stories of their experience.

Children of Japanese Americans interned during World War II have reported that their parents communicated so little about their earlier lives that they felt lonely, confused and burdened by the sense of a shameful secret, a "skeleton in the closet" (18). Some Holocaust survivor parents, in order to avoid having to discuss the horrific events they had lived through, would tell their young children that the tattoos on their arms were their telephone numbers. Now mature adults, children from such families recall having heard only "bits and pieces" of their parents' story, yet assert that they experienced the psychological presence of the Holocaust constantly, often in nonverbal ways (19). Studies indicate that in survivor families in which communication was indirect or "guilt inducing," adult offspring developed high rates of depression, anxiety, hypochondriasis, and impaired self-esteem (8). In other Holocaust survivor families, children found themselves a "captive audience" to unremitting recitations (19). Extremely detailed, uncontrolled communication has also been described in families of Vietnam veterans with PTSD, whose accounts of their experiences have produced symptoms of so-called secondary PTSD in their children (20). Thus, the literature suggests that trauma can lead to atypical modes of communication in families that may be directly painful and damaging and that may contribute indirectly to a range of adverse mental health outcomes.

II. BACKGROUND

In the 1980s, approximately 150,000 Cambodians came to the United States as refugees. They were the survivors of a series of highly traumatic experiences that have now been extensively documented (21,22). From 1969–1973, a Cambodian civil war between communist and noncommunist forces (secretly assisted by US bombing under then-President Richard Nixon) led to the deaths of 60,000 Cambodians and internal displacement of hundreds of thousands more (23). In 1975, the victorious Khmer Rouge faction, under the leadership of Pol Pot, imposed a program of radical agrarian collectivism aimed at purging Cambodia of all Western influence as well as all traditional sources of authority. Anyone with a history of power, education, or privilege of any kind (military leaders, government workers, police, Buddhist monks, doctors, teachers, shop owners) was targeted for torture and execution, often while family members were made to watch helplessly. All the society's institutions were shut down. People were herded out of cities en masse and sent to remote labor camps to perform long hours of backbreaking work. Children older than 6 years of age were separated from their parents and assigned to children's crews. The Khmer Rouge introduced their own calendar and designated the year of their ascendancy Year Zero. *Angka*, the term for their governmental organization, became the primary focus of loyalty and duty ("your mother, your father, your God") and demanded absolute obedience (24). Rules were enforced by teenage brigade leaders; children were recruited to spy on their own parents. Resistance was met with public torture.

The trauma enacted by the Khmer Rouge was as much symbolic and psychological as it was material and physical. It involved assaults on the integrity of the most sacred foundations of Cambodian culture: the family, Buddhism, the customs of courtesy towards neighbors and respect towards elders, and the notion of hierarchy that was traditionally understood as the basis of order (25). A small number of survivors of this period have published English-language first-person accounts of their experiences. The authors describe and name feelings of disorientation, pervasive fear, shame, humiliation, and degradation that marked their existence, and which they recognize the Khmer Rouge deliberately sought to engender (24,26–28).

The Khmer Rouge's agricultural plan was a failure and the harvests were inadequate to feed the population. In less than 4 years, 1 to 2 million people or nearly one quarter of the Cambodian population perished from starvation, disease, or murder. In 1979, in response to repeated border incursions, Vietnam invaded Cambodia and overthrew the Khmer Rouge. Tens of thousands of Cambodians saw an opportunity to escape what they feared would be another brutal regime and fled on foot to the Thai border. These escapes were harrowing, occurring at night, through mountainous jungle, in earshot of gunfire. Some families were resettled in western countries within a few months, while others waited for up to 10 years in refugee camps marked by higher and higher levels of crowding, banditry, domestic violence and demoralization. Mollica et al. (29) found that Cambodians experienced an average of sixteen traumatic events, including three episodes of torture, before arrival in the United States. In the inner-city neighborhoods in which most Cambodians have found housing in this country, many have experienced additional trauma as a result of crime, poverty, crowded housing conditions, and discrimination in their new minority status. Because most had been small farmers or unskilled laborers with little or no education, they have had difficulty finding work and learning English. The challenges of learning how to negotiate unfamiliar institutions, values, and behaviors are complicated by persistent physical and psychological symptoms.

Writers from various disciplines—anthropology, sociology, history—use various lenses and outcome measures to attempt to describe the enduring impact of such experiences on individuals and on the Cambodian community. For the most part, psychiatry has focused its approach on diagnosis and on demonstrating that the prevalence of *Diagnostic and Statistical Manual* (DSM)-defined PTSD in this population is extremely high, even many years after the original events—up to 90% in community samples from US cities (30); however, whether the diagnosis is meaningful in a setting of such widespread trauma, even when "culturally sensitive" assessment instruments are used, or whether it captures what is most important about posttraumatic experience for Cambodian patients is a matter of ongoing debate. The one study (31) that looked specifically at Cambodian parents found that 55%

of mothers and 30% of fathers met PTSD criteria. What is it like for children to be growing up with such symptomatic parents? Studies of functioning among Cambodian survivors are very limited and offer inconsistent findings, possibly because they have relied on "coarse-grained instruments" to look only at variables such as English-language ability, income, and welfare status (32). None has looked at how Cambodian adults function as parents, or how their role as parents intersects with their efforts to manage their distress and suffering and to overcome the discontinuities in their lives.

III. THE FUNCTIONS AND LIMITS OF NARRATIVE

One of the most universal ways people attempt to heal life disruptions and create a sense of order in their worlds is through the telling of stories or narratives (33). Chandler, a senior historian of Cambodia, notes that in pre–Khmer Rouge times, public recitation of well-known stories was used to symbolize the restoration of order in society after periods of hardship and destruction (34). Story-telling appears to be an innate human process that people in almost all cultures begin to learn about from early childhood (35). People naturally think of their lives as narratives, too, and in recent years, anthropologists, psychologists, and literary theorists have explored the important functions served by the stories people tell about themselves. Self-narratives help with the formation of identity; narrative transforms the "mere passing away of time" into a meaningful unity, the self (35). Because experience is reshaped in the process of forming a narrative, narratives represent agency; they are empowering (36). Pennebaker and a variety of colleagues (37), in a 20-year series of experiments involving a wide range of nonclinical subjects, have found that individuals who speak (or write) in a nondirected way about "the one or two most traumatic events" in their lives experience measurable improvements in mental and physical health. Participants have come from all socioeconomic levels and represented "all the major ethnic and racial groups" in the United States. Putting a complex life event into a narrative format, Pennebaker observes, allows one to integrate thoughts and feelings while organizing them in a coherent fashion. The mind doesn't have to work so hard to bring structure and meaning to the experience.

But what is the impact of extreme trauma on the impulse and capacity to make narratives? One of the few groups for whom Pennebaker's protocol has not proven beneficial was a small clinical sample of Israeli patients with PTSD. After talking about their experiences, these subjects reported increased physician visits and worsened avoidance symptoms (38). Herman (39) begins her now-classic *Trauma and Recovery* by noting the "twin imperatives" trauma survivors struggle between: the wish to tell the world about the horrific events they have experienced and the wish not only to conceal them, but also to banish them from consciousness. She notes, too, that the violation of human relatedness that trauma involves leads to loss of trust in the value of connection and communication with others. More recently, experimental and theoretical investigations into the neurobiology of PTSD have suggested an alternative way of understanding survivors' difficulties in telling their stories. One of the hallmarks of PTSD appears to be the inability to cognitively organize traumatic experiences despite continuous rumination and emotional responses to internal and external reminders. Probably as a consequence of dysfunction in multiple brain structures, the brain's natural ability to integrate experience breaks down. In a series of studies, van der Kolk (40) has shown that traumatic memory initially consists primarily of isolated sensory, emotional, and motoric imprints, with few autobiographical elements and a minimal storyline; the central nervous system appears to be unable to integrate the sensations related to the event into a whole semantic memory.

Auerhahn and Laub (14), who have worked for many years collecting oral histories from Holocaust survivors for the Fortunoff Video Archive at Yale University, draw on multiple paradigms (psychodynamic, social, neurobiological) in attempting to explain the complexities of what survivors can and can't communicate. They argue that along with survivors' unconscious defenses against knowledge and memory, survivors cannot fully "grasp trauma, name it, recall it, and, paradoxically, forget it" because severe trauma "creates a fragmentation of the self. . . . Trauma happens, often with no experiencing 'I'. . .its historical truth may never have been fully grasped by the victim or attained the status of a psychic representation."

Auerhahn and Laub feel that not only survivors and their children, but also all who hear about extreme trauma struggle with the attempt to "formulate" and hold such knowledge in mind, hence, for example, the disappearances and reappearances of the concept of trauma-related illness from psychiatric nosologies. They have described ten "forms of knowledge" of massive psychic trauma that fall along a continuum according to an individual's psychological distance from the trauma. These forms range from, for example, "Not Knowing" to "Fragments" to "Overpowering Narratives" to "Witnessed Narratives" to "Action Knowledge," and thus these forms of knowledge are also forms of communication. They have found that survivors tend to know/communicate mostly through two of the forms: retention of fragments of unintegrated memories and reliving such memories in what they call "transference phenomena," the grafting of isolated fragments of the past onto current relationships and life situations. Published first-person memoirs of survivors, such as those from the Khmer Rouge era referred to earlier, generally represent "witnessed narratives" in which the author's observing ego remains present, understanding itself to be "continuous with the remembered subject but currently at a different stage . . . a person who remembers and relates not only to the experiences that are recalled but to the experience of remembering as well." Children of survivors tend to know through the form of particular life themes that prove central to their identities or personalities. Auerhahn and Laub (14) note, however, that there is much individual variability; forms may coexist within an individual, and the process of healing can "open up the walls between the forms." Nevertheless they feel that because of the limits of knowledge and healing available to many of those who experience trauma, it often takes several generations for the story to be told fully.

Mollica (41,42), who co-founded one of the first culturally competent treatment programs for Southeast Asian refugees, notes that Cambodian patients presenting for care initially describe their traumatic experiences in ways which are reminiscent of several of the forms described by Auerhahn and Laub (14), and consistent with van der Kolk's findings (40). Their accounts are stereotyped, do not develop, progress in time, or reveal the storyteller's feelings or interpretation of events; they are "prenarratives." Many patients are so inwardly consumed by these stories that they are extremely isolated, even from their own families. In Mollica's view, mental health treatment can assist the patient to talk about the past in a different way, and this process of transforming the trauma story is central not only to integrating the trauma, but also to healing social disconnections. As the patient develops trust in the therapeutic setting and some comfort with the process of disclosing feelings (a significant challenge for an individual from a culture with no history of mental health treatment and a tendency towards interpersonal reserve), the storytelling forms a bridge between the patient and the therapist. As the patient develops more control over his or her narrative, feelings of shame and powerlessness decrease and the story comes to symbolize parts of the self that can be shared with those one is close to.

There appear to be two published studies that have peripherally explored the issue of communication about traumatic experiences in nonclinical samples of Cambodian families. One is the second report in Sack and colleagues' (43) series on the psychiatric status of a group of Cambodian adolescents who were resettled in Oregon in the early 1980s. These youth spent part of their latency years under the Khmer Rouge. The older ones had been in work camps and the younger with their parents; all had memories of the era. In separate interviews, the adolescents and their parents were asked to indicate with a yes or no whether they ever discussed the Khmer Rouge period together. A full 90% of the parents said yes, a somewhat surprising result, both because of the challenges of relating traumatic information discussed earlier, and because of the common characterization of Cambodians—and Asians generally—as highly reluctant to express negative information or affect, so as to avoid causing feelings of discomfort in a listener (44). However, only half the teens in Sack et al.'s study acknowledged such conversations. There are several possible explanations for this discrepancy: parents or teens may have been supplying what they thought was an expected answer, teens might have been involved in a discussion that had little impact and was forgotten, or they might have pushed an intense conversation from consciousness. More recently, Rousseau and Drapeau (45), as part of a larger study comparing adjustment in children of refugees from Central America and Southeast Asia, used a semistructured interview format to ask Cambodian children, adolescents, and their parents (N = 143) about the extent of communication about prior parental trauma. They found that, on the whole, parents rarely spoke to children of any age about their experiences, explaining that there was no point or that the children were not interested, as compared with Central American families, who communicated more openly. Many of the Cambodian adolescents expressed a wish to know more about their family's past, and struggled with a feeling of unreality about the snatches of stories they had heard.

This chapter will report on an ethnographic study undertaken in order to investigate in depth the following question: To what extent and in what ways do Cambodian parents communicate their traumatic histories to their adolescent children? An additional goal was to identify factors that influence these communication practices. Data relating to the impact of patterns of communication on teens' mental health and developing identity as well as on parent–child relationships were also sought. Whereas much of the work in the field of intergenerational transmission of trauma has involved studies of grown, adult offspring recollecting their childhoods, this study aimed to capture the perspective of young people and observe the phenomenon in process. As a consequence, it was hoped that the information obtained would not only enrich theoretical knowledge, but have relevance for clinical and community interventions with Cambodian families.

IV. METHODS

A. Study Design

This study was a focused ethnography. Developed by anthropologists, ethnography seeks to explore an unfamiliar culture by eliciting views of its own members. Information is obtained in order to illuminate systems of meaning from within the culture's own frame of reference (46). As a qualitative research method, ethnography uses techniques such as participant observation and in-depth interviews of key informants and primary informants to generate hypotheses rather than test an investigator's *a priori* hypotheses (47). Traditional ethnographic research typically takes several years; focused ethnography, which is being increasingly used in health sciences research, is a truncated version of this process, thought to be feasible because the question under consideration is much more limited in scope (48).

This study was approved by the Human Subjects Review Committee of the University of Washington. Washington state has the third-largest Cambodian population among the 50 states. Field work occurred over 18 months in 1994–1996 in the greater Seattle area, where about 6,000 Cambodians live. "Participant observation" included attending religious and secular holiday celebrations, senior breakfasts, and a women's quilting group; the first author also facilitated an ongoing support group for Cambodian adolescent girls in a community afterschool program. "Key informant" interviews were held with ten adult individuals thought to have important perspectives on the cultural questions under consideration, including bilingual health care and social service providers, teachers, and monks. Primary informants were parents and teens from eight families who were interviewed in depth.

B. Participants

Primary informants were recruited principally by key informants with the aim of achieving diversity and balance with respect to gender, English-language competence, employment status, neighborhood of residence, and health status of the parents. All parent informants were survivors of the Khmer Rouge period. To avoid bringing too much of a clinical flavor to the discussion, parents were not assessed systematically for symptoms of PTSD or other psychiatric disorders, although sometimes this information emerged from the interviews.

Seven mothers and three fathers were interviewed. Three of the mothers were single parents. All families but one lived in public housing; only one parent worked outside the home. Eight of the parents chose to be interviewed in Khmer, the Cambodian language, and stated they had little to no English language competence; two spoke English well enough that the interviews were conducted primarily in English, at their request.

The teens were 14 to 18 years old, and despite attempts to achieve gender balance, seven were female and one male. They were born in about equal numbers in Cambodia (during the last 2 years of the Khmer Rouge period), in the Thai refugee camps, and in the United States. None of those who were born in Asia had any memories of Cambodia, although some reported vague memories of the Thai refugee camps.

C. Data Collection and Analysis

Primary informants were interviewed on one or two occasions for from 1 to 3 hours at a time. Parents were interviewed in their homes and a Cambodian interpreter was present even if the parent chose to converse primarily in English. Teens were interviewed in community settings. Informed consent was obtained before each interview. Questioning was based on a list of questions compiled in advance; however, interviews were begun in a very open-ended way and, as much as possible, information was allowed to emerge naturally from the conversation to avoid unknowingly excluding anything that might be relevant. Parents were asked about the kinds of stories about their lives in Asia that they share with their children, about how such conversations occur, and the effect of the conversations on the children and themselves. To minimize the possibility of causing emotional distress, parents were not asked to directly recount stories of their traumatic experiences, although a few told such stories spontaneously. Teens were asked about stories they had heard, and about the impact of these stories; their sense of Cambodian identity was probed as well. Interviews were audiotaped and English was transcribed as spoken.

Analytic techniques were based on ethnographic practice. Transcripts were read carefully and repeatedly, then annotated. Important and recurring words, phrases, ideas, examples, and affects expressed by informants were coded, leading to the identification of several major themes. Themes were then studied for patterns of connection, and compared across subgroups of subjects.

Trustworthiness is the term used in qualitative research to approximate the ideas of reliability and validity (49). Multiple methods commonly used to establish trustworthiness were used in this study. These included verification of segments of audiotaped translation by a second Cambodian interpreter, independent coding of selected transcripts by two additional readers (a psychiatrist experienced in treating Cambodian patients and a Thai nurse with expertise in qualitative research), review of emerging findings with several of the key informants, and triangulation, which is comparison of findings with existing literature.

V. RESULTS

A. Contextualizing Issues

Several key issues emerged as background to all subsequent findings. First, adult informants indicated that it is not traditional in Cambodian culture for parents to share many details, particularly intimate details, of their life histories with their children. It was normative in prewar Cambodia, for example, for a teen to know nothing about how her parents met. This reticence seems to be a function of the hierarchical way the parent–child relationship is conceptualized. It was seen as particularly important to protect girls from too much knowledge of adult life so that they remain innocent and pure. Some informants reported that once they had married and had children of their own, their mothers in particular began to disclose more personal stories to them.

The reticence may also be connected to the relatively unchanging nature of life in rural Cambodia over the generations, which, our informants suggested, created little need to narrate or explain. One father reported,

> The old people in those times never. . .[told] children. . .what happened about their life because. . .you were born and you lived with them all the time so you kind of know what they are doing. . .they think like you. . .

and then he compared this to his present situation:

> [I] tell [my] children about my life more than my parents because what I've gone through is more difficult.

Another explanation raised by one key informant is that telling stories about the family was a role more typically played by grandparents than by parents, because grandparents weren't so busy with day to day management of the farm or the business and the home.

The type of stories that adult informants did recall hearing often from their parents were traditional stories, folktales, which always concluded with a moral teaching, especially stories illustrating proper behavior for boys and for girls. When asked about stories her parents had told, nearly every mother in the sample began to immediately recite the *Chbop Srei*, which is not a story but a didactic code in verse, first written down in the 19th century (25), specifying hundreds of rules of behavior for girls (e.g., girls should not make any noise as they walk, girls should always speak sweetly), which parents and teachers expected them to memorize, a task which they had clearly taken seriously.

This leads to the second contextualizing issue, which is the widening cultural divide between Cambodian parents and their children in this country and the intense intergenerational conflict this distance is causing. Cultural differences involve many aspects of life (e.g., gender roles, dating practices), but most germane to this discussion are differing ideas about the parent–child relationship itself. The parents in this sample were brought up in a world in which children were taught to respect their parents absolutely, to never question their authority, to never look their parents in the eye as a sign of differential status. When it came time for marriage, Cambodian youth were expected to allow their parents to choose their partners for them "out of gratitude to their parents for having raised them." The Cambodian word most often used to describe the proper relation between parents and children, *klaic*, represents a seamless melding of respect and fear. But the teens in this sample live at least part of their days in a very different world: they watch American television, attend coed public schools, have non-Cambodian friends and teachers, and are developing very different expectations about autonomy, choice, and relationships in their lives. This is infuriating, terrifying, humiliating, and heartbreaking to their parents. Not only do the parents feel out of place in this country in which they are underemployed, don't speak the language well, and therefore function less competently than their children, but on top of all their other losses—of family, friends, and homeland—they feel they are losing their children, losing the ability to raise their children to be Cambodian, to be, in their frame of reference, healthy, whole human beings (25,50). The mothers recite the *Chbop Srei* to their daughters and the daughters laugh and say, "No one can follow all those rules!" and the mothers are stunned. One reported,

> When I was teenager, I am so respectful to my parents, like when they talk, even good or bad, ok. But teenager here. . .it's not the way I expect them to be. It seem to me like they don't respect me at all. . .even I teach them how to say good, how to be good, they don't understand at all, they say, What is wrong with this? When I say, You do something wrong, honey, they say, No I'm not wrong, I'm right, you're wrong.

The third contextual issue in considering questions around narrative transmission is much more concrete and concerns the fact that parents and teens are usually not fluent in the same language. Although many parents understand a little English (all in this study having taken ESL classes at some point) and some appeared to understand more than they acknowledged, only two felt able to converse with us in English and they struggled a great deal to express complex concepts. Conversely, all the teens know at least a little Khmer, and many have attended Khmer language classes in the community, but few stated they felt capable of discussing important issues in Khmer. Many of the parents laughed about the mistakes their children make when they speak Khmer. Although parents and teens feel that they can get their ideas across to each other most of the time, they acknowledged that communication about abstract or complex ideas is difficult. Thus, whatever information about the past is shared between parents and adolescents is likely to lack subtlety and nuance.

B. The Parents' Perspective

All parents interviewed endorsed the idea of sharing with their children stories from what they referred to as "Pol Pot time" and from the refugee camps. The reason stated by most was a desire to help their children understand how much they have to be grateful for, growing up in the United States in peacetime, compared with the deprivations the parents had to endure. Recalling life under the Khmer Rouge, one mother said,

> [I] want [my] daughter to know. . .the difficulty that [I] went through, like [I] don't have food to eat, don't have clothes to wear, don't have school to go to, don't have any hospital to go when you're sick, and you have to work, work, and work. And then here you have food to eat, a place to live, clothes to wear, school to go, and the government help everything. . .so you should try to live nicely. . .

The parents' purpose in telling such stories is both spiritual (a lesson in gratitude) and practical; the stories are didactic, in the manner of traditional Cambodian folk tales, and are meant to motivate their children not to take for granted the opportunities that are available to them here, not to squander them.

> She want her to appreciate. . .to think. . .job is important, work is important, school is very important, then no playing around and wasting. . .time.

Education and career are important because they will enable the children to attain a higher socioeconomic status than the parents have been able to achieve:

> You children living now are much luckier than your mother. You have good luck, so you should study very hard. I tell my children. . .don't be uneducated like I am, it makes it difficult to live in the US. . . . I don't want them to eat welfare. . .like I have to. . .

Because education is highly valued in Cambodian culture, the children's imagined academic successes also provide a link with tradition, symbolize a link between the past and the present. Most of the parents, even those who came from poor, rural backgrounds, recalled prewar Cambodia in idealized terms, as a place where they had happy childhoods, everyone was "very young," enjoyed their siblings, attended New Year's festivities, and had time for fun. "I had a good life until the war came and took everything away from my family," one mother remembered. Some of the parents in the sample were students when the Khmer Rouge took over and shut down the schools; all saw their anticipated developmental trajectories destroyed, along with the world that gave them meaning.

Clinicians who work with Cambodian youth repeatedly hear them complain about how strict their parents are, how relentlessly the parents emphasize work and study, and denigrate all of the other ways in which teenagers commonly spend time, such as socializing or engaging in hobbies or just relaxing. Such attitudes do not appear dissimilar from those voiced by parents from other first-generation immigrant groups who came to America in search of a better life. But that is not the primary reason Cambodian parents left their homeland, and in these narratives it becomes clear that the parents' values and priorities are connected to the complex and pervasive losses they experienced under the Khmer Rouge. If the pressure with which parents exhort their children to succeed carries echoes of the ceaseless orders the parents heard from the Khmer Rouge brigade leaders—demanding they work even when ill, exhausted, and starving—it is because the parents so desperately hope that the children, by their attainments, will free the family from, or at least weaken the bonds of, this legacy. Although many parents speak of their children's "luck" in growing up in the United States, they rarely attribute luck to themselves for having survived. They tend to see themselves as forever damaged and broken. They see their children in Buddhist terms as having a different *karma*, having collected more merit in the course of their past lives. They see their children as free of the negative *karma* that for many parents is the only explanation for the destruction of their families and country. (51) But because individual identity and family identity are so intertwined in Cambodian culture, the children's accomplishments, while having their own intrinsic value, will also help restore the parents' dignity.

Three parents indicated additional reasons for sharing some stories about their traumatic past. One mother described the context in which she makes reference to her history:

> They ask me "Why are you here, mom? Why don't you live in Cambodia?" I said, because of the war. . .and they ask me, how do I get here? And I tell them that I was walking from Cambodia to Thailand for about a month. They said, "Oh how hard you are, walking from Cambodia to Thailand." And I said, "Yes, and now can you just make me happy, as the daughter can you make your mom happy now?"

In extended conversation with this parent, it became clear that her wish to be made happy refers not only to a particular behavior she desires from her daughter (coming home by curfew) but also unfortunately to a more diffuse expectation that her children can somehow compensate her for all her losses. While it is tempting to liken her statements to what has been called "guilt-inducing communication" noted in Holocaust survivors' families (8), it is also important to understand them in the context of traditional Cambodian culture and values, where duty towards one's parents is seen as a lifelong commitment, individual happiness and family happiness are virtually inseparable, and pity, compassion, and sacrifice are seen unequivocally as virtues.

One mother who suffers from flashbacks, nightmares, and emotional dysregulation consistent with a diagnosis of PTSD, and has been in psychotherapy, reported that telling her daughter her story brings her comfort in the moment:

> Sometimes I tell her, you know, make me feel better. . .when I tell her everything about my inside that I keep a long time, and sometimes I tell her a lot,. . .it makes me feel better. . . . She sit down by me and. . .she holds me. . . . She say, stop upset mommy, you know, nothing happen, no more, this country peace.

Not only does this mother confide in her daughter to a degree which is culturally anomalous, she also allows her daughter to take care of her emotionally, a reversal of their expected roles.

In this small sample, one father indicated in vague terms the importance of telling about "Pol Pot time" in order to deepen his children's sense of identity as Cambodians, "to have the story of the place where they come from, in order to tell if someone asks."

C. Fears about the Transmission of Trauma

Almost all the parents spontaneously expressed concern that hearing their trauma stories could negatively affect their children. They tended to express these fears using exactly the same images as they used to express their hopes; they worried that hearing the stories could hurt their children's potential:

> Maybe if I told everything to her, it would make her full of tension. . .she would have an upset. . .and then she couldn't study.
>
> I don't want them to feel sad, I don't want them to know all the sad things. I want them just to be happy and study and be good.

Most of the parents stated that they don't get visibly upset when they tell their stories to their children, and that it is not fear of emotional display that inhibits them from speaking; yet in talking with us, several suddenly began to cough or wheeze or sob when they began to talk about the Khmer Rouge period.

One mother, who experienced severe head trauma at the hands of Pol Pot's soldiers and now suffers from memory deficits and other cognitive problems, expressed reluctance to speak because she so easily loses her train of thought—a situation that is deeply frustrating to her. It is her story that would explain why she can't tell her story, but she can't tell it. Her daughter described what her mother's attempts at telling are like:

> My mom likes to talk about it once she remembers, [but] when she doesn't remember . . . you ask her and she doesn't want to talk about it. . . . Sometimes she remembers a little bit, then she starts over from the beginning again, then she says part of it, then she like forgets again.

All parents reported deliberately editing their accounts. One mother said,

> I tell some of it, but not all. I tell briefly, in summary, not in detail, some is not necessary.

Some parents indicated an intention to tell their children more as the children mature, and become capable of understanding "bad things," although most indicated that they still feel at a loss to understand all that happened in Cambodia.

Several of the parents used the rhetorical device of a list to describe their experiences, which seems to offer a way to both organize their memories and succinctly indicate the endlessness of their suffering:

> Sometimes we sit down and I tell her about that place. . .how I didn't have no food and no medicine, no clothes, no store, you know, everything, nothing.

In its sparseness, lack of emotion, and stereotypic quality, this type of communication is indeed a prenarrative, but its minimalism is also highly suggestive, creating space for the listener's imaginings to fill.

Ironically, the parents' reticence can serve to heighten the impact of the little that is said. One teen asserted several times that she never heard Cambodian stories from her parents, but as the interview was ending, she remembered this:

> If my mom eat a certain stuff, she would think about it. Like if she ate a soup with a fish in it, she wouldn't eat it. If it had a head in there, she wouldn't eat it.

Does she say why? we asked.

> She says she could remember the Khmer Rouge killing people, chopping off their heads.

This might be called an antistory, a story that silences the wish to know more.

D. The Teens' Perspective

Teens expressed a variety of attitudes toward hearing stories and information about Cambodia, ranging from innocent curiosity to apparent indifference to muted hostility. Some of the younger girls want to know all about the kind of clothing people have worn in Cambodia through the ages, and they are sure that the study of ancient Cambodia would be as interesting as the study of ancient Egypt, which they learn much more about in school. One girl reported that in her social studies class, each student was required to choose a foreign country to research. Although she wanted to study Cambodia, her teacher rejected the idea, mistakenly assuming that she knew too much about the topic already. Several teens expressed interest in knowing more about contemporary Cambodia and the kind of life people lead there: "Can you buy milk and bread?" "Do they really use outhouses?" they asked. Most, but not all, said, but only when asked, that they wanted to know more about modern Cambodian history, and about how it was that their families came to be living in the United States. Two girls mentioned the need to learn more about their own heritage so that, in time, they could pass it on to the next generation. As they spoke, several teens became aware of gaps and inconsistencies or problems with the knowledge they possess, and turned to the interviewer for help: "Was that the same war, or a different war then? When the Americans bombed Cambodia, it was a mistake, right?" Two teens appeared to have so little familiarity with events that had shaped their parents' lives that talking with them about these things felt almost surreal. "What's a refugee camp?" one 15-year-old honors student asked, and when the interviewer translated "refugee camp" to the Khmer equivalent, it did not clarify the concept for her. "Pol Pot? I think I heard of that. That was a guy, right?"

Several teens described how the process of learning about Cambodia's traumatic history began almost imperceptibly, overhearing their parents' conversations, which may have been the parents' intent. One girl recalled:

> We go over to my friend's house, my mom and her mom, they're. . .kinda like best friends. . .and so usually they talk about Cambodia, and then tell about their childhood. . . and I hang out with my friend but then I hear, like, stories, because they talk loud. So I hear like little specks, like walking through the forest and then, something, I don't know. Like little, teeny little specks.

Just as the parents indicated that they tell only a portion of their stories, most of the teens reported that they know only "a little" or "a teeny little bit", and that they ask their parents only "some," not "too much" about their former lives. Their statements betray the teens' awareness that there is more to the stories. The minimizing labels appear to be attempts to cope with their own anxiety over knowledge that they sense to be in fact dangerous, overwhelming, infinitely terrible. The first time the first author heard a Cambodian teen talk about the Khmer Rouge period, she referred to it, with a nervous smile, as "the Pol Pot thingy."

Teens openly expressed conflicted feelings about listening to their parents' stories, which paralleled the conflict parents expressed about telling them. One teen's concerns were a direct echo of her mother's worries that to transmit the information could transmit the trauma:

> My mother doesn't want to put all the bad stuff into my mind, she doesn't want me thinking about it too much. She's scared that it might affect me too, [giggling awkwardly] I don't know, in some way.

But most of the teens have their own reasons for ambivalence, born out of their own experience. Several described the intense grief that overtakes their parents when they talk about the past:

> My mom she cries when she talks about it. That's why I don't want to talk about it, I don't want my mom to stress. That's why I don't want to ask her. . .because she's really sad and she's crying and I have to watch her cry. . .

There are two levels of experience described here that the teens would prefer to avoid: seeing their parents suffer, and feeling so helpless in the face of the parents' suffering, as helpless as the parents themselves.

One teen very sensitively described how in the process of telling her story, her mother loses control of the narrative, the narrative takes on its own life:

> Sometimes she cries when she talks about the past, and other times she just goes deeper and deeper into it. And I don't really like it because I don't really want to hear those things in a way. She keeps going, she makes the story like how she really sees it . . . she doesn't just say . . . she tells me more . . . more than what I asked her. I ask her a question she tells me my question. . .she answered it already but she keeps going.

An older teen described the disturbing experience of her father having what is probably a flashback, when the boundaries between present and past disappear:

> He'll talk about the past, and it's as if it's happening now, you know, just talking about it, it seems like he's there right now.

Teens described how they attempt to rescue and reclaim their parents at such moments, for example by distraction:

> I try to get her mind off it. I change the subject. I usually talk about my grandpa, my mom's dad, because she loves my grandpa.

E. Failures of Communication

Some teens seem to resist hearing their parents' stories not just because they are so painful, but also because of the demand that hearing threatens to place on them. Especially in families where there is a lot of struggle over rules and appropriate behavior, and where many of the Cambodian stories are didactic, teens begin to suspect that any mention of Cambodia will lead to a disciplinary lecture, to the criticism that they are becoming too American. Anything Cambodian thus becomes negatively valenced for these youth. One mother reported:

> I tell them the story how hard it is to raise them in the place that don't have enough food, don't have good place to sleep, no water to shower, no bathroom. . . . And they say they understand, but why do you want to tell me, I don't want to know. . . . They talk back to me just like that. They don't want to hear, they don't want to see, they don't want to know anything about the past. . .They say, You just want us to stay home and follow your rules. . . . This is America, not Cambodia. . . . Why don't you forget all the past, mom? . . . And come into the new life right now. . .It's just the past. It ought to be past.

The process of sharing stories often seems to bring parents and teens only minimally closer. Even parents who share a great deal of their experience are left with the feeling that the teens have not really understood very much, and they tended to express this in another image that conveys smallness in the face of enormity, a surprisingly quantitative image: they estimated that their children have understood "only about ten percent." Ironically, the teens described being deeply, indelibly affected by what they hear. When we asked our teen informant how she feels when her mother says she can't eat soup containing fishheads, she responded quietly, "I guess I can't eat it either."

Another girl said,

> I watch a movie sometimes, like a sad movie, and then. . .that brings up the subject of my mom. Like how she survived in the war. . .the people in there, like, they're experiencing the same [feeling] and so I. . .think about it and I feel bad about it. . .cause I can feel how. . .she felt, so I have the same feeling too.

One teen described recurrent intrusive memories of her mother's recounted traumatic experiences

> I think about it, but I don't let [my mother] know that I'm thinking about it. She doesn't know that I know as much as I do. . . . She thinks that I don't really understand because I'm young and young people are stupid and just want to have fun. . . . When she tells me these things she probably thinks that I don't keep it. . .in my mind like I just kind of let it go. . .like it's just for the time being.

F. The Killing Fields

One of the most surprising themes that surfaced in this study was the role of the film, *The Killing Fields*. Every family had watched it together on television or video, and many had watched it several times. This activity proves to be one of the most successful ways in which the history of the Khmer Rouge period is shared. Although this was a Hollywood movie, the parents have no difficulty embracing it as their own. "That was my story, that was what happened to me," one mother declared. Watching the film returns the parents to their lost world while providing them with some distance from the terrible events unfolding before them. They all emphasized that the film portrays only a fraction of the terror. "It is not even ten percent of the real story," they said, but this was not offered as a complaint. Watching the film with their children is successful exactly because the story is edited and less personal. The primary question that arises when parents and children watch the film together is very basic, very simple. Not "How could the Khmer Rouge kill their fellow Cambodians?" or "How could Pol Pot have come to power?", the kinds of questions we thought teens might ask their parents. These young people want to know, "Is it true, mom? Did it really happen?" Because it is on television, a medium they favor, it is not only safer, it is also more relevant, more convincing. One girl explained,

> It really opened my eyes. I was just stunned just right there just sat down, watched it. . . . I really didn't know. . .like how hard it was during the time of Pol Pot. . .I never saw anything so brutal like that. . . . When they kill people it's like right there in front of you. . .

The film helps the teens start to make sense of their parents' lives, to put the fragments together. In the moment of watching it together, the parents are seen as people possessing knowledge, as people with answers. One mother reported,

> They start to ask me, Is it true, mom? Yes it is true. And they start to ask me about it, about the story, and I tell them.

VI. DISCUSSION

It appears that there is substantial variation among Cambodian families in the amount of information about past trauma that is shared between parents and children. The combined impact of trauma and resettlement has led some parents to disclose a great deal, which constitutes a break with Cambodian cultural inhibitions about communicating negative information and with traditional notions of parent–child relations. Other parents speak of the traumatic past rarely, or very indirectly. In either case, there is often a substantial gap between what parents think they have conveyed and what children recall and know. Some teens were startlingly ignorant of the most basic outlines of recent Cambodian history.

Parents express ambivalence about the experience of telling and teens express ambivalence about the experience of listening to stories about Cambodia. Both are inhibited because of fears about the transmission of trauma. Some teens resent the criticisms of their Americanized behaviors which their parents' accounts sometimes detour into. For some parents, language limitations and the physical and psychological injuries they sustained during "Pol Pot time," such as head trauma and PTSD, greatly increase the difficulty of communicating their stories. Some convey their experiences in "prenarratives" and others use forms described by Auerhahn and Laub: unintegrated fragments (a memory of witnessing decapitation), transference phenomena (presenting hard work to one's children as a life-or-death matter), or overpowering narratives ("she just goes deeper and deeper into it . . .") (14). Yet they would like to construct a meaningful story that would inspire their children to achieve educationally and financially, providing the family a more secure future and symbolically undoing some of the traumas of the past. The compromise that most parents arrive at, a strategy of editing, shifting emphasis, and in some cases (which will be detailed in another publication), even altering crucial facts, succeeds only in part. Often both parents and children are left with a sense of isolation, and need to struggle alone with the information that what they know or sense lies outside the boundaries of what has been shared.

The advantage of watching the film *The Killing Fields* can be understood in terms of Pennebaker's work. The film presents a more coherent, organized, sensory-rich narrative than most of the parents can generate themselves. In the process of watching, it is as though their own stories are blended into the film's recounting, so that their stories become easier to hold, offering to the parents and teens some of the benefits and relief that Pennebaker believes a good narrative offers. To paraphrase what Kirmayer (52) has written about accounts of the Holocaust in literature and film, aesthetic devices succeed in muting and containing "the chaos that persists closer to the experience."

These data offer several examples of how the stories Cambodian parents tell their children can in fact reveal "the chaos" and, one might say, transmit the trauma they have experienced. For example, teens describe symptoms that parallel their parents' symptoms: they mirror and identify with their parents' sad affects evoked by telling their stories, have intrusive memories of their parents' stories, and display avoidance behavior (e.g., not eating fish soup) at narrative reminders of their parents' victimization. Listening to their stories can involve teens in a traumatic reenactment of their parents' experience when they find themselves as helpless as their parents at seeing a family member suffer, or see a parent lost to them as he is caught up in a flashback of the past.

The "transmission" that stems from story-telling about the past also seems to take the form of roles these youth are asked, implicitly or explicitly, to take on in the family. A minor child is asked to care for a traumatized parent (by listening to her stories, or by distracting him from his intrusive memories); to single-handedly raise the family's socioeconomic status through absolute commitment to school or work, regardless of her abilities; to take on the burden of a parent's suffering (to be responsible for making him "happy"). These roles are derived from, but involve subtle distortions of, traditional Cambodian conceptions of familial duty. Interestingly, very similar roles (as well as others) have been described in children in other survivor populations (4,9). Designated roles are problematic because they foreclose teens' needs to develop their own identities. While in Cambodia, individual identity may have had little meaning apart from the family, these teens are growing up in the United States, where separation and individuation play a prominent role in adolescent development, and many will feel their loyalties divided between the parents they want to please and protect and the peers they wish to emulate.

"Transmission" as a consequence of storytelling plays itself out, too, in the mixed feelings about their Cambodian identity some teens appear to have developed. When their parents identify "Cambodian-ness" primarily with rigid and archaic codes of conduct, and with unspeakable pain, the children seek to distance themselves from this association. Some teens, however, appear to have developed a more positive sense of Cambodian identity, buttressed, for example, by positive images from stories about life before Pol Pot time, and the fun they experience celebrating Cambodian holidays in the traditional way with their families. Some clearly envision themselves passing on a story about their Cambodian heritage to their own children, even if they still lack details of its content.

The results of this study are consistent with the findings of Sack and colleagues (43) and of Drapeau and Rousseau (45) regarding trauma-related communication in Cambodian families, but they also reveal a broader range of practices that can be understood as communications and provide additional information regarding the motivation of parents and impact on their children. Like all qualitative research, the results of this study are not necessarily generalizable. The subjects were not a random sample and no conclusions regarding prevalence can be drawn from these data. This was a very small sample. Having more subjects might have introduced more themes or complicated the themes. In particular, the fact that almost all the adolescents were female may have affected the findings, because in studies of Holocaust survivor offspring, gender appears to play an important role in determining responses to parental communication as well as vulnerability to transmitted trauma (4). No attempt was made to categorize the amount or type of trauma exposure experienced by each parent or to assess for parental PTSD. It is likely that these variables influence the types of communication that occur in individual families as well as their impact.

Kirmayer (52) has written that the context of retelling is crucial to the nature of memory. Self-narratives, he notes, are "context-sensitive reconstructions," and cultural context is crucial in determining the kind of narratives survivors have available to them. When Holocaust survivors arrived in their new countries, they felt an inner compulsion to share their stories, yet listeners tended to recoil from them in shock and incomprehension, withdrawing into what Danieli (1) called a "conspiracy of silence." It wasn't until the 1960s, when the first scholarly history of the Holocaust was published and received widespread public attention, that survivors began to tell their stories again.

This study occurred at a particular time in both the history of Cambodia and in the life of these teens, and these contexts undoubtedly had an impact on the data elicited. Not long after these interviews were completed, Pol Pot, aged and infirm, agreed to a series of interviews with an American journalist and video crew from his hideout in the Thai jungle; shortly afterwards he died. The events were well-covered by the Seattle media and the major newspaper ran several related stories in the ensuing days about Cambodian history and resettlement. In the support group for Cambodian girls that the first author ran, few members brought up Pol Pot's death spontaneously, but when asked, many acknowledged having discussions with their parents or teachers about the event. Those who hadn't yet heard the news then excitedly asked their peers for information. "It is easy to forget when there are no collective occasions for remembering," Kirmayer notes (52). This event occurring in their American world may well have altered what our teen informants could tell us if we were meeting with them today.

In thinking about the context of these findings, it is also important to keep in mind the developmental level of the teens at the moment in time the data were collected. Most of these youth were in early to mid-adolescence, and it is very likely that as they progress into late adolescence and young adulthood, their interest in their parents' experience and its relevance to their personal and ethnic identities will shift and deepen. Although children are able to recognize and label their own ethnic group from a very young age, it is not until adolescence that a clear sense of ethnic identity begins to emerge. Researchers have suggested that there is a sequential progression in the formation of ethnic identity, beginning with an "unexamined" phase in early adolescence that leads, with cognitive maturation and increased life experience, to a phase of "exploration and questioning" in mid-to-late adolescence and may later culminate in an "achieved" ethnic identity; this model has been validated in immigrant Asian American youth in the United States (53,54). In addition, 5–10 years after these interviews were completed, most of these teens will be nearing the age their parents were at the time the Khmer Rouge came to power in Cambodia and this, too, may affect what is told and what is asked and what is understood and remembered.

REFERENCES

1. Danieli Y. The treatment and prevention of long-term effects and intergenerational transmission of victimization: a lesson from Holocaust survivors and their children. In: Figley CR, ed. *Trauma and its wake: the study and treatment of post traumatic stress disorder.* New York: Brunner/Mazel, 1985: 295–313.
2. Nagata DK. The Japanese American internment: exploring the transgenerational consequences of traumatic stress. *J Traum Stress* 1990;3:47–69.
3. Aarts P. Intergenerational effects in families of WWII survivors from the Dutch East Indies: aftermath of another Dutch war. In: Danieli Y, ed. *International handbook of multigenerational legacies of trauma.* New York: Plenum Press, 1998:175–187.
4. Felsen I. Transgenerational transmission of effects of the Holocaust: the North American research perspective. In: Danieli Y, ed. *Intergenerational handbook of multigenerational legacies of trauma.* New York: Plenum Press, 1998:43–68.
5. Op den Velde W. Children of Dutch war sailors and civilian resistance veterans. In: Danieli Y, ed. *International handbook of multigenerational legacies of trauma.* New York: Plenum Press, 1998: 147–162.
6. Solomon Z. Transgenerational effects of the Holocaust: the Israeli research perspective. In: Danieli Y, ed. *International handbook of multigenerational legacies of trauma.* New York: Plenum Press, 1998:69–84.
7. Rosenheck R. Impact of posttraumatic stress disorder of WWII on the next generation. *J Nerv Ment Dis* 1986;174:319–327.
8. Lichtman H. Parental communication of Holocaust experiences and personality characteristics among second generation survivors. *J Clin Psychol* 1984;40:914–924.
9. Ancharoff MR, Munroe FJ, Fisher L. The legacy of combat trauma: clinical implications of intergenerational transmission. In: Danieli Y, ed. *International handbook of multigenerational legacies of trauma.* New York: Plenum Press, 1998:257–276.
10. Kupelian D, Kalayjian AS, Kassabian A, The Turkish genocide of the Armenians: continuing effects on survivors and their families eight decades after massive trauma. In: Danieli Y, ed. *International handbook of multigenerational legacies of trauma.* New York: Plenum Press, 1998:191–211.
11. Solkoff N. Children of survivors of the Nazi Holocaust: a critical review of the literature. *Am J Orthopsychiatry* 1981;51:29–42.
12. Solkoff N. Children of survivors of the Nazi Holocaust: a critical review of the literature. *Am J Orthopsychiatry* 1992;62:342–358.
13. Simons RL, Johnson C. An examination of competing explanations for the intergenerational transmis-

sion of domestic violence. In: Danieli Y, ed. *International handbook of multigenerational legacies of trauma.* New York: Plenum Press:1998:553–570.
14. Auerhahn N, Laub D. Intergenerational memory of the Holocaust. In: Danieli Y, ed. *International handbook of multigenerational legacies of trauma.* New York: Plenum Press, 1998:21–42.
15. Nader KO. Violence: effects of parents' previous trauma on currently traumatized children. In: Danieli Y, ed. *International handbook of multigenerational legacies of trauma.* New York: Plenum Press, 1998:571–583.
16. Krystal J, Nagy L, Rasmusson A, et al. Initial clinical evidence of genetic contributions to posttraumatic stress disorder. In: Danieli Y, ed. *International handbook of multigenerational legacies of trauma.* New York: Plenum Press, 1998:657–668
17. Yehuda R, Schmeidler J, Elkin A et al. Phenomenology and psychobiology of the intergenerational response to trauma. In: Danieli Y, ed. *International handbook of multigenerational legacies of trauma.* New York: Plenum Press, 1998:639–656.
18. Nagata D. Transgenerational impact of the Japanese internment: clinical issues in working with children of former internees. *Psychotherapy* 1991;28:121–128.
19. Danieli Y. History and conceptual foundations. In: Danieli Y, ed. *International handbook of multigenerational legacies of trauma.* New York: Plenum Press, 1998:1–20.
20. Rosenheck R, Nathan PN. Secondary traumatization in children of Vietnam veterans. *Hosp Commun Psychiatry* 1985;36:538–539.
21. Chandler D. *The tragedy of Cambodian history: politics, war, and revolution.* New Haven: Yale University Press, 1991.
22. Chanda N. *Brother enemy: the war after the war.* New York: Harcourt Brace Jovanovich, 1986.
23. Shawcross W. *Sideshow: Kissinger, Nixon, and the destruction of Cambodia.* New York: WW Norton, 1979.
24. Hin C. *When broken glass floats: growing up under the Khmer Rouge.* New York: WW Norton, 2000.
25. Ledgerwood JL. *Changing Khmer conceptions of gender: women, stories, and the social order.* Ann Arbor: University Microfilms, 1990.
26. Criddle J, Mam TB. *To destroy you is no loss.* New York: Atlantic Monthly Press, 1987.
27. Ngor H. *Haing Ngor: a Cambodian odyssey.* New York: Macmillan, 1987.
28. DePaul K, Pran D, eds. *Children of Cambodia's Killing Fields: memoirs by survivors.* New Haven: Yale University Press, 1997.
29. Mollica RF, Wyshak G, Lavelle J. The psychosocial impact of war trauma and torture on Southeast Asian refugees. *Am J Psychiatry* 1987;144:1567–1572.
30. Carlson EB, Rosser-Hogan R. Mental health status of Cambodian refugees ten years after leaving their homes. *Am J Orthopsychiatry* 1993;63:223–230.
31. Sack WH, McSharry S, Clarke GN, et al. The Khmer adolescent project: I. Epidemiologic findings in two generations of Cambodian refugees. *J Nerv Ment Dis* 1994;182:387–395.
32. Sack WH, Clarke GN, Kinney R, et al. The Khmer adolescent project: II. Functional capacities in two generations of Cambodian refugees. *J Nerv Ment Dis* 1995;183:177–181.
33. Becker G, Yewoubdar B, Ken P. Health, welfare reform, and narratives of uncertainty among Cambodian refugees. *Culture Med Psychiatry* 2000;24:139–163.
34. Chandler D. Songs at the edge of the forest: perceptions of order in three Cambodian texts. In: Wyatt DK, Woodside A, eds. *Moral order and the question of change: essays on Southeast Asian thought.* New Haven: Yale University Press, 1982;53–77.
35. Polkinghorne DE. *Narrative knowing and the human sciences.* Albany: State University of New York Press, 1988.
36. Mishler E. *Research interviewing.* Cambridge: Harvard University Press, 1986.
37. Pennebaker JW, Seagal JD. Forming a story: the health benefits of narrative. *J Clin Psychology* 1999;55:1243–1254.
38. Gidron Y, Peri T, Connolly JF, et al. Written disclosure in posttraumatic stress disorder: is it beneficial for the patient? *J Nerv Ment Dis* 1996;184:505–507.
39. Herman JL. *Trauma and recovery.* New York: Basic Books, 1992.
40. Van der Kolk BA, Fisler RE. Dissociation and the fragmentary nature of traumatic memories: overview and exploratory study. *J Traum Stress* 1995;8:505–525.
41. Mollica RF. The trauma story: the psychiatric care of refugee survivors of violence and torture. In: Ochberg F, ed. *Post-traumatic therapy and victims of violence.* New York: Brunner/Mazel, 1988: 295–314.

42. Mollica RF, Lavelle J. Southeast Asian Refugees. In: Comas-Diaz L, Griffith EE, eds. *Clinical guidelines in cross-cultural mental health.* New York: Wiley, 1987:262–304.
43. Sack WH, Angell RH, Kinzie JD, et al. The psychiatric effects of massive trauma on Cambodian children: II. The family, the home, and the school. *J Am Acad Child Adolesc Psychiatry* 1986;25: 377–383.
44. Uba L. *Asian Americans: personality patterns, identity, and mental health.* New York: Guilford Press, 1994.
45. Rousseau C, Drapeau A. The impact of culture on the transmission of trauma: refugees' stories and silence embodied in their children's lives. In: Danieli Y, ed. *International handbook of multigenerational legacies of trauma.* New York: Plenum Press, 1998:465–486.
46. Agar MH. *Speaking of ethnography.* Thousand Oaks, CA: Sage Publications, 1986.
47. Spradley JP. *The ethnographic interview.* New York: Harcourt Brace Jovanovich, 1979.
48. Muecke MA. On the evaluation of ethnographies. In: Morse JM, ed. *Critical issues in qualitative research methods.* Thousand Oaks, CA: Sage Publications, 1994:187–209.
49. Inui TS, Frankel RM. Evaluating the quality of qualitative research: a proposal pro tem. *J Gen Intern Med* 1991;6:485–486.
50. Mortland CA. Cambodian refugees and identity in the United States. In: Camino LA, Krulfeld RM eds. *Reconstructing lives, recapturing meaning: refugee identity, gender, and culture change.* Amsterdam: Overseas Publishers Association, 1994:5–27
51. Mortland CA. Khmer Buddhists in the United States: ultimate questions. In: Ebihara M, Mortland CA, Ledgerwood J, eds. *Cambodian culture since 1975: homeland and exile.* Ithaca: Cornell University Press, 1994:72–90.
52. Kirmayer L. Landscapes of memory: trauma, narrative, and dissociation. In: Antze P, Lambek M, eds. *Tense past: cultural essays in trauma and memory.* London: Routledge, 1996:173–198.
53. Phinney JS, Chavira V. Ethnic identity and self-esteem: an exploratory longitudinal study. *J Adolesc* 1992;15:271–281.
54. Ying Y-W, Lee P. The development of ethnic identity in Asian-American adolescents: status and outcomes. *Am J Orthopsychiatry* 1999;69:194–208.

10

Language in the Cross-Cultural Encounter

Working with and without Medical Interpreters

Siobhan M. O'Neill

Department of Psychiatry, Massachusetts General Hospital, Boston, Massachusetts 02114

I. INTRODUCTION

English speakers residing in the United States may easily overlook the importance of language in everyday life because we take for granted that we will be understood. In the United States, one can travel thousands of miles without having to negotiate language differences and the fear of not being understood. However, this is not a fact that millions of people living in the United States can take for granted. The 2000 census counted 20 million inhabitants with "poor English" skills and 10 million inhabitants with no ability to speak English. This represented a significant increase over the 1990 census.

Imagine being in a foreign country and not speaking the language well enough to know that you can communicate. Then imagine being sick, and having to seek medical or psychiatric care under these circumstances. Even for patients from another culture who have some command of English, seeking psychiatric care is complicated. For patients who speak little or no English, it can be a tremendously stressful and frightening experience.

Conversation is at the heart of all human relationships, and is the foundation of the physician–patient relationship. What happens when the physician and patient have no common words to carry on a conversation? What happens when we clinicians are deprived of our most useful tool and the raw material of our art? Verbal communication takes on greater significance in the psychiatric evaluation of patients no matter what the cultural background of the patient. The complexity of the role of language in the physician–patient encounter is even greater in cross-cultural psychiatry.

Writing about the psychodynamic experience of migrants, Grinberg and Grinberg (1) say of language, "One's own language, the mother tongue, is never as libidinally invested as when one lives in a country where a different language is spoken. All childhood experiences, memories, and feelings about early object relations are connected to language. Special meanings become embedded in it." It is a fundamental part of life. Schaff, as cited by the Grinbergs, considers language the most traditional element of culture, and the most resistant to change, that is, the element of culture which migrants find the most difficult to give up. In the study of cross-cultural psychiatry, therefore, it is crucial to consider the role language plays in people's lives and development and how issues of language arise in working with patients who are from cultures other than the dominant local culture. Whether these patients have become proficient in the dominant language or require interpreter assistance, the very fact that there is no shared mother tongue between clinician and patient has dramatic implications. Language is a central, and embedded, part of culture.

In the first section of this chapter, I will discuss the clinical and psychodynamic implications of work with cross-cultural patients who have learned to speak English, including the developmental and defensive aspects of speaking a second language. In the second section I will address the technical, clinical, and psychodynamic implications of working with patients with limited English proficiency in collaboration with medical interpreters. Throughout I will outline strategies for optimizing the clinical encounter with patients from both groups. I will use English as the reference language given that it is the language of the culture in which this book is being written and published. However, the concepts discussed may be applicable to other cross-cultural and cross-language settings. Indeed, the ideas presented here derive not only from my own clinical experience, but also from that of other clinicians writing about their cross-cultural work all over the world.

II. WORKING WITH PATIENTS FROM OTHER CULTURES WHO ARE PROFICIENT IN ENGLISH

Communication difficulties between patients and clinicians may be due to problems of language (understanding English, speaking English, or both) or to cultural misunderstandings not easily negotiated through language, or to both language and cultural differences. A thorough discussion of the impact of cultural differences is beyond the scope of this chapter; however, it is important to note that Western medicine and psychiatry themselves are cultures within the larger culture, and hence may engender misunderstandings due to conflicting cultural values. In this section, I will consider the issues of language arising in work with patients who have learned to speak English, and will touch briefly on some of the cultural issues that arise through language.

A. Challenges to Communication

It may not be at first apparent that there are significant differences in communicating with people whose mother tongue is the same as our own, and people who speak

English fluently, but who acquired their English secondarily. In ordinary conversation, these differences may or may not matter much. In the psychiatric evaluation of a patient, the differences are important, yet may easily go unrecognized by the clinician unfamiliar with this issue.

The nonnative speaker of any language is automatically at a disadvantage when engaged in conversation with native speakers. Rapid speech and variation in local accents may interfere with language comprehension of nonnative speakers, and even of native speakers who learned English in a different part of the world. Idiomatic expressions, slang, and cultural allusions are used often in day-to-day speech, and may vary significantly from one region of the country to another. Even a nonnative speaker who has spent significant time in the United States may not understand all such expressions and allusions. For example, it is remarkable how many allusions there are to *The Wizard of Oz* in day-to-day conversation. Consider the following expressions: "the yellow brick road," "This ain't Kansas," "ruby slippers," and "the Wicked Witch of the West." Many people who did not grow up in the United States are not familiar with these and many other expressions, which refer to elements of American culture. In quotidian conversation, the references to a shared heritage of literature, music, film, and television are endless. In psychiatric work with patients who were not raised in the United States, it may be important to avoid slang, idiomatic expressions, and culture-specific allusions as much as possible, and to speak slowly with clear enunciation. This will minimize some of the problems in comprehension.

Communication between clinician and patient may be adversely affected by the patient's inability to express himself fully in English. A person's ability to comprehend a second language is always greater than his ability to speak that language. A patient may understand complex questions, and thus seem to be proficient in English. Because of the usual discrepancy between comprehension and speaking skills, she may not be able to form complete, complex answers, especially if it involves abstract issues such as emotional or inner experience. Studies and experience have shown that patients who speak English as a second language may be judged to be exhibiting paucity of speech and thought, and even thought disorder when the real issue may simply be one of spoken language ability (2,3). If a patient appears to comprehend well, it is important not to assume that his ability to reply will be equal. If in fact the patient's replies are brief, simple, and not what would be expected given the questions, assessment of the language skills must be made first, before the quality of the responses are interpreted as symptoms and translated into psychopathology. If a clinician suspects a patient's speaking ability may be limiting the interview, an interpreter should be used.

In addition, an individual's ability to speak a second language can fluctuate with mental state. For example, when fatigued, frightened, or under emotional distress, a person's ability to speak a second language is often diminished (4,5). When distressed, a person naturally returns to the language of childhood (1). Significant pain, delirium, dementia, depression, mania, and psychosis may diminish or completely impair an individual's ability to speak a second language. In the case of reversible conditions, ability to speak the second language should improve with recovery from the condition (6–8).

Case Example: A young woman presented to the emergency room complaining of insomnia for many nights. She initially spoke in English rapidly and fluently with little accent, and it seemed appropriate to interview her in English. Soon she began to switch between English and French, eventually speaking mostly French, with little apparent awareness of her language switching, and little awareness that those evaluating her may not understand her. Subsequent evaluation with an interpreter revealed further history and symptoms of racing thoughts, tangential thoughts, distractibility, grandiosity, impulsivity, and hypersexuality. This was consistent with the patient's history of bipolar illness and her prior episodes of mania.

In this case, the patient clearly had the ability to speak and understand English, but she was floridly manic, and was not able to stay focused enough to maintain a conversation in English. It is important to consider this issue in evaluating patients who can usually speak English, but who show signs or symptoms of any of the conditions mentioned earlier. In these cases, it may be important to use an interpreter in the evaluation and treatment. Even if the patient initially declines the offer to have an interpreter present, it may be clinically indicated to have one standing by.

B. Psychodynamic Factors in Working with Patients Who Speak English as a Second Language

Language is a means through which humans not only communicate, but also form identity, articulate reality, and form and articulate relationship to others. The infant's acquisition of language is concurrent with and used in the service of the development of identity and separation from the mother. Language is therefore intimately tied to these early psychological tasks, as well as to development throughout life. Greenson has said that language is the means by which a child both separates and remains connected to his or her mother (9). Later in life, language is an essential skill through which adults relate to other adults, and a central means through which individuals remain connected to their cultures.

A number of psychodynamic factors may affect a patient's ability to articulate aspects of inner experience and emotion in a second language. Theorists such as Buxbaum, Greenson, Fenichel, and Marcos have addressed the dynamics of patients who speak English as a second language in psychiatric treatment. Major themes from this literature include identity formation, regression, and language-specific defenses.

When people migrate to a country where their mother tongue is not spoken, they may reexperience the affectively charged infantile situation of not being able to understand others, and not being understood. The Grinbergs write about this regression to childhood or infantile frustrations, which can occur when an individual is once again in a situation where he is "preverbal" in the second language. The migrant who is struggling with the new language may feel a childlike dependence on others that he would not feel could he speak for himself. This dependent position may engender passivity, or a less questioning reliance on authority, or conversely anger, resentment, and rebellion. Anger may impair comprehension, and may make it even more difficult for the person to make herself understood. The same authors relate the ease or difficulty with which immigrants acquire a new language and function in that language to how they experienced their preverbal stage in infancy. The more frustration that a person experienced learning to speak as an infant, then the more difficulty he will have understanding others and making himself understood in a new language and culture (1).

In addition, as language is an expression of and link to culture, immigrants who have had a traumatic separation from their countries of origin (such as those forced to emigrate due to political oppression) may also experience as traumatic the loss of their mother tongue, and may find it nearly impossible to acquire the language of the country where they have relocated. "Giving up" or "replacing" the mother tongue with a new language may be experienced as too devastating a loss to be tolerable, especially in the face of loss of home, country, and in many instances family. Many traumatized refugees will continue to speak their own language rather than learning English for years or even decades after resettlement.

Grinberg and Grinberg (1) and Greenson (9) have written about identity formation as a process intimately tied to language acquisition and use. As words are learned, they are used to articulate the evolving image of the self and essentially become an integral part of the sense of self. Words also represent the individual in relation to others. All languages have an inherent structure to distinguish "I" from "you" and "he" (1,3). An individual generally accomplishes identity formation in the mother tongue. When faced with a new culture where the mother tongue is not spoken, it may be experienced as lost, and a corresponding sense of loss of identity may ensue. This may be a devastating experience resulting in depression, and if the disintegration of identity is severe, even psychosis (1).

As the individual incorporates the new language, it is an opportunity to reconstruct the identity in that language, or to develop a new sense of identity. This may be to the adaptive advantage of the individual, but may also cause a split in the identity, and make the formerly accessible sense of self less accessible through the acquired second language. Greenson, a psychoanalyst, writes of this phenomenon in his article "The Mother Tongue and the Mother," in which he describes the psychoanalytic treatment of a German-speaking patient, which was conducted primarily in English, and sometimes in German. He quotes the patient, "I have the feeling that talking in German I shall have to remember something I wanted to forget. . . . In German I am a scared, dirty child; in English I am a nervous, refined woman." He goes on to explain, "The new language, in this case English, offered this patient an opportunity to build up a new defensive system against her past infantile life. . . . A new language offers an opportunity for the establishment of a new self-portrait. This may supplant the old images, or new images may co-exist along with the old, which might lead to a kind of 'multiple' personality" (9).

This division in the personality may persist as a useful adaptation, or may be maladaptive. If the clinician does not entertain the possibility that there may be separate defenses functioning in each language, then this difficulty may be missed entirely. Such a division in the personality may be difficult to integrate in treatment unless the issue of language is addressed. For example, it may be useful to ask patients, when they seem hesitant, or stuck, if there is something they feel they could better express in their mother tongue. Even if the clinician does not speak that language, having the patient express herself in her mother tongue may free up the content to then be expressed in English (6). I have used this technique with positive results. Greenson addressed this issue in his treatment (described earlier) by using both languages in the treatment in the service of integration of the patient's experiences, which were segregated by language.

Many people have difficulty to express affect when speaking a nonnative language (2,10,11). This may be related to several factors. First, verbalizing in a second language requires greater intellectual focus if one must mentally translate while speaking, and then back translate while listening. The amount of energy this requires displaces the affect associated with the content (2). Furthermore, new language acquisition is an intellectual endeavor, requiring effort and concentration in a way which the development of the mother tongue did not (10). The mother tongue is learned by imitation and incorporation of the mother (9) and is concurrent with emotional development, and mastery. Emotions are experienced and named in the mother tongue. The two evolve together and foster one another. The emotions then become closely associated to the words of the mother tongue, and are not easily translated. Affect may be inaccessible in the second language, that is, isolated to the mother tongue.

In treatment, the second language may even be used as a defense against affect (9). The use of the second, more intellectualized language fosters the defenses of intellectualization, and reaction formation (2). In my own clinical experience, native speakers of English occasionally express something in a foreign language, often something emotionally laden, or uncomfortable. The use of the second language creates an emotional distance from the content, and serves the purpose of splitting off or isolating the affect. If this is not recognized, the affect may be displaced into behavior, acted out (2). In these instances, I encourage patients to say in English what they have said in a foreign language, and then inquire about the affective associations, and how it feels to express in English.

Conversely, some patients may experience greater access to affect in English as the second language.

Case Example: A young female graduate student of Chinese origin presented to the psychiatric emergency department with complaints of depression and suicidal thoughts. She had been living in the United States for some years and was proficient in English. An interpreter was offered to her because language proficiency can be affected by mental and emotional state. She declined, explaining that she was not accustomed to talking about her feelings or emotional experiences in Chinese, as this was not done in her culture, in her experience. She felt much better able to explain what was troubling her in English, rather than needing to "translate" this experience into a language that had never been for her a language for the expression of internal experience and emotion. The interview proceeded and the patient appeared to have no difficulty explaining her situation, responding to questions fully, and engaging in a conversation about treatment options.

In this case it was not the mother tongue to which the patient had affective associations, but to the acquired language. The use of the second language facilitated a therapeutic encounter. Use of the second language to facilitate a therapeutic effect has been observed by others as well (2,9).

I have explored some of the major difficulties encountered in the assessment and psychiatric treatment of cross-cultural patients who speak English fairly well, and how to facilitate treatment under the circumstances. It is important to remember that it is not the same as working with native speakers of English, and that careful attention to this fact may be enormously helpful.

III. WORKING WITH CROSS-CULTURAL PATIENTS WHO DO NOT SPEAK ENGLISH

In many instances, cross-cultural patients speak little or no English at all, which produces an entirely new set of challenges. Medical interpreters must be used to make clinical evaluation and treatment of these patients possible. In the second part of this chapter, I will focus on the use of interpreters in clinical medicine and psychiatry, and present the evidence supporting use of professional interpreters and the dangers of using untrained interpreters. I will then explore the special difficulties and psychodynamic implications of treating non–English-speaking patients working through interpreters. Recommendations will be made for optimizing the clinical evaluation and management of psychiatric patients who are not primarily English speaking.

A. The Argument for Trained Medical Interpreters

The fundamental goal of interpretation is faithfulness (12). To be able to achieve this goal the interpreter must understand the task at hand, its purpose, and the means for achieving it. Most trained interpreters have had instruction in medical terminology, have passed rigorous language-proficiency tests, and have hours of practice interpreting in clinical settings. Professionals are adept not only in this technical aspect of their work, but are also educated about the importance of maintaining as neutral a role as possible, patient confidentiality, and professional boundaries.

Years ago, in many hospitals, it was the expectation that patients with limited English proficiency would provide their own interpreters, such as family members or friends. Revision of civil rights laws, in particular the 1964 Civil Rights Act Title VI, which prohibits discrimination based on national origin, began to bring attention to the need for interpreters in medical settings as a means for assuring equal access to care.

It is obvious to most clinicians that there would be significant and potentially dangerous consequences of evaluating and treating a patient if the patient and physician were unable to speak to one another. It is impossible to diagnose a condition and treat a patient without first taking a thorough history. Without an adequate medical history, the risk of misdiagnosis, unnecessary tests, incorrect treatment, and adverse outcomes is high. It is less obvious to most clinicians that professional interpreters are far superior to family members, friends, or volunteer interpreters—including untrained clinical or ancillary staff—though many studies support this conclusion. Diagnostic accuracy is higher, patient outcomes are better, and patient satisfaction is greater when trained interpreters are used (7,13–19). In addition, sensitivity to cultural issues that may affect the physician–patient interaction is higher among trained interpreters than nontrained interpreters (4,7).

Accuracy rates with family-member interpreters were demonstrated by a 1988 study in Britain using videotaped interviews of Gujarati-speaking patients being interviewed by physicians with family members acting as interpreters. The four recorded interviews were subsequently independently translated and analyzed by the investigators for accuracy. Raters concluded that 16% to 29% of simple questions were misinterpreted, and 25% to 82% of complex questions were misinterpreted. Finally, they concluded that 70% accuracy was the best that could be expected, and that all interviews were badly misleading for linguistic or cultural reasons (20).

There are a number of reasons why family members do not, in general, make good medical interpreters. The most basic difficulty is inadequate language skills; furthermore, language ability may be difficult to assess. Stress and family dynamics compromise the ability of a family member to function as an interpreter for a patient. Family members are affected by the illness of a patient, and must continue in their roles as family members. Asking family to perform another function can add further stress, which can cause a dramatic decline in the ability to function in a second language. It is particularly stressful and even frightening for a young child to interpret, because children usually lack the sophistication of language to be able to convey complicated information, and may be overwhelmed by having to convey emotionally laden information (4). A clinical case report has even documented the occurrence of a posttraumatic stress syndrome in a young girl who acted as the medical interpreter through the extended serious illness of a younger sibling (21).

Family dynamics of hierarchy, propriety, and cultural beliefs may interfere with the ability of a family member to interpret well (4). A patient may not want to speak of embarrassing symptoms in front of a family member and may feel unable to ask for another interpreter. Haffner (4) gives the example from her experience of a Spanish-speaking patient whose son acted as the medical interpreter. The patient fabricated symptoms for three visits to her physician because she was too embarrassed to say in front of her son what the real problem was, and felt unable to request an interpreter when none was offered. Only when the son was not available and an interpreter had to be called was the patient able to express the true nature of her complaints. Psychiatric symptoms may be particularly difficult to assess because of the guilt and shame that many people feel about psychiatric illness. The patient may be reluctant to talk about the symptoms, and if he does, the family may be reluctant to interpret what the patient says. If the cultural beliefs of the patient and their family conflict with the customary practices of American medicine (e.g., telling patients directly about their illness and involving the patient in treatment decision making), the family may modify or leave out a great deal of what the physician says to the patient, even if not consciously (4). For these reasons, most authors in this field caution against using family members as interpreters, and make even stronger recommendations against expecting children to perform this function (4,7,13,15,21).

Using other untrained staff as interpreters presents problems as well. For example, if bilingual staff members are asked to volunteer as interpreters but have full-time responsibilities in other roles, such as patient care, maintenance, housekeeping, or clerical duties, then interpreting may conflict with their primary duties. Also, they may lack the medical sophistication necessary to perform the role of interpreter or the appropriate training in the importance of boundaries and confidentiality, and may not appreciate the purpose of the clinical encounter. Westermeyer (7) gives an example of this that is humorous, but illustrates the potentially serious consequences of using an interpreter with no training. A hospital janitor was asked to interpret in an emergency room setting for a patient who was brought in by police for bizarre behavior. With this interpreter, the patient's mental status was found to be normal. When a trained staff interpreter arrived, the janitor was heard to say to the patient, "don't tell them that, they'll think you're crazy." Evaluation with the staff interpreter revealed psychosis.

When a clinician is truly bilingual, he or she may be in the best position to evaluate the patient who is non-English speaking but shares another common language with the clinician. However, it is important to be aware of the risks of this approach. If the common language is the maternal language of both clinician and patient, this presents no problems. If the primary language of the patient is a second language for the clinician, then the clinician must rely on his own assessment of his language skills, and unless he has had practice in doing evaluations in the second language, may find it more difficult than he supposed (4,7). If a clinician would like to conduct the interview in his second language, the native language of the patient, then it is advisable to have an interpreter included so as to minimize unrecognized miscommunications. There is significant risk of poor communication where both patient and clinician are speaking in a language that is a second language for them both. In this case, it is far better to use a professional interpreter.

Growing recognition of the problems associated with volunteer interpreters, or family members and friends of patients, and of the superiority of professional interpreters, has led to new standards for hospitals, and even to legislation in some states calling for availability of competent qualified interpreters for non–English-speaking patients. For example, in July 2001, Massachusetts passed a law to ensure effective communication between healthcare professionals and non–English-speaking patients; it specifies that competent interpreter services be available at no cost to all emergency and psychiatric patients.

Despite the recognition of the superiority of professional interpreters, there are clearly shortfalls in their availability. A 1995 National Public Hospital Institute survey of 83 public and private hospitals cited by Baker (18) showed that 11% of all patients needed language interpreters, and 27% required interpreters in one third of the hospitals surveyed. Despite this need, this same survey showed limited interpreter availability, little or no standardization in interpreter training and no training for hospital professionals in how to collaborate with interpreters. In this survey hospital staff, family members of patients, or other staff did most of the interpreting (18). Studies conducted in Geneva, Switzerland, and South Africa show similar findings (3,13–15,17,18).

Major barriers to use of interpreters include economic support, lack of availability of trained professional interpreters, and lack of clinician recognition of the dangers of not using interpreters. Thus, even if excellent interpretation is available, it is not so useful if clinicians are not taught how to recognize the need for interpretation, and how to work with interpreters most effectively.

B. Challenges in the Clinical Interview with a Medical Interpreter

Although the challenges inherent in the clinical evaluation of the non–English-speaking patient are minimized when professional or trained interpreters are used, they are nonetheless significant. The interpreter is not a mere conveyor of messages. This oversimplified view does not take into account the cultural interpretation that may be an implicit function of the interpreter, nor does it take into account the dynamics of introducing a third person into what is usually a dyadic situation (7). Technical, cultural, and dynamic issues can all create potential difficulties while working with interpreters. This section will address these potential difficulties.

There are three basic models of interpretation: simultaneous, line by line, and summarization. All three models have advantages and disadvantages. The simultaneous model is the most time efficient and most accurate. It is the model used by the United Nations. The interpreter listens and interprets simultaneously, staying a few words behind the speaker. It requires highly skilled interpreters and is very difficult to do. It is more exhausting for the interpreter who must maintain exquisite focus.

In the line-by-line model, the speaker says one line and pauses for the interpreter to render the communication into the language of the listener. This method is time intensive, and if complex sentences are used, information may be missed or lost. In the summarization method the speaker states a complete thought, and then the interpreter summarizes the information for the listener. This method is time efficient, but much less accurate. Seemingly unimportant details may be lost, or facts may be distorted (22).

Technical difficulties arise for both clinician and interpreter. Interpreters may distort factual information due to summarizing or paraphrasing. This may limit the accuracy of the interview and cause the need for more clarification. In addition, there is an inherent tendency to normalize or to make sense of what does not make sense (7,12), which may especially affect the integrity of the psychiatric interview. The following example illustrates both the problem with summarizing and with normalizing. Marcos (12) described the following exchange when a patient was asked if he had any worries:

Patient:. . .I know that God is with me, I'm not afraid, they cannot get me [pause] I'm wearing these new pants and I feel protected, I feel good, I don't get headaches anymore.

Interpreter: He says that he is not afraid, he feels good, he doesn't get headaches anymore.

It is clear to someone with psychiatric training that the message conveyed by the interpreter misses very important information, which would influence the assessment of the mental status. Interpreters who have more experience and training in psychiatric interviewing tend to be more aware of these risks, but they are nonetheless present, and omission of information may happen unconsciously.

Differences in cultural expectations or ethical values may also challenge the clinician and interpreter interaction. Many authors describe that conflict and ethical dilemmas may arise for the interpreters when they realize that the clinician's approach makes cultural assumptions which may not apply to the patient, and then must decide to interpret accurately and risk adversely affecting the interaction, or to interpret what may seem more culturally appropriate, but is technically less accurate. For example, Putsch (23) described the following interview:

Psychiatrist: "Ask her how long she thinks she'll need to take these medications."

Interpreter [in Vietnamese]: "He says you should take this medicine for two weeks and then come back and see him." The return date and appointment were discussed in Vietnamese.

Interpreter: "She says she'll take the medicines for two weeks and then she'll come back to see you."

In this situation, the interpreter thought it culturally appropriate to be more directive to the patient rather than asking for the patient's input in the treatment planning process, which was what the psychiatrist was doing. The interpreter made the decision to change what was being said on both sides. Though technically this is not how interpretation should be done, one could easily argue that it was in the best interest of the patient. In this case, the interpreter could interrupt the interview and suggest to the psychiatrist that there may be a more culturally appropriate way to handle the discussion with the patient.

For the past several years, I have worked with the interpreter service at Massachusetts General Hospital (MGH), leading debriefing and process groups. This issue also comes up frequently in those group discussions, regarding the clinical context of obtaining informed consent, and discussing treatment options and prognosis with patients. In the United States, informed consent usually involves fully disclosing all of the risks inherent in treatments and procedures, and patients are actively included in discussions about treatment options and prognosis. The interpreters argue that, in some cases, to interpret all the details is culturally inappropriate and perhaps even detrimental to the patients. For example, they describe a common scenario in which a patient, who is from a culture where medicine is more paternalistic, needs to give consent for a diagnostic or treatment procedure. When all the potential risks are disclosed, including, as often is the case, the risk of death, some patients refuse the procedures altogether. They do not expect to be told they could die from that which is supposed to be beneficial for them.

Similarly, the MGH interpreters have described conflicts about informing patients of treatment options or prognosis, particularly when the prognosis is poor. In general, it is the practice in medicine in the United States to inform patients and to include them in medical decision making. The interpreters explain that, in some cultures, families are informed and make decisions, but information is kept from the patient. This is in conflict with the Western medical model, and yet if interpreters are to be accurate they must interpret exactly what health care providers say to patients. Kaufert and Putsch (24) describe similar dilemmas, and further discuss the ethical dimension of interviews with interpreters. They suggest that some of the dilemmas and conflicts may be untenable within the currently widely accepted model of medical interpretation in which accuracy is the main goal.

Cultural conflicts impacting the evaluation of patients may also arise between the interpreter and the patient (7). The following is a composite case based on the experiences of interpreters and clinicians at MGH.

> *Case Example:* An interpreter was asked to participate in an interview on the inpatient psychiatric unit. The female interpreter and male patient were from the same region of the world, though not the same country, and shared the same mother tongue. In the patient's culture of origin, a woman would not be in the position of "speaking for" a man, nor would she be expected to dress in the American style that this interpreter had adopted. Throughout the interview, the patient was making disparaging remarks to the interpreter, which were not interpreted to the clinician. Eventually, the interpreter was so upset that she had to stop the interview and leave the room. Afterwards she explained to the clinician what had happened.

In this case, if the interpreter had followed the principle "interpret everything," this conflict could have been identified earlier and action taken to address the conflict which was interfering with the evaluation process.

C. Psychodynamic Factors in Working with Interpreters

In any encounter between two or more people, dyadic or group dynamics arise. Usually in the psychiatric interview the clinician listens for the dynamics to emerge in the content and process, and pays attention to transference and countertransference dimensions to further understand the dynamics at play. In the interview involving an interpreter, most writers on the subject note that the principal difference is that the dyadic situation becomes a triadic, or group situation (7,25). As such the clinician has the more complicated task of monitoring three relationships instead of one and the dynamics involved become much more complex. Some of the most commonly encountered dynamic issues will be discussed in this section.

In the triadic situation, a power dynamic is inherently present and may have a detrimental effect on the patient evaluation if not recognized and managed. The interpreter is in the most powerful role, as she holds the keys to the communication; both other participants are essentially helpless to communicate without her. The clinician, who is accustomed to being in charge, is suddenly no longer able to use his usual abilities to assess meanings, emotion, and mental status because he must depend on the interpreter (23); yet, the clinician still holds all the responsibility for the clinical situation. This raises the potential for the clinician to resent the interpreter, and to feel left out by the interpreter/patient pair. The patient is the least powerful in the situation, being both dependent on the interpreter for communication, and being in the vulnerable role of patient. Some patients may feel overwhelmed by this two-on-one situation, especially if they are paranoid.

Clinicians and interpreters can negotiate the power dynamic by understanding their roles and their interdependence, and by appreciating the position of the patient. Often the emergence of anger can be a clue to the presence of a power differential and the resulting feeling of helplessness. For example, if the clinician begins to get annoyed or angry with the interpreter, or vice versa, it would be time to consider a power dynamic at play and to address it. Ultimately it is the responsibility of the clinician to notice and to manage these dynamics. Often it is helpful for the clinician to stop the interview, and leave the room to confer with the interpreter about what is happening.

Just as in any group, other dynamics may arise in the clinician-interpreter-patient grouping. As discussed earlier, there is a powerful emotional attachment to the mother tongue, which the patient may project onto the interpreter who speaks and understands it, and thus she may experience the interpreter as "good," as more understanding and more empathic than the clinician, who may seem "bad," or more distant due to her inability to speak the same language. Clinicians, too, may experience a feeling of distance from the patient (26). Not only can this splitting interfere with the clinician–patient alliance, but it may also lead to further complications. The interpreter, sensing the emotional attachment the patient feels toward him, may feel pulled to get involved with the patient. For example, the interpreters at MGH describe that patients frequently appeal to them for advice about what they should do, what medical decisions they should make. At other times, patients may even confide in the interpreter information they do not want the clinician to know, and ask that the interpreter not share the information. This is another set up for splitting, and can only be avoided by clear communication between interpreter and clinician, and by a clear definition of roles. In another scenario, the patient engages the interpreter in an ongoing conversation, and pretty soon the clinician is standing by, completely out of the loop. Again, it is crucial here for the clinician to interrupt, and confer with the interpreter about the goals of the interview and the roles of clinician and interpreter.

If the interpreter's identification with the patient is significant, then the interpreter may feel compelled to respond differently than she might usually, if even unwittingly, by advising the patient or distorting or leaving out information, or by arguing with the clinician's recommendations to the patient (26,27). A helpful way to address this type of countertransference enactment is to be alert to the possibility and for clinicians to educate interpreters about transference and countertransference phenomena. Mellman (27) has suggested that a useful signal for both clinicians and interpreters is to note when they find themselves doing something out of the ordinary for a patient. The following case example illustrates a transference/countertransference enactment but which could also be viewed as a difference of cultural expectations.

Case Example: A young female interpreter at MGH had interpreted many times for an elderly woman who was originally from the same country that she was from. The elderly patient became fond of the interpreter, would refer to her as "like a daughter," and would greet her with kisses, as she would a relative. The interpreter noted that ordinarily in her job she would not greet patients in such a way, but concluded that because this was the custom in their home country, she would allow it. She too had become fond of the patient.

In this example, the interpreter noted that she was doing something out of the ordinary. She attributed it to cultural custom from the home country and did not consider it further. It is useful to look at such examples, which may seem insignificant, but may interfere with the ability of the interpreter to do her job as well as usual. Mellman noted that, "While blatant errors in translation can be obvious, subtle countertransference errors can go unnoticed" (27). Although the interpreter's involvement with the patient may seem culturally appropriate and not blatantly problematic, the real potential for subtle unconscious errors is a strong argument for discouraging such involvement.

The MGH interpreters describe another common phenomenon, of feeling like they are emotional filters or "affect sponges" between clinician and patient. As previously discussed, emotion is most expressed in the mother tongue, and does not always translate. Interpreters strive to convey emotion as well as content, though in the process of interpretation in both directions the affect may not get transferred with the linguistic messages. In effect the interpreters may end up holding the affect of the interaction, which can leave them feeling burdened or overwhelmed. This is particularly true when the interview with a patient is emotionally laden, as when the content includes grief, life tragedy, poor prognosis of an illness, or loss.

Case Example: A young interpreter was involved with the care of a patient who was dying and had to inform the family members of the prognosis. She had interpreted for the patient many times, and felt she had come to know the family well. The information was shared with the family, and the interpreter was present as the family processed the news. Immediately afterwards she was called to see another patient, but felt so overwhelmed by the previous encounter that it was difficult for her to focus on the next interview.

A survey of Red Cross interpreters in Geneva assessed the emotional impact on interpreters of difficult patient interviews. Many of the interviews were of refugees who were traumatized. The study found that overall 83% of interpreters surveyed (n = 22) had a strong need to talk and to share feelings with the doctor after the patient interview (28). The article concludes that not enough attention is given to the emotional impact on interpreters of the work they do. I concur with this assessment based on my experience doing process and debriefing work with interpreters.

D. Optimizing the Clinician-Interpreter-Patient Interview

I have suggested in the previous sections some of the ways that specific difficulties in the interpreted interview can be avoided or mitigated, and will expand on that in this section. I will review the points as they would arise in conducting an interview, that is, beginning with deciding to call an interpreter, and ending with concluding the interview with the patient, and debriefing with the interpreter.

At the outset, it is important to be clear about when an interpreter is needed for a cross-cultural patient. In general, always call one when it is evident that the patient has limited understanding and/or speaking ability in English. Always request one when a patient asks, even if he seems fluent in English. Have a low threshold to request an interpreter when a patient's chief complaint may suggest depression, psychosis, a significant medical illness, or another alteration in mental status.

Next, it is important to request an interpreter who can interpret in the patient's mother tongue. This may sound obvious, but it is striking, for example, the number of times the MGH Spanish interpreters are called to see Portuguese-speaking patients. This usually occurs because Spanish interpreters are more readily available than Portuguese interpreters, not because there is confusion about the patient's mother tongue. The MGH interpreters must often explain to clinicians, who assume Spanish and Portuguese are similar enough that a Spanish interpreter will suffice for a Portuguese-speaking patient, that Spanish and Portuguese are different languages, and that it is not appropriate for Spanish interpreters to interpret for Portuguese-speaking patients and vice versa. Many hospitals display large posters indicating in multiple languages the availability of interpreters. This is helpful for identifying the appropriate interpreter as long as the patient can read her native language. If a patient is unable to read, and is unable to convey what language he speaks, interpreter services may be able to assist.

Once the interpreter arrives, it is helpful to spend a few minutes discussing the purpose of the interview, the goals to be accomplished, and any other information that may be relevant. For instance, it can be helpful to say, "the patient may not make sense, but it will be helpful to me if you interpret everything as closely as possible even if it does not make sense to you." I also prepare interpreters, when applicable, for the possibility that patients may be agitated, or otherwise uncooperative. It is important to clarify what type of interpreting method will be used (simultaneous, line by line, or summarization); simultaneous and line by line are more accurate. The clinician should also encourage the interpreter to interrupt the interview when clarifications are needed, or to stop the interview and confer outside the room when necessary. This is particularly helpful when conflicts in cultural expectations or dynamic issues arise.

Before beginning the interview, introductions should be made and the chairs arranged. Most writers on this subject recommend a triangle arrangement (29) so that all parties can easily see one another. During the interview, the clinician should address the patient directly, in the second person, and maintain eye contact with the patient. This will optimize forming an alliance.

It is helpful for the clinician to speak slowly, to use simple sentences, and to pause frequently. Avoid jargon, technical terms, and overly complicated language. If patients are speaking too quickly for the interpreter to keep up, interrupt and clarify when necessary.

Finally, when the interview is concluded, spend a few minutes debriefing with the interpreter. Ask if there is anything important that she noticed and would like to point out, if there were any cultural issues which may have affected the integrity of the interview, and also, ask if the interpreter would like to discuss her personal response or to process feelings that may have arisen during the encounter.

IV. CONCLUSION

With the increasing numbers of non–English-speaking residents in the United States, hospitals and clinics are facing the challenge of providing equal access to care for non–English-speaking patients. Meeting the challenge will require not only increased availability of trained professional interpreters and training for clinicians who will be working with them, but also a better understanding of the implications of diagnosing conditions and treating patients in collaboration with medical interpreters. In addition, increased sensitivity to the language issues that exist in working with patients who speak English as a second language will optimize clinical work with this population.

REFERENCES

1. Grinberg L, Grinberg R. *Psychoanalytic perspectives on migration and exile.* New Haven and London: Yale University, 1989.
2. Marcos LR, Urcuyo L. Dynamic psychotherapy with the bilingual patient. *Am J Psychother* 1979; 33:331–338.
3. Drennan G, Swartz L. The paradoxical use of interpreting in psychiatry. *Soc Sci Med* 2002;54: 1853–1866.
4. Haffner L. Translation is not enough: interpreting in a medical setting. *West J Med* 1992;157:255–259.
5. Diaz-Duque OF. Overcoming the language barrier: advice from an interpreter. *Am J Nurs* 1982;82: 1380–1382.
6. Oquendo MA. Psychiatric evaluation and psychotherapy in the patient's second language. *Psychiatr Serv* 1996;47:614–618.
7. Westermeyer J. Working with an interpreter in psychiatric assessment and treatment. *J Nerv Ment Dis* 1990;178:745–749.
8. Nicassio PM, Solomon GS, Guest SS, et al., Emigration stress and language proficiency as correlates of depression in a sample of Southeast Asian refugees. *Int J Soc Psychiatry* 1986;32:22–28.
9. Greenson RR. The mother tongue and the mother. *Int J Psychoanal* 1950;31:18–23.
10. Cheng LY, Lo HT. On the advantages of cross-culture psychotherapy: the minority therapist/mainstream patient dyad. *Psychiatry* 1991;54:386–396.
11. Marcos LR. Bilinguals in psychotherapy: language as an emotional barrier. *Am J Psychother* 1976; 30:552–560.
12. Marcos LR. Effects of interpreters on the evaluation of psychopathology in non-English-speaking patients. *Am J Psychiatry* 1979;136:171–174.
13. Bischoff A, Tonnerre C, Eytan A, et al. Addressing language barriers to health care: a survey of medical services in Switzerland. *Soz Präventivmed* 1999;44:248–256.
14. Bischoff A, Tonnerre C, Loutan L, et al. Language difficulties in an outpatient clinic in Switzerland. *Soz Präventivmed* 1999;44:283–287.
15. Drennan G. Counting the cost of language services in psychiatry. *S Afr Med J* 1996;86:343–345.
16. Woloshin S, Bickell NA, Schwartz LM, et al. Language barriers in medicine in the United States. *JAMA* 1995;273:724–728.
17. Baker DW, Parker RM, Williams MV, et al. Use and effectiveness of interpreters in an emergency department. *JAMA* 1996;275:783–788.

18. Baker DW, Hayes R, Fortier JP. Interpreter use and satisfaction with interpersonal aspects of care for Spanish-speaking patients. *Med Care* 1998;36:1461–1470.
19. Ngo-Metzger Q, Massagli MP, Clarridge BR, et al. Linguistic and cultural barriers to care. *J Gen Intern Med* 2003;18:44–52.
20. Ebden P, Carey OJ, Bhatt A, et al. The bilingual consultation. *Lancet* 1988;1:347.
21. Jacobs B, Kroll L, Green J, et al. The hazards of using a child as an interpreter. *J R Soc Med* 1995; 88:474P–475P.
22. Brooks TR. Pitfalls in communication with Hispanic and African-American patients: do translators help or harm? *J Natl Med Assoc* 1992;84:941–947.
23. Putsch RW III. Cross-cultural communication. The special case of interpreters in health care. *JAMA* 1985;254:3344–3348.
24. Kaufert JM, Putsch RW. Communication through interpreters in healthcare: ethical dilemmas arising from differences in class, culture, language, and power. *J Clin Ethics* 1997;8:71–87.
25. Baxter H, Cheng LY. Use of interpreters in individual psychotherapy. *Aust N Z J Psychiatry* 1996; 30:153–156.
26. Musser-Granski J, Carrillo DF. The use of bilingual, bicultural paraprofessionals in mental health services: issues for hiring, training, and supervision. *Commun Ment Health J* 1997;33:51–60.
27. Mellman LA. Countertransference in court interpreters. *Bull Am Acad Psychiatry Law* 1995;23: 467–471.
28. Loutan L, Farinelli T, Pampallona S. Medical interpreters have feelings too. *Soz Präventivmed* 1999; 44:280–282.
29. Phelan M, Parkman S. How to work with an interpreter. *BMJ* 1995;311:555–557.

11

Prejudice and Institution, Change and Resistance

Dismantling the Children's Psychiatric Hospital of Attica

[*,†]Stelios Stylianidis, [‡]M-G Lily Stylianoudi, and [†]Panayiotis Chondros

[*]*Children's Psychiatric Hospital of Attica,* [†]*Scientific Association for Regional Development and Mental Health (EPAPSY), and* [‡]*Research Center for Greek Society, Academy of Athens, Athens, Greece*

I. INTRODUCTION

In this chapter, we attempt to describe the mechanisms set in motion by psychiatric reform in Greece by using our experience with the Children's Psychiatric Hospital of Attica (CPHA; also known as Daou) as an example. Psychiatric reform encounters a plexus of resistance translating all the prejudices that exist and are created in places like asylums. This chapter consists of the gathering and recording of the experience of the three authors—each of whom has a different relationship with and position in the CPHA—through participant observation and open interviews, using discourse analysis methodology. Stelios Stylianidis, a psychiatrist and psychoanalyst, is the current director of the CPHA. Panayiotis Chondros, a psychologist, is a volunteer participant on the CPHA Work and Planning Team. M-G Lily Stylianoudi, a jurist-anthropologist, collected the material for this chapter within the context of a planned study of the deinstitutionalization of the CPHA. Together, we are attempting both to combine our experiences and to overcome our own prejudices and resistance.

Three writers, three readings, and three texts form the mosaic of this chapter using four different approaches: social and cultural psychiatry, psychoanalysis, social anthropology, and psychology. This meeting occurs in the field of experience, the common locus of living experience formed by human suffering, where people come—wittingly or not—to reconcile their differences. Human suffering forms a space where communication takes place (1), because it can function as and at the same time create a *nonlieu* (2), in the sense that a *nonlieu* does not house any organic society and is where the hazy play of identity and relation is eternally inscribed. The *nonlieu* constitutes "the locus of the inscribed and symbolized meaning" (2). The translation of this experience, the verbalizing of the researchers' personal grief so that the written text could be published in the form of a chapter, came into conflict with our individual history and brought us up against a double prejudice: On the one hand, each of us had to set aside the tools of our specialties and meet at a locus where discussion would be feasible, which meant putting aside stereotypical representations each had of the others' fields. Moreover, we also needed to set aside our prejudices toward what was said by CPHA employees. So, throughout the process of writing, our presentation of the context and of individual, intrapsychic problematics had to call into question both our scientific ideology and how scientific we were being, so that this meeting could be possible and meaning be advanced.

Yet, a true process of participant observation cannot, by definition, be neutral. The emotions and the prejudices of the researchers—especially during this period of psychiatric reform and changes within the asylum—remained and remain in the background of our scientific analysis and attempt to understand the psychic reality of the research team. The fact does not escape us (indeed, it was a running conversation among the writers) that the necessary distance and *a posteriori* analysis of the meanings of the psychic actions and behavioral patterns of CPHA employees were essentially not feasible. Consequently, the underlying tone of this chapter may be interwoven with intense feelings of anger, fear, and indignation. It is possibly laced as well with psychic and social representations of the idea of Self, including the savior syndrome, in which one must prevail over the corruption, the organized practice of exclusion, and the ignorance of patients' suffering that are imposed by the domination of asylum logic. We tried not to allow the inevitable idealization of the act of change to lead us, at least *a posteriori*, to reject the existence of blind spots and scapegoat mechanisms as well as to engage in splitting between the "good" (change) and "evil" (corruption, homoeostasis) of the asylum reality.

II. PREJUDICE

This chapter takes a psychodynamic approach to prejudice, along with elements of a cognitive framework. Prejudice could be more generally defined as an apparently unjustifiable negative behavior, an undesirable and unfair attitude toward an individual or a particular group. We consider prejudice to be the result of defense mechanisms, such as projection and displacement, that are activated to settle an intrapsychic conflict, whereas a stereotype is a cognitive structure containing the knowledge, beliefs, and expectations an individual has about a group. We attempt to synthesize the psychodynamic and cognitive approaches using a psychoanalytical method to interpret the phenomena conceived by the researchers as prejudices operating within the employees of the CPHA.

In English, as in other European languages, prejudice (3) refers mainly to a point of view (predecision, prejudgement) or an opinion (preconception) formed well before the adoption of associated elements; thus the opinion or point of view is based on inadequate or even imaginary elements. In Greek, prejudice is a derivative of the verb *prokatalamvano*, whose first historical citation meant "to seize beforehand or occupy in advance, *particularly by use of military force*" (emphasis added)—to outrun, to anticipate, and to dominate and possess (4). In rhetoric, it appears with the meaning "to pre-empt someone or something through speech, anticipate" and "to have a preconception of, understand beforehand" (4). In more contemporary language, a metaphorical meaning of prejudice is to persuade a person to form an opinion in advance of any adequate examination, to predispose a person toward someone or something. Consequently, the word *prejudice* has four basic dictionary meanings: (i) advance occupation, seizure; (ii) a rhetorical form by which the speaker preempts and then refutes potential objections from opponents; (iii) preliminary perception or learning; and (iv) (in modern Greek) an opinion, especially pejorative, formed and influenced without experience or a thorough examination of the matter, *especially when related to a perceived evil* (emphasis added). Correspondingly, an encyclopedic dictionary (5) gives the meaning as a "roughly formed opinion, without the required assessment of the matter due to the influence of personal motive or other factors." It is worth noting that publication of this dictionary predates the research on prejudice, and the definition is in line with the scientific data of the period (see La Pierre, 1934 [6]), remaining succinct and precise to this time.

Greek semantics seem to be isolating the basic characteristics of prejudice as being *seizure* and *occupation*, where one subject suffers as a result of the belligerent actions of another hostile agent. *Seizure in advance*, an action that precedes another, places the recipient of prejudice in a position of terrifying weakness against, and possible reaction to, the agent of prejudice. *To overtake and dominate* seems to form the basic characteristic of prejudice, because the prejudice is directly linked with the expression of hostile behavior. However, prejudice also means *perception* and *learning,* corresponding precisely to the idea that firstly, prejudice is learned behavior vis-à-vis the Other, who is unknown, different from the agent, and thus particularly frightening and threatening.

Prejudice encompasses a specific position either for or against a corresponding positive or negative value, as well as an accompanying emotional state. The social sciences primarily examine the perceptual or cognitive element of prejudice, one of many in a phenomenon this complex. This element contains the ideas and opinions we have of those individuals or groups who are the object of premature judgment. This point of view resulting from premature judgment is also called a *stereotype.* At the same time, as ready as the carrier of prejudices is to express him or herself in action, so too is the sufferer of those prejudices. There is, in other words, also an inner readiness for action, the behavioral aspect of prejudice. Both the carrier and the object of prejudice react to whatever they think or feel by behaving in a way reflecting the acceptance or rejection of others. The resulting acts of prejudice constitute varying degrees of *discrimination*, a term closely associated with prejudice and stereotyping.

As seen from the earliest attempts to measure and give meaning to prejudice, it is a complicated phenomenon interacting on various levels of analysis with quite different terms, dependent on or identified with them, interpreted or explained by them, without this interaction always constituting a two-way relation. So, apart from stereotype and discrimination, prejudice also encompasses particular attitudes and behaviors. If prejudice is considered to be the negative dogmatic view of groups different from those to which we belong, and by extension, of individuals from those groups, then we can distinguish, at least theoretically, between prejudice as such and discrimination. Prejudice refers to negative attitudes whereas the behavioral aspect of prejudice constitutes discrimination—behavior directed against those offended by prejudice. Links between the two are not self-evident, as already shown in La Pierre's classic 1934 study (6).

Subsequent research led to the concept of ethnocentrism (7), used to describe the way an "ethnically" focused individual rigorously accepts those culturally similar to him or her and rejects those who are dissimilar. This rejection also includes individuals and groups from within his or her own culture who, nonetheless, deviate from the culture in some way. Thus, it could be seen that prejudice is a general, discriminatory, ethnocentric attitude, creating a "syndrome of attitudes" that also includes the phenomenon of the "scapegoat." What especially distinguishes the study of prejudice by Adorno's prewar team, known as the German Institute for Social Research, is a series of psychoanalytically oriented interviews during which they attempted to interpret the "syndrome of attitudes." They presented a personality theory to explain this phenomenon as resulting from individuals being raised within families with autocratic, tyrannical parents, producing mixed, conflicting feelings. Splitting is produced in the soul of the person with prejudices: these ambivalent feelings toward the parents are distinctly positive and negative. The positive feelings become directed toward the parents, but the negative, hostile feelings are levelled at other targets, such as members of other ethnic groups or those believed to be offending against the status quo and the laws. This fundamental cognitive state is considered dependent on the psychological mechanism of repression, coinciding with Freud's hypothesis of repressed desires. All desires that cause shame and are thus denied are transferred to other individuals. These negative feelings toward the parents remain repressed even throughout adulthood.

A world that produces an individual with prejudices is one that allows him or her to express whatever would otherwise be forbidden. Other people, those who are different, become easy scapegoats, accepting the sentiments originating from prejudiced people "who unload their own guilt in creating these scapegoats, in other words, psychologically transferring their sins onto others" (8). This idea of purification, integrally associated with the scapegoat phenomenon, has been developed considerably in the latest studies and is considered a significant mechanism of self-justification for the transferred aggression that accompanies prejudice (9).

III. DEINSTITUTIONALIZATION AND THE PERSISTENCE OF ASYLUM CULTURE

In the last 50 years, the dominant role of the psychiatric hospital in a psychiatric health care system has been fundamentally challenged, due to various historical, institutional, cultural and scientific circumstances. In many cases, this challenge did not result in an alternative network of psychiatric health care facilities to completely replace the former dominant role of the psychiatric hospital as, for example, happened in certain regions (*regioni*) of Italy. In some countries (e.g., France and Germany), a parallel network of community psychiatric care services was developed; however, no decisive limits were placed on either the continuing investment of essential human and material resources in the perpetuation of the psychiatric hospital or on the symbolic function of the science of psychiatry, as creator of psychiatric institutions. In other cases (e.g., the United States), "deinstitutionalization" was linked with dehospitalization. The number of psychiatric beds were drastically reduced for administrative and financial reasons, without adequate networks of community housing facilities and primary and secondary psychiatric health services having been anticipated and organized. In such cases, we would always maintain that the symbolic, imaginary, actual nexus, as defined by the psychiatric hospital/asylum, remains the same. From the *empty matrixes* of Foucault's leper-houses to the *orthopedic* notion of confronting the uncertainty of the psychopathological phenomenon arising from the asylum culture, from Falret's *moral therapy* to Rotelli's asylum as a *place of zero interchange*; the suffering subject's loss of the ability to negotiate (emotionally, psychically, financially, as a citizen); undifferentiated spaces and time; the sum of rules and rituals denying the body—all are *tesserae* in the same asylum mosaic. So, the critical opportunity and will to abolish psychiatric hospitals, such as the CPHA, does not, as Saraceno (10) notes, simply constitute an "opportunity of charity and humanitarianism, but a technical and scientific one as well (the conversion of the prohibition of therapy to the possibility of therapy)."

IV. BACKGROUND: THE CHILDREN'S PSYCHIATRIC HOSPITAL OF ATTICA AND PSYCHIATRIC REFORM

The CPHA is the only children's psychiatric asylum in Greece. From 1932 until 1961, the hospital's 114 acres operated as a sanatorium. In 1932, the Association for Destitute Sufferers of Tuberculosis built the Zoodohos Pigi Sanatorium, which came under state administration in 1943 and was renamed the State Nursing Sanatorium for Civil Servants. It was subsequently converted into the Public Children's Psychiatric and Neuropsychiatric Hospital with a capacity of 350 beds, and was not known by its current name until 1986.

As with all asylum-type psychiatric institutions, the CPHA once received children from all over Greece with all forms of affliction: severe developmental disorders, childhood psychoses, complex mental and behavioral problems, neurological syndromes, and social problems (e.g., orphans, those abandoned by families in difficulty). Finally, the CPHA received, and in certain cases still receives, children under the age of 18 from welfare institutions throughout the country that are unable to treat cases of complex psychopathology, because they do not possess the adequate infrastructure and essential training. The CPHA staff consists of about 438 employees, of whom 43 hold administrative positions, 35 are doctors, 147 are in nursing, and 44 are technical staff. The remaining 169 belong to various auxiliary categories. There are a total of 132 patients still receiving CPHA services, of whom 96 are male and 36 female, with ages ranging from 15 to 40. The various facilities spread across the CPHA's grounds house 102 individuals, 75 boys and 27 girls.

It should be pointed out that only 15 of the inpatients currently treated at the CPHA are younger than 18 years. Indicatively, the average age of the patients in Annex A is 35 years, and their average length of treatment at CPHA is 25 years! It seems as if the "immobility" of the institution, identified with the "immobility" of time, brings out and crystallizes the fundamental antithesis between the function of the hospital as a children's psychiatric institution (according to its founding charter) and the long-term hospitalization of young adults (no longer children) within it. We observe a refusal, mainly by the professional staff and less so by the nursing staff, to treat patients who from the point of view of their age do not fall under the purview of their specialties. It is as if the evolution and the present state of this children's psychiatric hospital have taken place without their participation, and the guilt and anger resulting from this denial are, almost always, transferred to the inconsistent and slow Ministry of Health.

In the early 1980s, the form and function of the hospital changed and new facilities were established both within the hospital and in the broader community. In 1981, construction of small housing units was completed, with "annexes" intended for patients with low functional and self-help levels, and "lodges" for those with higher degrees of function. 1985 saw the creation of Special Occupational Training Workshops, a Department for Autism in Children, and Outpatient Medical Centers serving the wider public. In 1986, the Special School was formed within the Hospital under the Ministry of Education. The Emergency Unit, also established in 1986, still receives patient referrals from all over Greece. In 2002, the Emergency Unit treated 158 patients, the majority of whom were 17- and 18-year-old boys from Attica not under court order, for stays of over a month.

Between 1984 and 1987, Child Guidance Centers were successively created around Attica in Neo Iraklio, Nea Smyrni, Athens, Rafina (as part of the CPHA) and finally in Pallini. The establishment of these facilities was influenced by community pressure as well as by the need for access to services that could provide psychiatric care without the stigma of the CPHA. Other facilities that continue to provide services to children and adolescents in the community under the umbrella of the CPHA are the Special Therapy Unit for Autism, the Center for Dyslexia, based in Pallini, and *To Litharaki*, a children's day treatment program. *To Litharaki*, along with the Pallini Adolescent Group Home and Pallini Sheltered Living, were all founded between 1984 and 1986, created within the framework of deinstitutionalization directives under EEC regulation 814/84. In these intermediate care facilities, Pallini Group

Home and Pallini Sheltered Living, there are nine individuals younger than age 18 years, six boys and three girls. In the Autism Unit and the Day Treatment Center, 21 individuals receive treatment, of whom 15 are boys and 6 are girls. It is perhaps worth underlining the fact that these community mental health facilities receive a disproportionately large volume of children's psychiatric cases and related requests for counselling, relative to the infrastructure and staffing available. Lastly, we should mention the Foster Family Program, part of the Department of Social Work, which has recently suffered considerable reductions.

There are multiple measures still planned within the context of the ongoing deinstitutionalization of the hospital. These include the transfer of functionally restructured clinics to modern child psychiatry departments at pediatric and general hospitals in Attica, the restructuring of the Emergency Unit in cooperation with community care facilities, and the creation of new community treatment facilities and halfway houses, while reinforcing and upgrading existing community facilities. In particular, four clinics will be transferred to form Departments of Child Psychiatry at regional hospitals in Attica. The Emergency Unit will be reorganized into the Emergency Receiving Division (taking patients up to the age of 14 years), the Adolescent Crisis Center, and the Admissions Unit for emergency community problems. In the community, creation has already begun of a group home serving children with autism-spectrum disorders, and of a short-term residential treatment program. Subsequently, five more short-term residential programs will be built, the occupational workshops will be transferred and upgraded, and the Child Guidance Centers, the Day Treatment Centers, and the Special Therapy Unit for Autism will undergo improvement and operational upgrading.

V. ASYLUM LOGIC AND THE CHILDREN'S PSYCHIATRIC HOSPITAL OF ATTICA

It could perhaps be claimed that, historically, institutionally, and on an operational level, the CPHA has far more in common with the Leros Psychiatric Hospital than with other psychiatric hospitals in Attica. In 1990, international media attention to the inhumane conditions for patients housed at Leros caused an uproar, leading to deinstitutionalization and reform. Similarities with the CPHA include:

- Its location on the eastern fringes of Mt. Pendeli is particularly isolated despite booming development in the area.
- Staff hiring procedures are dependent on a network of patronage relationships (involving various chairmen and local parliamentarians of whichever party is in power) and incorporate hardly any objective assessment criteria.
- There is limited liaison with other medical, psychological, and welfare services.
- Local and broader market networks have been formed specifically to supply goods to the CPHA.
- The inpatient and outpatient facilities of the CPHA emerged more from staff needs and preferences than from an assessment of the needs of those using the services.

- There has been no systematic planning whatsoever for humanizing the CPHA.
- The multiple breached promises of restructuring from Health Ministry leaders over the past 15 years form a colorful mosaic of a distinctive human topography of patients, personnel, stigmatization, and social exclusion of the entire institution from the local community, and social, political, and financial mechanisms—all maintaining and striving for the homoeostasis and immobility of the asylum.

The natural setting for the CPHA could be described as idyllic. Before the great fire on Mt. Pendeli, its slopes were wooded; and there is a wonderful view of southern Evia Bay and the Cyclades. Once, the hospital included special areas such as the gymnasium, Special Primary School, occupational workshops, the Club, a small theatre, and a chapel. All these buildings evoke a sense of nostalgia and loss in many employees, especially those from the administration: "In the good old days, the hospital throbbed with life. Now it's on the wane and they are taking our patients." In the past, a number of child psychiatrists, progressive for their times, had roughly sketched in their minds the creation of an informal "therapeutic community" with diversified treatment activities and areas of care, nursing and housing. The small scale of the Lodges lent itself to such a humane and less impersonal operation. The originality of these attempts at humanizing the asylum is highlighted by the fact that not one of the directors at that time, themselves child psychiatrists, actively questioned the use of locked wards, bars, electroshock therapy, or the enforcement of legislation prescribing "therapeutic measures" for children and teenagers by order of the public prosecutor. It is clear, we believe, from the gradual evolution of the institution, that significant attempts at democratizing and humanizing the CPHA have already been made. However, what has never been substantially called into question, either practically or theoretically, is the core of asylum logic and practice.

The propagation of the institutionalization of asylum logic and for decades, the absolute domination of the doctor-centered model has not been substantially doubted by anyone. The tip of the iceberg is the strictly hierarchical structure of the CPHA administrative team. The director of child psychology at the CPHA, Dr Anna Yioti, notes in her 1999 study on the administration of the CPHA that "they are considered privileged by other employees, and the aim of the majority of employees, professional staff aside, is to be transferred to an Administrative Clerk's position" (11). Administrative clerks systematically avoid all physical and emotional contact with patients; this despite drawing hazard pay for working in unhealthy conditions, based on written verification from each and every administration that they come into contact with patients! As will be seen below, this differs from the position of those who do in fact come into daily contact with the patients.

VI. ASYLUM LOGIC AND CHANGE

The year 2001 was one of important pronouncements on health reform in Greece, with the creation of hospital managers among the multitude of institutional, legislative and administrative changes enacted. Since November of 2001, the Minister of Health has directly appointed hospital directors. In addition, this year saw the institution of regional Periphery Systems for Health (PSH).The chairmen and policy advisers of these local health care catchment areas act as "mini-ministries" of health in their particular district (12). It is worth mentioning that under this system, the hospitals lose their legal and administrative independence and become decentralized units of the PSH. This legal stipulation at first may seem of particular interest for the prospect of modernizing and decentralizing health services in harmony with contemporary Europe. In practice, however, it has created complicated administrative and management problems stemming from a new form of bureaucracy and a re-negotiation of the limits of power and intervention between the PSH and the hospitals.

Within the broader context of calls for reforming the dysfunctional National Health System, attention should be given to the declared political will to implement a 10-year national mental health plan, code named *Psychargos* (13,14). National mental health policy under *Psychargos* follows World Health Organization guidelines and has financial backing from the European Union, under whose rigorous administrative and managerial supervision it falls. The plan, which seems to have secured its requisite financial means, calls for an accelerated dismantling of all asylums in psychiatric centers throughout the country. Five asylums, including the CPHA, are to be gradually abolished before 2006, with the simultaneous development of community mental health facilities throughout the country. Based on an assessment of needs, resources, and the institutional framework of the CPHA by the Management Plan, there are expectations that once the CPHA has been dismantled in 2006, its grounds will house a Center for Physical and Medical Rehabilitation and an upgraded Urban Health Center with a 15-bed Short-Term Care Unit.

International experiences with deinstitutionalization, as well as pilot attempts at psychiatric reform in Greece, demonstrate how many adverse conditions such attempts encounter. To begin with, we know that change in itself is difficult, because any change in any system, *a priori*, sets off reactions, resistances, and insecurity; increases stress, upsets routines and operations that over the years have become entrenched in vested interests; threatens small and large self interests; and calls into question the prevailing, repetitive, asylum culture and rationale and, consequently, the continued operation of every institution. In short, change comes up against and provokes conflicts with the incumbent regime, which creates models due to the years-old entrenched routines; these models have replaced whatever value system once existed and attempt to achieve the institution's founding aims. Change provokes a continual confrontation with the individual's sense of personal continuity affected by unsought change. At a personal level, this transforms the confrontation into personal inquiry in relation to the organizational stability and inflexibility of institutions. This is because change "demands a system based on continuous training and feedback through exchanges and consultation between members of inter-disciplinary groups" (15), which, at least in Greece, only occurs fragmentally and superficially.

VII. INHABITANTS OF THE ASYLUM

The arrival of the new director of the CPHA in November 2001 is typified by the following fundamental paradoxical nature. As he stated himself:

> Unlike other directors designated to modernize, develop and improve the existing functions of a hospital, I was appointed Director of the CPHA not to develop and improve the state of the hospital, but to dismantle its current form as a psychiatric asylum. The restructuring of the CPHA, the aim of the next stage of this dismantling, rang in the ears of employees as a deliberately misleading and unfeasible promise, as being utopian, threatening and insulting. Consequently, my appearance signalled a destructive threat to the present and uncertainty for the future, within the broader unreliability of the State. (Stylianidis, November 12, 2002)

Before analyzing the paradox, it must be pointed out that beyond any fantasies one might have had of the "appointed director," in reality, perhaps the director can be seen as a "messenger" for administration—the far-off center of decision making—and as saddled with change, whatever that change may be. (Here, at this historically significant point in the change, "director" refers to the role and position within CPHA's organization, not to the individual holding that position.) What the messenger conveys may be of positive or negative content and, at least until it is announced, he conveys this ambiguity. Seen this way, the ambiguity of the announcement cloaks the role of director in the corresponding ambiguity, inducing a subsequent ambivalence toward him, a process involving the reinforcement and intensifying of prejudices and resistance, becoming the nexus for the projection of all the prejudices and resistance of hospital employees. This director, appointed from on high, charged with the mission of change, could be in the distinctive position of miracle worker, like the trickster in mythological narrative, a singular character in the myth able to keep the myth rolling. Instead, he becomes an ambiguous, "genderless" figure, thus susceptible to all manner of projections and people's interactive investments with him; he is neutered in the sense of not being recognized as male or female, with this situation reinforced by the sexual/libidinal homoeostasis of the asylum. It must be borne in mind that such enormous changes in institutions assume the proportions of a myth of origin for the social group in whose collective unconscious it is recorded as such, while the protagonists "act" their respective roles, in the sense that they become enmeshed in all the subconscious mechanisms the situation brings into play. The moment of change could become a privileged historic moment permitting participation and psychic investment in it, so that the asylum staff, or at least a large number of them, could become "co-founders" of this myth of origin [see Stylianoudi-Stylianidis (16)]. In this particular case, exactly the opposite is happening. The way in which dominant institutional mechanisms interact and become entwined reinforces the repression of desires in the subject. The institutional environment prevents individuals from being subjected to their desires, substantially shrinking any libidinal investment or reinvestment in other objects of pleasure and creativity. The social and unconscious structure of the institution virtually allows only negative and destructive psychic processes; the death drive seems to outweigh the life drive. At the same time, the director is also the ever so foreign and frightening Big Other:

> I noticed an activation of "conspiracy theories" coming into play from various power sub-centers and other para-institutional interferences, which were decisive in the outcome of issues. When a system cannot basically contain such paranoid mechanisms, deterministically, it propagates their ramifications: envy toward whatever the Other represents,

> destruction and nullification of the Other's ideas and actions, frustration, withdrawal, a sense of futility, meaninglessness and discouragement for a significant proportion of employees who refuse to take part in these long-standing factions and splitting. (Stylianidis, November 12, 2002)

In Greek mythology, the stranger, the different, unfamiliar one on your doorstep, can always turn out to be one of the gods. And despite all the psychoanalytical interpretations this may allude to, it is at this point worth mentioning that Greek society in a way remains rural in structure, despite its apparent urbanization. Most often, this urbanization is, in essence, symbolic, traceable to the social reproduction strategies of Greek families (17). Rural social structure, being traditional, manifests what could be termed "magical" thinking with its equivalent symbolism. At this point it is worth commenting on an event from October 2002, the *thyranoixia* or "opening" of the CPHA's chapel, which provoked a high degree of interest among employees, who came to the ceremony *en masse*, and caused considerable activity throughout the hospital. The delay of the opening ceremony had been linked by employees to a series of misfortunate events, triggered by the arrival of the new director, rendering their ceremony more urgent. One might say the ceremony had become an "exorcism of evil." This self-perpetuating religious patina, which produces certain behavior in the subject on whom it acts and through symbolics operates against those at whom it is directed, is reinforced by its appreciation on the part of the director:

> After my two-month orientation period, I found a common denominator, two common defense mechanisms permeating staff relations and conflicts: multiple dichotomies were at work, good versus evil, between the "insiders" (those from departments within the Hospital and the central administrative structure) and the "outsiders" (those from Medical Pedagogical Centers), each a threat to the other. (Stylianidis, November 12, 2002)

This dichotomy, good versus evil, is the consequence of a Christian ethic that incorporates this dichotomy to give meaning to the world. At the same time, it reinforces the distance between us and the Other. This Other, not belonging to the group, "has all those unacceptable features attributed to the group" (18). This reinforces the collective mechanism of projecting the negative features, inadmissible thoughts and intentions, and unmentionable desires of employees onto someone else, the foreigner, the outsider, the unfamiliar.

So, on the employee level at the CPHA as a whole, we observe a rigid, immobile structure, resulting from the asylum system, permeated by "mythical, magical thinking," wherein the religiosymbolic and the real are inseparable. Fear of the Other, of the "foreigner" easily creates a state where the Other becomes the "scapegoat," against whom any form of excessive behavior (hostility, violence, illegitimate behavior) expiates its agent of any deviance. The "foreign" and "alien" aspects are also intensified by an inability to pinpoint or categorize the Other in specific stereotypical forms, thus intensifying the confusion and disruption, strengthening the imaginary threat from the foreigner and subsequently fuelling existing paranoid mechanisms.

At the CPHA, the director's professional background, family status, tax declaration, and participation in the nongovernmental organization, EPAPSY, remained for considerable time the subject of unrelenting interest and the source of various hypotheses—even in the press—of the "dark motives" behind his appointment (19). There was also a break-in at the office of the director's secretary, presumably to uncover documents containing important information relating to the hospital's reorganization that was hidden from the employees by the administration. These constitute serious penal offences under Greek law. On an individual level, the personal career and history of the present CPHA director, characterized by his participation in the movement for deinstitutionalization and alternative psychiatry, both in Greece and internationally, without political party affiliations, have triggered all these mechanisms through the inefficacy of stereotyping. This cautious, even hostile attitude of employees toward the new "boss" also has a basis in a history of successive appointments of directors, resulting in, among other things, swift, politically based transfers of staff. The fact that the position of director does not mean advancement to anyone already part of the hospital hierarchy possibly strengthens this attitude. Reflections such as: "Directors, like party chairmen and government ministers, are incidental," that "planning takes place in a vacuum, becoming a scenario for despair," that "we are victims of an untrustworthy government," and even personal reflections such as "We employees are to blame for what's happening. Why don't we leave?" constitute a reality which transforms the daily routine of the employees into torture, indicating also the degree of hostility toward appointment holders. The same cautious, suspicious attitude was also seen toward the child psychiatrists, especially those who acted as directors, playing out in relation to any initiatives or innovations they might organize. The basic conviction of nursing staff and administrative heads is that doctors "build their careers on the backs of employees" and "have their little shops," that is, the Medical Pedagogical Centers, where they fulfill their ambitions through the scientific teams they supervise. To all this, we should add a 1995 television program that publicly exposed the prevailing conditions within the institution. The resulting general outcry seems to have strengthened existing paranoid mechanisms and the "conspiracy theories" that dominate both fanciful and realistic discussions among employees. Under these conditions, then, the advent of a new director with an anti-institutional, social psychiatry past, represents, if unjustifiably, a threat to the system.

Returning to the paradoxical nature of the mission of the director entrusted with change at the CPHA, it is clear why discourse around its restructuring into a modern general hospital serving the needs of East Attica residents or a modern physical and medical rehabilitation center sounded like the repetition of false and impracticable promises to employee ears. The significant paradox (perhaps the most "maddening," according to one of the authors), clear to anyone called on to be the bearer of change, is that whereas the overwhelming majority of employees were especially displeased with the status quo, virtually no one wanted to make the least change to operational methods or to the plexus of interactions and "back scratching" that, in the final analysis, make up an institution's world. This translates into an exceptionally complex and elaborate network of mutual support and "patron–client" relationships, woven over the years into the hierarchical structure. It begins with shift and overtime allocations, and ends by crushing any psychic or emotional investment toward the "theoretical" object of any activity within the asylum.

Apart from a number of shining exceptions among the nursing staff, who are constantly in contact with the institutionalized children, and "give their very soul for the best care possible," the remaining staff seem to be totally without incentive or commitment, concerned only with trying to "secure their own survival" by withdrawing to other duties outside the hospital. These exceptional members of the nursing staff are trying to effect a fundamental upgrading of the supply of quality care to patients and taking various initiatives to elevate their role in therapy, including operating as a team, using individualized care planning, and developing socialization programs. However, these initiatives were found to be antithetical to the nursing service leadership team because they drew attention to gaps and inadequacies in their own performance. The main hindrances faced by each motivated employee are the endless bureaucratic procedures ("we must cover ourselves"), which result in the denial of any employee expectation and the downgrading of the care provided.

VIII. THE INFORMAL ORGANIZATION

All that has been cited so far obliges us to examine two important parameters: the *formal* and *informal* organization of the CPHA (20–22), because:

> The size and nature of this informal organization of the CPHA is such that, if the formal organization of the CPHA resembles some huge monster, the informal organization is the shadowy (and thus more frightening) reflection of that freak, and, I daresay, the employees live and work under the cover of that shadow. (Chondros, October 9, 2002)

By *formal organization* we normally refer to what can be recorded on an organizational chart and what relates to the official functioning of a system, administrative procedure, regulations and hierarchy. The CPHA seems to have a sluggish and impersonal bureaucratic system of organization. For example, offices and departments are named using numbers and codes, such as P1 and 319. All administrative staff assume that each request "must have the director's okay and signature," whether it be for boiler maintenance or a child's therapy program. Finally, it is bureaucracy that defines and imposes the pace at which decisions are formally received and implemented, irrespective of the particular weight attached to the office of "director." Thus, a basic inconsistency can be seen in how employees view the position of director and the person holding that position. Let us not forget that the formal organization determines the duties, rights, and obligations of every hospital employee. Bureaucracy imposes a brutal order on the system, often to the detriment of the very patients using the services offered by the CPHA.

The *informal organization*, like the *formal organization,* an integral working part of an operation, refers to relationships between employees and the unofficial methods mobilized to detour official, bureaucratic procedures. Forms of informal organization are unofficial employee communications networks, gossip, and the creation of small groups with similar aims or methods:

> I found the employees are not uninformed, as I had mistakenly believed, but that there is a profuse flow of information related to subjects of immediate concern; however, it is fragmentary and to a large extent either erroneous or distorted. It seems this information especially helps in supporting their position that no change can yield positive results, neither for the patients, nor for the employees, in which case there is no reason for it. For example, according to one nurse's information in relation to dismantling the asylum, the responsibilities of facilities established in the community are being assumed by "quasi-private" companies [nongovernmental organizations], which, by definition, according to her opinion and information, do not provide suitable services and necessary care. The transfer of children from their unit to the community could only be expected to cause disruption to the children by a change of environment and would be to the disadvantage of those working with the children. Another typical example both of wishing no change to the status quo and of how information is distorted, is a phrase in an administration document stating that "the administrative entity will exist until 2006." We were informed that it immediately spread throughout the hospital that "the hospital will continue to exist until 2006." (Chondros, December 11, 2002)

Under normal conditions, informal organization assists in the smooth running of the organization and is legitimate. However, in this particular example, the informal organization has assumed excessive proportions:

> My experience of the Administration of the CPHA has led me to form an image of this form of organization at the CPHA as highly bloated and distorted in the particular form it takes, in relation and correspondence to the formal organization of the hospital. (Chondros, October 9, 2002)

If the formal organization, the bureaucracy, allows the impression to be formed that the hospital is operating as it should, as defined by laws and the standing orders of the organization, the informal organization allows the employees to function as they themselves wish. On an official level, it may be difficult for an outside observer (such as a researcher or evaluator) to collect information on the hospital; it was once said the CPHA "is not on the map." But inside the hospital, any piece of information—decisions, rumours, gossip—goes into immediate circulation and can take the form that any individual or group of individuals desires, to be used in accordance with the self-interests of each.

The size of stifling bureaucracy within an organization is what often renders it necessary for each employee to follow a series of unofficial, informal procedures to cope with his or her duties. However, in an institutional context where inaction prevails, the informal organization can be used to cover this inaction. At the CPHA, this informal organization has brought about an entrenched perception of work relationships and a particular mode of operation. Disturbance of this corporate mode leads to the creation of stresses concealed behind the apparent calm and, ultimately, to a series of conflicts and destructive behavior toward others, and also to self-destructive withdrawal.

Changes proposed and promoted by hospital administration upset the stagnation brought about over many years, not only by bureaucracy, but also by the informal employee organization. This results in procedures directed toward deinstitutionalizing the asylum being met by continual suspicion and the total nullification of the director's power. It is not uncommon to hear from CPHA employees the expression "we're eating our own flesh." The director himself, in an official meeting with employees, expressed fear of an "extensive 'phagocytic' phenomenon consuming people, relationships and patients" within the CPHA.

There are indicative instances of strained relations between, on the one side, the director and the reforming team, and, on the other, a portion of the employees. Between June and October 2002, four meetings were held to inform employees about the formation of a hospital corporate plan, to encourage the participation of employees in decision making, and to give them an update on similar measures being implemented in the country's other large psychiatric hospitals. Officials from the Ministry of Health and principal administrators from three other psychiatric hospitals attended the third meeting only. While the first two meetings were confrontational, the third was more like a scientific seminar characterized by waning interest from employees, who showed low attendance and departed before the meeting was over, drawing strong negative comments from the guests from the ministry and other hospitals. The fourth meeting was held after the circulation of anonymous announcements, and declared "solidarity" with the director. This meeting was organized by the CPHA Employees' Union and the Union of Doctors of Hospitals in Athens and Piraeus and gave support to the entire reform effort, leaving the disclaimers silent, and in a twilight zone.

A final characteristic feature emerging from administration is the continual partition and splitting into subgroups or even rival camps, between:

- the administration, as a united whole, and employees;
- the director and administrative clerks;
- administrative clerks supporting change and those who do not—the director's immediate colleagues, having formed a "Work and Planning Team," were seen several weeks later by other staff members as the "confidantes" who "would divide up the hospital booty" with the director;
- administrative clerks and those who come into contact with patients, be they doctors or nurses;
- employees and patients; and
- ultimately, the entire workforce and the environment beyond the hospital, the community.

One particular example of splitting, among doctor–managers, forms a category where the ambiguity of their roles—being both medical and administrative personnel—allows them, as we have seen, to be transformed into recipients of discriminative treatment. The creation of subgroups within the hospital with different expectations, hopes, self-images, and modes of communication raises basic questions regarding the operation and the climate of cooperation, two highly significant factors in the deinstitutionalization and restructuring of the CPHA.

IX. AND THE CHILDREN?

The relationship between employees and patients demands careful and expert study. Patients are the group of individuals whose desires and needs should have greatest weight, for it is they who are least capable of expressing those needs or defending those desires. The state of the children's housing is an indicator to any visitor of relationships between employees and patients. The visitor's first impression of the annexes and lodges where the patients are housed is that they are more important than the individuals for whom it is assumed they exist. This is quite clear; from the moment one entered a lodge or annex, discussion was invariably taken up with the problems and needs of the units, and, by extension, of employees (i.e., work conditions, relationships with administration) and not with the needs of the patients themselves, the children whose care has been entrusted in each hospital facility:

> I visited the units as a volunteer wishing to come into contact with and meet the children housed there and to see how the units functioned. It seemed particularly difficult for the employees to accept that my sole reason for being there was for personal contact with the children, and so the visit took on a formal character, unrelated to my intentions—it could be said I had the air of the "inspector" about me.
>
> I sadly discovered that one of the Annexes visited had all the features of asylum management. The space was arranged so that the children were gathered in their own area away from the nurses, where they spent their entire day. At one point a child came out from behind the benches defining their "area" and approached us, and although this is what I wanted, I was advised that it was better for the child to stay in his area, that he was filthy and could be carrying contagious diseases (as, indeed, some were) or could become violent and hit someone without meaning to. Moreover, the door to the unit was locked and, as mentioned by the matron and a social worker, although this practice had been abandoned, it was re-instituted after the death of a child. Without the cause of death being specified by those employees present, though some were certain it had happened, locking the unit was seen as basic security, also protecting them from the dangers of the outside world, such as the exposure of a child to chemical cleaners. (Chondros, December 11, 2002)

Contact with the children outside their care and housing facilities, for example, in the playground or on the service bus, shows that they know changes will take place (e.g., "Will our school be moved?" or "Will the hospital be closed?"). Yet, whenever they expressed their opinion, it was done clearly ("Yes, I want it to change;" "I don't.") and far more soberly than the employees did. The children displayed what could be called "simple interest" and "anticipated stress" toward the possible changes to their lives. Communication with them outside was totally different from that experienced in the units, without the persistent presence of all those clearly in charge. As cited earlier, all employees working closely with the children mentioned how difficult it was to communicate with them, to take an interest in their opinions. And this was from nurses who actually gave daily reports on their care and condition. Employees working closely with the children believe they do understand the desires and points of view of those children who have and can express them. Contact with the children is especially pleasant, without fear or upsets.

These staff opinions and behaviors raise the question of prejudice with regard to two very basic issues. First, in relation to patients, the plausible question arises as to whether and to what degree it constitutes prejudice toward psychiatric patients in general and not toward these ones in particular. Is the way in which employees work determined more by prejudice toward "craziness," which requires the patients to be dangerous and the illness to be contagious? Employees whose duties are associated with the care of the children, and so come into daily contact, thus claim there are "objective" reasons for their attitude vis-à-vis the children they take care of. For the reasons cited, that the children could involuntarily become violent; that, because they cannot talk, they cannot communicate; that, despite constant effort the children are filthy, it was therefore better not to have physical contact with them. Avoidance of contact for certain reasons seems more to assist in establishing a particular way of working that "suits" certain employees, than to be the result of anxiety and fear caused by the patient. Restricting children to specific areas of their unit seems to facilitate the supervision of the children and to reduce the workload of employees, rather than protect them from the "craziness."

A second level on which we observed the existence of prejudice again concerns the attitude of employees toward the change. Just as the change has definitive and immediate bearing on the future of these patients, there is an indirect effect on the relationship between employees and patients. People working in the annexes and lodges have strong doubts as to the feasibility of the changes proposed by the administration and how these changes will benefit them and the children being treated at the CPHA. These attitudes seem to correlate, firstly, with the reasons leading them to work at the hospital, with the education and training they were given for this position, as well as with the perceptions they have formed as to how their work should be carried out. Of interest is that these attitudes and behaviors do not differ from those of employees in the wider public domain. The same phenomena are also observed in the corporate world. According to writers describing changes in the business sector, the basic sources of people's resistance to the process of change are (not in order of importance) nostalgia for the past, life routines, lack of self-esteem, fear of the unknown, and financial insecurity. Indeed, the extent to which the object of change involves values makes the justification and support for change even more difficult and arduous (23).

Our reason for conducting an in-depth examination of the formal and informal relationships between individuals at the CPHA and the possible existence of instances of prejudice is that we believe this constitutes an area where one can and should intervene to effect improvements and to create a climate and framework that will permit efforts at change to proceed to the benefit of all, both patients and employees. It seems that these negative attitudes and prejudices, products of learning and social constructs, can change through regular daily contact and interaction based on specified terms, such as equality and honest communication between representatives of the various factions, and by identifying common goals and interests, as well as differences (24–26). An example of efforts in this direction would be the promotion and support of daily cooperation between a member of the Work Team, whose goal is the implementation of reform, and a representative of employees who are "doubtful and negative" toward change. This process demands a lot of time, patience, will, and care. Experience has shown, however, that it is always preferable and of greater benefit to all than constantly reacting and avoiding dialogue and cooperation.

X. NARCISSISM, SUFFERING, AND THE DENIAL PACT

All of this empirical material on the CPHA allows us to comment on certain aspects of this institutional world, beyond all that has been cited so far, through the prism of psychoanalytical validation. These points of view relate to narcissism in the subject, narcissism in the institution, and psychic suffering. It is basic that we understand, both theoretically and clinically, the extent and nature of psychic suffering within the institution as the product of a constant interaction between individual psychopathology, the psychopathology of the institution, and social reality related to the institution in question (social representations, stigma, prejudice).

According to Kaës et al. (27), we can discern three sources of suffering within an institution, beyond the fact that it seems interwoven with complaints and the determination of the causes of those complaints. The first source of suffering is integrally tied to the very existence of the institution. The next source is the special and distinct circumstance of each institution, with its particular social and unconscious structure. The third source is the psychic structure and functioning of the individual in question. Kaës et al. isolate suffering associated with life itself; this is the consequence of restrictions, resistances, the frustrations each person has. In other words, it relates to the distance separating the object from desire, to stress, and to the individual's relationship with truth. In favorable circumstances, this suffering leads the individual to a psychic process, especially in the development of defense mechanisms with sufficient compromises and in pursuit of realizing higher aspirations and goals (sublimation).

The deficiency and dysfunction of defense mechanisms, and sublimation in particular, often result in the destruction of the subject (physical and/or psychic) and the destruction of objects and the bonds with them. This suffering, expressed and experienced through uncontrolled anxiety, is pathological. Both within the institution and elsewhere, it paralyzes and often breaks down the specific and unique individual psychic reality of the subject, as well as the common space shared by the subject and objects, within the various expressions of bonds.

As described earlier, institutions use such defense mechanisms so as to strengthen the individual's existing defenses, and to keep the individual at a distance from the various painful experiences generated in institutional life. These mechanisms are linked to the functioning of the "denial pact" and to all agreements made in the face of the negative between individuals and groups. These processes of "encystment" of the individual's suffering within the institution result in, among other things, the nonregistering of painful experiences in the individual's psychic process and the gradual destruction of the pleasure of thinking, especially collectively.

Certain aspects of this suffering are articulated in the common life of the institution, but it must be stressed that the institutional space is also the space of psychic suffering of individuals with their particular history and psychopathology. The institution is a common psychic object; to be precise, the institution does not suffer. *Individuals suffer in relation to the institution; they suffer within this relationship with the institution.* By often referring to the institution's psychopathology as the "object," perhaps unconsciously we are inventing a way of externalizing our suffering as active or passive objects. In this way, we are able to project what exists and is experienced as suffering onto the individuals who constitute the institution: *It is the institution within us that is represented within us as a suffering institution.*

Psychic suffering in the institution also stems from not understanding the cause, the object, the defense mechanisms triggered, the meaning and content of the suffering we feel. The undifferentiation, the isomorphy and the consequence of failing to distinguish between body and space, the limits of the Self and the Other, create an atmosphere of confusion, of anomy, and of diffuse, indeterminate anxiety. The suffering in question originates from and is retained in the undifferentiated nuclei we all have within us, our "well-guarded" psychotic part, which represents for us an unspeakable danger and threat to our psychic integrity. In the final analysis, this undifferentiated "magma" constitutes the fear of our own identity, alluding to a nonidentity, to a painful void of psychotic experiences (28).

In the psychoanalytical perspective, a prerequisite for this understanding of psychic suffering, as just described, is the acceptance of the problematic of narcissism; according to Freud, "the recognition of the achievements of civilization is extracted violently, and with so much suffering, from narcissism" (29). Clearly, we never disclaim narcissism, which ensures the continuation of generations, of groups, and of institutions, and constitutes and structures the identity of the genealogy and the bonds with it. In this way, the individual's dual existence is emphasized: his or her own psychic reality and interpsychic relationship with other members of the social group. An institution is structured on the dual basis of narcissism and intermediate formations, which can be called transpsychic, to the extent they support the necessary bond between the subject and the whole. These intermediate formations "can be identification, or better, multiple identifications, the commonality of symptoms, defenses, collective ideal, cosupport, as well as the "narcissus pact" and "denial pact" (*pacte dénégatif*) among the members of the group" (27).

Essentially, the denial pact is an unconscious one—an agreement between subjects involved in an institution—and is intended to secure the continuation of investments and the benefit accompanying the structure of bonds (groups, institutions). Moreover, it is intended to maintain psychic areas necessary to the maintenance and reproduction of certain functions articulated through intersubjective or more collective forms of communication: the function of the ideal, collective organization of defense mechanisms. As an example of this process, we can refer to the case of a CPHA patient who, in a short space of time, became the "scapegoat" for the entire asylum system and paradigmatically revealed the collective defenses of the institution: denial even of the institution's treatment function, splitting among hospital departments, disorder and annulment, mutual accusations with a negative attitude, and destruction of bonds and relationships between units in the hospital. Very often, the "denial pact" itself is repressed. The members of the institution repress—through the pact—the differentiation, violence, abandonment, splitting, and unbridgeable disputes between individuals. In practice, the denial pact is transformed into a pact of silence and oblivion toward all elements that form the history of the institution. It consists of a pact whose terms can never be laid out or expressed publicly.

The denial pact operates in complement to the narcissus pact, to the extent to which institutions are formed by people unconsciously both acting as organizers and participating in mixed groups. For those who constitute the institution, these formations attempt to secure bonds, investments, representations, satisfaction of people's needs and desires, and, as has been mentioned, the activation of collective defense mechanisms. An especially important aspect of the narcissus pact (30) is the hypothesis that "the ideal of Self" is a common formation constituted by the subjective psychic function and social groups including family, institutions, and nations. The narcissus pact is involved in each institution's formation and inactivity, and, in the final analysis, it is a part of the process of its demise.

The architecture and psychic material of the institution consist of its "myth of origin." Through the narcissus pact and the denial pact of its members, this "primary" myth offers a common identifying matrix and a code, allowing the members who constitute the institution to confront uncertainty, the unknown, and change. The threat or disruption, whether external or internal, to this "mythical matrix"—which includes everything that regularly organizes the homeostasis of the institution and the psychic economy of each of its members—can provoke catastrophic reactions, even psychotic defenses. When the institution no longer supports the narcissism of the subjects who form it, the institution becomes the object of aggression, self-destructiveness and the destruction of the sum of its operations.

In psychiatric institutions, the analysis of an organization's crisis and the narcissistic suffering that disconnects it ultimately reveals the disconnection of the two components of narcissism: the individual-subjective dimension of narcissism and its collective dimension. The threat of this bond's rupture and the questioning of both institutional support for the individual and individual support for the institution seriously calls into question the common order (symbolic, real, imaginary) on which the continuation of each subject is narcissistically based. Consequently, the ground is fertile for the creation of manifestations of confusion, discouragement, withdrawal, and, particularly, all the varied expressions of psychotic function (splitting, projection, projective identification), which take possession, virtually without differentiation, of most of the psychic scene of the psychiatric institution. (Here, we use the term "psychiatric institution" rather than "mental health institution" because it includes all the conflictual dynamics between the science of psychiatry, based on the medical model, and the social mandate of social control, which by definition possesses the psychiatric establishments.) The aim of any institution is to generate "mental health," but in most cases, in practice, it disconnects—rather than connects—feelings, thoughts, and representations between individuals. That is, it operates as a mechanism that destroys culture, sublimation, and the prerequisites needed to structure an intermediate, transitional space, as described extensively by Winnicott.

It is also of interest to note that, in this domain of crisis and collective uncertainty, the psychic suffering of employees finds refuge in intense psychosomatic reactions (which in some individuals touches on psychosomatic dislocations), in severe reactive depressions, chronic dysthymic states, and outbursts of maladaptive character traits. When attempts at this sort of pathological "settling" of psychic conflicts do not advance, we often notice the appearance of political and ideological actions that have more the character of "acting out" than of political and ideological analysis. For example, we see the circulation at the CPHA of anonymous slanderous proclamations couched in pseudoideological nuances as indicative of the collective acting out of fear and anxiety in reaction to the looming changes.

XI. THE THREAT OF CHANGE

We believe that the unknown aspect of change, or novelty itself, does not provoke fear or paranoid anxiety. These can, however, be provoked by the unknown that coexists with the already known. For example, the "unknown" or unforeseen reactions of a chronic "quiet" patient may cause crises and mutual accusations of incompetence among the staff. A similar mechanism is at play in the differentiation of opinions regarding support for reform efforts.

In this context, the substantial threat comes from the fear of being unable to react to regulations already enacted and the fear of encountering a different social "milieu" that places the previous identity of the individual and institution in doubt. The process of forming a new collective identity, in juxtaposition with the old, provokes manifestations of paranoid reactions, regression, or rationalized resistance amid enormous administrative obstacles. In this way, despite the continually proposed involvement and participation of its staff, each attempt to modify the existing administrative mechanisms of the CPHA was initially met with "insurmountable" bureaucratic impediments. Of course, when these did not constitute an adequate wall of resistance, the threat of overprecise compliance with procedures and concomitant accusations of corruption was evoked. What drives bureaucratic ossification in an organization is not only its tendency to maintain the interactions and balances that already exist and to maintain compulsive, repetitive behavior, but also essentially its tendency to support the existing disintegration and splitting among elements of the system. Ultimately, bureaucracy attempts to cover up or impede any change in the existing symbiotic-type balances.

It should be made clear that all these elements form a strong blend of unelaborated prejudices, inadmissible both psychically and intellectually, which creates fantasies of the destruction and annihilation of the institution and its staff. The asylum, as a closed structure, produces chronic states of illness, in patients and staff. It also produces the characteristics of all closed systems; in other words, repetitive behavior, reinforcing endless bureaucratic feedback, with duplication of normative procedures, agreements, and administrative requirements. It produces the outcomes of bureaucracy: the lack of any initiative, the need to consolidate the slightest assumption of responsibility, the acquisition of practical skills at creating and inflicting bureaucratic obstacles, and the prevalence of a perverse use of bureaucracy to the apparent detriment of any creative or exploratory inclination of employees.

In the final analysis, the established tendency to break down relationships, affiliations, and feelings, to negate every pleasure taken in meaning, thinking, and acting, increases the entropy of the system, the anomy, the disarray, the disruption, and produces—if not imposes—a freezing process, a process of psychic death. The attempt by employees of the asylum to reduce the conflicts and tensions that accompany any attempt at vision and change results in a weakened connection between the ideal and the real, the diffusion of endeavors, the undoing of investments, the proliferation of activity deprived of meaning, the total inability to elaborate conflict. This leads clearly to the repression of all desire, as well as hate toward any desire, and hate toward taking pleasure in thinking and the object of their work.

We could distinguish two powerful "strategies" for the employees in their relationships with patients. The first is to suppress, completely, and from the beginning, the object of their work, in other words, the care of patients. The second is to directly, and almost openly, use the patients in order to settle their own problems and conflicts as a group. Everyone is "in danger of dying": physically, psychically, and occupationally. It seems that the lack of an institutional space operating transitionally, able to incorporate all Bion's (31) beta elements, often with disarming naturalness, ends up in the destruction of affiliations and connections, a prerequisite for forming what Hochman (32) termed "institution mentale." These institutions, as systems and formations—cultural, symbolic, imaginary, and social—function as incorporating wholes, and so impress their mark on the bodies, souls, and thought of each of their members. The predominance of such an operation of disintegration and psychogenic function obviously has a very high cost, both to the individual and on the collective level, through the functioning and reproduction of the institution as a generator of violence, destructiveness, and annihilation, as a vehicle of the perpetual process of negation, hate, and the death process toward any living form and operation.

XII. CONCLUSION: BEYOND THE ASYLUM?

Any attempt at opening up the asylum to the community only has meaning once it has been incorporated into the prospect of its dismantling and restructuring within a network of community mental health facilities. For many years, this basic working hypothesis for any attempt at reform could not become an object of real scientific, psychic, and emotional elaboration, and thereby allow a rational strategic plan for moving beyond asylum ideology to mature. In such a vacuum of knowledge and elaboration, the asylum culture of abandonment, of splitting between patients and everyone else, of groups of employees and families being excluded, with the users of the psychiatric health services and members of the community being excluded from involvement in decision-making processes, constitutes a culture of confusion, misery, and personal maneuvering. This culture is diffused, reinforced, and supported by the plexus of intense beliefs we call prejudices, which, during the process of reproducing this culture, are constructed by it and simultaneously create and reinforce the character of the culture.

The absence of a collective vision and of a strategic development plan for the psychiatric hospital reduces the functional ability of any administration to settle conflicts, projections, disinformation, and, ultimately, the management of asylum misery and the consequent prejudices. When many of the corporate demands that originated from the microculture of competing groups of employees could not be satisfied, they were reproduced, with counterparts at virtually all levels, resulting in the creation of splitting and the backlash of already-existing prejudices. This splitting extended to every category of employees (e.g., administrative staff against physicians and professional staff, technical services against nursing staff, social workers against physicians' authority, secondary personnel against all others) and was expressed through various patronage obligations.

Moreover, institutions are formed through unconscious organization and mixed formations that ensure, for the individuals within them, the bonds, the vital processes of investment, the satisfaction of desire, the requisite defenses, and the corresponding support for their psychic, mental, and social functioning. The common base offered by this "denial pact" is interesting to the extent that required *zones of shadow*, the *ineffable*, the *pockets of toxicity*, and the *garbage bins* (which we all know exist) make up the common denominator of the psychic-mental function and social behavior within the institution. In this way, what is commonly known and accepted is inhibited and neglected because everyone realizes that a real process of reform and examination of any phenomenon can open a Pandora's box and endanger the homoeostasis of the entire system. The "denial pact" also includes defective controls that propagate the long chain of complicity that exists, while making everything seem legitimate. The existing suffering of the members of the institution can overflow in some instances so that the members are driven to "legitimize" themselves in not carrying out their proper mission: to treat and care for the patients. Finally, all of the institution's internal mechanisms (political, administrative, union, inquiries about proper management) come into play to prevent its members from accomplishing their own basic duties.

In closing, we should mention one basic fact arising whenever and for whatever reason one comes into contact with such institutions. Institutions, pervaded by an intertwining of the psychic defense mechanisms of both their patients and employees, leave no psyche intact or unchanged. It is a well-known fact that in clinical work with psychotics, the person involved might experience psychotic moments such as depersonalization, a sense of detachment from reality, diffuse psychotic anxiety, "irrational" feelings of hate and destruction, and sudden raving. Each writer of this chapter, depending on his or her degree of involvement with the CPHA, experienced corresponding states. These experiences could be discerned on two levels, first as a feeling of alienation and disconnectedness, not simply observation or self-observation, to the point of feeling "as if" one is not there. Second, we experienced a paranoid construction, as if continually trying to protect ourselves from the destructiveness and negative thinking projected toward us through the activation within ourselves of these paranoid mechanisms. A significant part in the day-to-day relationships with our closest colleagues is identification with the enemy: psychotic defense mechanisms instantly protect one's psychic integrity from the pervading destructiveness.

Reform, or change, is felt as an absolute threat to the continuation of the psychiatric hospital and its estate. Perhaps the asylum constitutes an extension of the homes of all employees, the melding of their bodies with that of the institution, which all must be maintained by any means necessary. Each threat to the internal psychic order of the asylum is tantamount to a lethal threat. It is self-evident that the process of change and transformation of the institution's homoeostasis triggers all the mechanisms described in this chapter. The lack of transitional space for thought, play, creativity, relationships, and the psychic processing of this suffering seems at times to be the only possible response to the expression of bonds being destroyed, of states of obsession and tension, of invalidating any positive proposal, of declaring the anxiety of breaking up, and of the sense of self-composure that is threatened.

The training process, supervision, contact with "third parties" as well as the community and other institutions and services, the participation in the formation of a common strategic development plan, and the formation of groups with well-defined frameworks, rules, and purposes can all potentially act as islands that safeguard creativity within a psychic space that interacts, plays, and does not destroy because it is threatened. These recent positive indications of change and the creation (per Winnicott) of *intermediate experience spaces* by members of the Work Group and the Nursing Service are especially heartening as examples of their investment in and interpretation of the change process.

In this chapter, we have attempted to describe from within facts and events that more typically are examined in terms of macrosocial and general theory. This effort constitutes a task that is arduous, lengthy, controversial, and ambivalent precisely because the "interior" of the institution reflects and is reflected in the "interior" of all individuals concerned, including the writers of this chapter. The historic moment at the CPHA is creating such a mass of reactions as to propagate in its own idiosyncratic way the change that is taking place. Nonetheless, by writing this chapter, the team hoped to reorganize and understand the psychic and mental processes and psychopathological phenomena that appeared and continue to appear against the process of change, and in this way give meaning to these representations. Giving meaning to the narratives of the "Others" led us to another way of understanding our own participation, roles, and *ethos*: in a field of research, and through the complicated process of at "once changing and understanding" (33).

REFERENCES

1. Stylianoudi MGL. *I therapevtiki diastasi tis sinentevxis* [The therapeutic dimension of the interview]. *Epitheor Koin Ereun* 2002:107[A].
2. Augé M. *Non-Lieux: Introduction à une anthropologie de la surmodernité*, Paris: Seuil, 1992.
3. Sills DL, ed. *International encyclopaedia of the social sciences, vol 12.* New York: Macmillan Company & The Free Press, 1967.
4. Dimitrakou D. *Mega Lexikon olis tis Hellenikis Glossis* [Great dictionary of the Greek language, vol XII]. Athens: Ekdoseis DOMI, 1964.

5. *Epitomon Othografikon kai Egkyklopaedikon Lexikon "Heliou"* [Abridged orthographic and encyclopaedic dictionary of 'Helios']. Athens: Ekdoseis Heliou, 1930.
6. LaPierre RT. Attitudes versus action. *Soc Forces* 1934;13:227–237.
7. Adorno TW, Frenkel-Brunswik E, Levinson DJ, et al. *The authoritarian personality*. NewYork: Harper & Row, 1950.
8. Moscovici S. *Psychologie sociale*. Paris: PUF, 1988.
9. Riga AB. *Prejudice*. In: *Paedagogiki Psychologiki Egkyklopaedia, Lexikon* [Pedagogic and psychological encyclopaedia]. Athens: Hellinika Grammata Publications, 1991;7:4111–4112.
10. Saraceno B. *La fine dell' intrattenimento*. Milano: ETASLIBRI–Res Medicina, 1995:44.
11. Yioti A. *Diadikasies yia tin metexelixi tou Pœedopsychiatrikou Nosokomeiou Attikis sto plesio tis Psychiatrikis Metarythmisis* [Evolution processes of the children's Psychiatric Hospital of Attica in the context of psychiatric reform]. Dissertation in Social Psychiatry, University of Ioannina, 1999.
12. Greek Law 2889/2001: Improvement and modernisation of the National Health System and other directives, art. 1: establishment of periphery health systems, art. 5: Administration of Hospitals.
13. Ministry of Health and Welfare. *Psychargos* 2001–2010: development program for facilities and aux. Facilities within the Department of Mental Health. Athens: MYPEP/EPIPSY, 2001.
14. Greek Law 2716/1999: Development and Modernization of Mental Health Services.
15. Stylianidis S. *Modela psychokoinonikis apokatastasis kai provlimata metaforas tous ston choro tis Psychiatrikis Metarrythmisis stin Ellada: theoretikes, klinikes kai praktikes paratiriseis* [Models of psychosocial rehabilitation and problems in applying them to psychiatric reform in Greece: theoretical, clinical and practical comments]. *Tetrad Psychiatr* 2001;75:12–32.
16. Stylianoudi MGL, Stylianidis S. "Maria: Her Body and Her Stare": imprinting of evil and re-investment of body image. In: Frykman J, Seremetakis N, Ewert S, eds. *Identities in pain*. Lund: Nordic Academic Press, 1998:108–125.
17. Gizelis G, Stylianoudi MGL, Kalpourtzi E, et al. *I Oikoyeneia stin Kentriki Makedonia: Stratigikes Koinonikis Anaparagogis* (Family in Macedonia: Strategics of Social Reproduction). *Helliniki Koinonia: Epetiris tou KEEK*, (Yearbook of the Centre for Greek Society) 1998;4.
18. Allport GW. *The nature of prejudice*. Reading: Addison-Welsey, 1954.
19. Tsapogas G. Commercialization of health on "high functional budget". *Rizospastis*, 2003;8:14.
20. Morgan G. *I opseis tis Organosis. Eisagogi stis theories Organosis kai Diikisis,* Athens: Ekdoseis Kastanioti, 2000. [Greek translation from *Images of organization*. Thousand Oaks, CA: Sage Publications, 1998.]
21. Zianikas HA. *Diikitiki Epistimi kai Praktiki sto Dimosio: Dynamiki Eksighronismou* [Management theory and practice in the public sector: modernization dynamics]. Athens: Sideris, 1996.
22. Kontis TH, Mantas N. *Epharmosmeni Organotiki kai Diikitiki* [Applied management]. Athens: Sighroni Ekdotiki, 1993.
23. Quimet G, Dufour Y. Vivre et gérer le changement ensemble. *Rév Fr Gest* 1997;113:22–40.
24. Brown R. *Prejudice: its social psychology*. Oxford: Blackwell, 1995.
25. Howestone M. Contact and categorization: social psychological intervention to change intergroup relations. In: Stangor C, ed. *Stereotypes and prejudice: essential readings*. Philadelphia: Psychology Press, 1999.
26. Wilder DV. Koinoniki Katigoriopiisi: Nixeis yia ti Dimiourgia kai ti Meiosi tis Diomadikis Strevlosis. In: Papastamou S, ed. *Diomadikes Scheseis* [Intergroup relations]. Athens: Odysseas Publications, 1999. [Greek translation of Wilder DV. Social categorization: implications for creation and reduction of intergroup bias. *Adv Exp Soc Psychol* 1986:19:291–355.]
27. Kaës P, Bleger J, Enriquez E, et al. *L'institution et les institutions. Études psychanalytiques*. Paris: Ed. Dunod, 1988:32–35.
28. Racamier PC. *Les schizophrènes*. Paris: Payot, 1990.
29. Freud S. *Pour introduire le narcissisme*. In: Berger D, Laplanche J, et al., trans. *La vie sexuelle. Col. Bibliothèque de psychanalyse*. Paris: PUF, 1969. [Reedited in 1986.]
30. Castoriadis-Aulagnier, P. *La violence de l'interprétation. Du pictogramme à l'énoncé*. Paris: PUF, 1976.
31. Bion WR. Attaque contre la liaison. In: Bion WR. *Réflexion faite*. Paris: PUF, 1983. [Original: Bion WR. Attacks on linking. *Int J Psychoanal* 1959;40.]
32. Hochmann J. L'institution mentale : du rôle de la théorie dans les soins psychiatriques désinstitutionnalisés. *Inf Psychiatr* 1992;68:985–991.
33. Taylor SJ, Bogdan R. *Introduction to qualitative research methods*. New York: John Wiley and Sons, Inc, 1998:82.

12

The African Renaissance and the Struggle for Mental Health in the African Diaspora

Frederick W. Hickling

Department of Community Health and Psychiatry, University of the West Indies, Kingston, Jamaica, West Indies

EDITORS' NOTE*: From November 17–21, 2002, an historic conference, "Psychiatric Issues in the African Diaspora," was convened in Boston, Massachusetts, by the Massachusetts General Hospital Department of Psychiatry's Division of International Psychiatry. At the invitation of conference chairman Dr. Chester Pierce, professor of psychiatry at Harvard Medical School, psychiatrists from Africa, the Caribbean, Central and South America, the South Pacific, Canada, the United Kingdom, and the United States engaged in a wide-ranging dialogue on the mental health challenges facing people of African descent, searching for mutual solutions to common problems. The 25-member host national committee included psychiatrists of African descent living in the United States and practicing psychiatry in a wide variety of clinical, academic, research, and administrative settings. Presentations were accompanied by small- and large-group discussions facilitated by Dr. Felton Earls of Harvard University and Dr. Ezra Griffith of Yale University and attended by international presenters, advisors, and consultants as well as host national committee members.

Psychiatrists of African descent from 20 countries presented vivid descriptions of the mental health problems, services, and human and material resources currently available within their home countries along with examples of issues they face as

*Adapted with permission from Executive Summary. In: Organ PG, ed. *The African Diaspora: psychiatric issues. Proceedings from the African Diaspora Meetings, Boston, Massachusetts, 17–21 November 2002*. Boston: Massachusetts General Hospital, Department of Psychiatry, Division of International Psychiatry, 2002:6–7.

individual clinicians. The diverse and complex topics covered the full range of mental illness and mental health, from clinical concerns such as the treatment of homeless, immigrant, or traumatized populations to the systemic issues of governmental health policies, resource allocation, and the training and support of mental health care professionals. Much of the dialogue focused on distinguishing the universal aspects of mental illness while understanding the specific and unique clinical manifestations found among people of African descent around the world. In addition, many of the international presenters outlined theoretical and empirical constructs that attempted to understand the current clinical manifestations and etiologies of mental illnesses among people of African descent within a historical framework that includes genocide, colonization, enslavement, and oppression.

Two recurrent topics of particular concern and discussion were the need for relevant evidence-based, empirical research and clinical intervention projects related to the mental health issues of African-descended people, and the need to diagnose and treat the insidious and destructive effect that racism continues to have on the mental health and well-being of people of African descent. By the end of the 5-day conference, the participants had identified several recommendations, including:

1. Creating and developing the infrastructure, organizational framework, and financial support for short- and long-term, international collaborative research and intervention projects focused on the mental health needs of people of African descent throughout the world, with the goal of "thinking globally, acting locally."
2. Creating short- and long-term research agendas to address the immediate and ongoing needs of African-descended people around the world. These agendas should focus on community-based, culturally relevant research and on interventions addressing the mental health issues and problems of displaced and disadvantaged populations, particularly elders, children and adolescents, the homeless, immigrants, and those suffering from HIV/AIDS and other preventable infectious and medical diseases.
3. Creating and maintaining an international organization of psychiatrists of African descent to embrace the issues and challenges identified at this initial conference and expeditiously develop and implement the appropriate policy initiatives, public education and outreach efforts, and research and intervention projects necessary to address and resolve the devastating mental health problems and issues that affect people of African descent, over one quarter of the world's population.

This chapter by Dr. Frederick Hickling, adapted from the conference proceedings, is only one example of the work presented at this landmark conference. We hope it will prompt readers to explore further the range of issues raised by the conference participants. To read the full text of the entire proceedings or to print a copy, go to *www.massgeneral.org/diaspora* and click on "Proceeding & Directory."

I. INTRODUCTION

The mental health challenge for African people in the Diaspora at this time is to make sense of the psychology of racism and colonization, to challenge the psychosociological constructs of slavery and underdevelopment, and to catalyze the transformation process that will move the African Diaspora into freedom, prosperity, and psychological stability. The challenge for African mental health professionals at home and abroad is to create a blueprint for mental health in the African Diaspora. This chapter attempts to meet this objective by revisiting the developmental history of the world using a psychopolitical analysis with race as the primary dialectic construct. This challenges the conventional political analysis of Karl Marx, which uses class as the primary dialectic construct, and rejects the postmodern constructs of Foucault (1) and others as the latest form of Western philosophical orthodoxy, which facilitates globalization.

This thesis negates these analyses using a historical and political methodology called psychohistoriography developed in the Caribbean island of Jamaica and grounded within a postcolonial philosophical perspective. It concludes that historical events of the past 500 years have systematically confronted the European imperative to own the world and the people and resources contained therein. These challenges of world history have forced the systematic transformation of world mental health systems, based on the negation of the Eurocentric concept of white supremacy and the confrontation of the European delusion of world ownership by Divine Right. The concept and praxis of the African Renaissance, which has emerged since the fall of apartheid in South Africa, represents a recent phase of the historiographic negation of the racist European social system that has dominated the history of the world for the past 500 years. Makgoba (2) defines the African Renaissance as follows:

> The African renaissance is a unique opportunity for Africans to redefine ourselves and our agenda according to our own realities and taking into account the realities of the world around us. It is about Africans being agents of our own history and masters of our own destiny.

The African Renaissance and the struggle for mental health in the African Diaspora must also be seen in the context of Pan-Africanism and the great Pan-Africanists of the recent century. Frederick Douglas, Harriet Tubman, and W. E. B. Dubois in the United States and Marcus Garvey, George Padmore, and C. L. R. James in the Caribbean join Jomo Kenyata, Kwame Nkrumah, and Nelson Mandela to represent some of the great Pan-Africanists of the 20th century, who have helped to chart the emergence of the African Renaissance and the necessity for African people to redefine themselves.

This chapter argues that the African Renaissance must be seen in the context of mental health in the African Diaspora. It also argues that African mental health must incorporate the phenomenological perspective of psychiatry within the prism of the psychological, political, and philosophical experiences of African people. It posits a thesis that demands the rethinking of African epistemology from an interdisciplinary and philosophical repositioning, and the fusion of such thought with the dream of a United Africa and the Pan-Africanist vision of cooperation and justice. The thesis takes off from the writings of another Caribbean psychiatrist, Frantz Fanon

(3), using race as the primary dialectic for analysis, and repositioning class as the secondary dialectic antipode.

II. PSYCHOHISTORIOGRAPHY: METHOD

The ideas and concepts in this chapter have come from a number of psychohistoriographic large-group experiences over the past 25 years. The technique of psychohistoriography (4) was developed in Bellevue Mental Hospital, Jamaica, in the late 1970s. The process was developed in response to the major changes that were taking place in that mental institution as a result of the intense decolonization process that had been triggered by the political climate in Jamaica in that decade (5). The technique was adapted from the concept of historiography, which is a method of analysis of historical documents that had been described initially by Thomas Becker (6) and by the Caribbean historian Elsa Goveia (7). Historiography is a method of analysis of historical documents used to determine a given society's outlook, ideology, and beliefs and to identify dynamics and social forces that compel change.

Historians have used historiography to analyze the writings of the period in a particular region, in order to identify the vectors of change in a given society. Often, there have existed conflicting views between historians and psychiatrists, as psychiatrists have tended to make exclusively causal (biological) explorations, whereas historians have tended to address themselves exclusively to the understanding of actual experiences in all their detail. The time has now come for such sciences to include, within both fields of enquiry, the evidence from psychopathology to work for their mutual advancement.

The investigation of psychopathological phenomena in society and in history must be of prime importance to the realistic perspective on our total human reality. For therapy to progress and for change to take place, the patient must internalize insights to facilitate transformation by dealing with forces that block action. The marriage of psychiatry and history through the investigation of psychopathology must promote problem solving and reality testing and facilitate the mastering of anxieties. The process must reinvest normal life goals within the acceptance of personal limitations and handicaps, while fulfilling the development of the highest degree of human creative potential.

Thus, the technique of historiography was incorporated in a graphic technique called psychohistoriography, an analytic methodology designed to produce insight in a group situation by the examination of psychopathology within the historical perspective of that group. The method incorporates historical material garnered from anecdotes and knowledge within the oral tradition, and presents this material in a graphic form within a dialectic perspective to identify reality-based themes and trends, and to facilitate productivity and change for the individuals and group. Psychohistoriography was developed in the mental hospital in Jamaica within the context of helping people from various socioeconomic and educational backgrounds, with underdeveloped political and psychological constructs, to debunk the myths of colonization and to establish reality as a framework for future action.

Psychohistoriography uses group psychological dynamics in the collective analysis of the group's history and behavior as recorded in the person's memories, exemplified in the oral tradition that is so common in the culture of the African Diaspora (8). A major contributor to the components of the process has been the Martiniquan psychiatrist Frantz Fanon, one of the first psychiatrists to recognize the importance of politics in the understanding of the psychopathology of human beings, particularly black people. Fanon demanded that the historical perceptions of the world be seen within a dialectical framework and that psychological analysis is incomplete without this component. The analytic work of Fanon has given us a platform for contemporary analysis, and locates this work firmly on the shoulders of the ancestors who have gone before.

The psychohistoriographic analysis occurs in a large-group setting with a designated chairperson and analyst. Using a blackboard or a large flip chart, the analyst begins by drawing a horizontal line across the center of the chart, constituting the time line or time continuum. The group then decides collectively the period of history under consideration and the analyst charts the initial year of that period on the extreme left edge of the time line. The present year is charted at the extreme right-hand edge of the time line and the line between these two points is subdivided, with equidistant points each representing equal time periods.

A dialectical matrix is then established above and below the time line. The conventional dialectical continuum used in the context of Marxist dialectic materialism is the social class continuum. This dialectic continuum is charted on the extreme left-hand side of the graph and the dialectical antipodes of the class are placed on the top and the bottom left hand corner of the chart, respectively. In this context, the primary dialectical matrix identified was the racial dialectic, with the anecdotal historical material serving the interests of the white and the black people involved being charted. The social class dialectic, those of the rich and the poor, was also charted, but as the secondary dialectic antipode. Central to this understanding of the separation of these dialectic analytic continua was the identification of the coterminous relationship between race and class (9). The third matrix, which is important for the analysis, is the dialectical matrix of the mad and the bad. Once the psychohistoriographic matrix is completed, it is then ready to receive historical data either from anecdotal materials within the group or the reports of written work characterized in particular times on the graph.

Using conventional group dynamic techniques, the group discusses its history by eliciting the individuals' free associations. Each historical fact is verified by the group and is referenced wherever possible or necessary. Once consensus is achieved regarding each historical datum, the group establishes its class relationship. The datum is then entered on the chart at the point corresponding to the time when the datum occurs and which has been collectively agreed on as the racial/class position. As many historical facts as possible are discussed by the group and recorded in the manner stated. Very soon the chart becomes filled with consensual historical material.

The analysis continues by the process of visual inspection by the analyst and the group, identifying specific clusters of charted historical data. Around these clusters, vertical theme lines are drawn and horizontal trend lines are established, again by group consensus. The theme and the trend lines are then labelled by the group using single words or single phrases that express the group's perception or insight of the theme or the trend. The theme lines represent a cross-sectional analysis at a particular point in time, and are represented by labels at both dialectical ends of the chart, either at the top or the bottom, respectively, representing the race/class/psychopathologic perceptions of the historical themes. The labelled themes are then listed on separate sheets of paper and used within the process of "insight bringing," to allow the group to understand the development of their attitudes and behavior through this particular analysis of the dialectical perspective of their history.

III. PSYCHOHISTORIOGRAPHY: RESULTS

This chapter will now identify specific and repetitive theme lines that have emerged from a number of different collective analytic processes in different group settings during the past 25 years.

A. The Discovery Grande: Invaders—"Come Outta Mi Land" (Circa 1492)

The European encounter with the New World began as an accident, with Christopher Columbus endeavoring to find passageway to the Far East. Instead of finding that pathway, he encountered millions and millions of human beings, unknown to the European world, who inhabited North and South America and the Caribbean. The dialectic perception of this discovery by the Europeans is strongly contested by the perceptions of the indigenous Caribbean and American people, who regarded the European "discovery" much more as an intrusion and, in reality, an invasion of their personal, social, and geographic space by marauding white pirates. The early 16th-century writings of the Spanish monk, Las Casas (10), identify the dialectical processes involved in this period. The Europeans were particularly interested in plunder and the exploitation of the mineral and other treasures of the lands that they had found. The principal insight of this theme line was the recognition that the Eurocentric concept of white supremacy, which identified European ownership of the world and the people and resources therein by Divine Right, were elements of a collective delusion that we have called the European psychosis. Essential to this delusion was that people of color, indigenous inhabitants of the rest of the world, were subhuman, only slightly superior to domestic animals.

B. Ethnic Cleansing: Genocide—"Dem a Kill We" (Circa 1520)

By definition, a delusion is a fixed, false belief, contrary to rational argument, that is out of keeping with the cultural beliefs of the time. Clearly these delusional ideas of owning the land and the people of the world was out of keeping with the belief systems of every culture in the world, with the exception of the European culture.

By the systematic eradication of all opposition of the indigenous people by mindless and ferocious genocide, by systems of cultural imperialism, the European was able to impose the madness of European colonization on the world. Las Casas describes the voracious genocide of the Spanish Europeans on the native Arawak and Taino Indians of the Caribbean. Millions of people were wiped out not only by disease brought to the New World by the Spaniards, but also by a systematic genocidal destruction of these people who were hunted down by bounty hunters paid for by the State. The Spanish were excited by the prospect of gold and other mineral riches to be found in the New World. By the middle of the 17th century, the Taino Indians in the Caribbean had been virtually decimated. Thornton (11) estimates that there were 72 million native people in the Western Hemisphere, but that they were reduced to less than 6% of that number, slightly more than 4 million people, in the following two centuries. The European delusion had been dragged into reality by the genocidal negation of the cultural opposition. The gun had become the midwife of the madness.

C. The Rights of Europeans—"Dem Wipe de Slate Clean" (Circa 1655)

The Americas and the Caribbean represent a slate wiped clean by Europe—a template for European social engineering. Having removed the original inhabitants, Europe proceeded to re-engineer these countries and populate them with Europeans and then with black people enslaved from the continent of Africa. Millions of African people from West Africa and Southwest Africa were brought across the Middle Passage to feed the plantation system developed by the Europeans. The British Merchant Navy was the main agent of transportation of the African slaves, who were sold on the auction blocks from Barbados in the East to Jamaica in the West; Charleston, North Carolina in the North; and Palmares, Brazil in the South. The physical and mental cruelty of the process of enslavement, the period of enforced labor, and the passage across the Caribbean is a story that has not been completely told. The dismembering of Africa and the Holocaust of African slavery certainly does not impinge on the memory of European people in the same way that the Jewish Holocaust of Nazi Germany has impinged on the collective psyche of white people at this time.

D. Fueling the Plantation: The Birth of Capitalism, Forced Migration, African Slavery—"Dem Tek We from We Lan" (Circa 1700)

The horror of the imposition of the European psychosis on the New World and on the mental health of the African people must have been profound. The concept of a mad slave was unheard of in that period, and European slave owners would have executed African slaves with mental and physical disability like sick animals. But suicide and other forms of mental illness have been well documented among African people who were enslaved in the New World (12). The European lie that mental illness was unknown in African slaves has recently been summarized elsewhere (13); Halliday (14), for example, wrote in 1824 that mental illness rarely occurred among West Indian slaves, African heathens and pagans, and Welsh and Irish peasants.

The ferocity with which the ideas of white supremacy and European ownership of the world were imposed can only be likened to the irrational violence of psychosis. The essence of this psychohistoriographic theme underlines the epiphany that the collective delusion of a race, a psychosis of racism, can be imposed on whole nations of people, if the lunatic enslaver holds the instruments of superior military power. Nonetheless, "the horrors of the African experience in the New World did nothing to diminish the African cunning for survival, wisdom for regeneration and reinvention of self, penchant for adaptation, and courage to resist the enslavement" (13).

E. Emancipation from Slavery—"Fight Down de White Oppressor" (Circa 1830s)

European colonization of the New World virtually wiped out the indigenous populations of North and South America, but the stubborn ferocity with which African slaves in the Americas resisted the slavery imposed by the European madness soon triggered the emancipation of African slaves. This retreat by the European slavemongers to concede emancipation in essence represented the first major collective psychological encapsulation of these delusional ideas within the sweep of history. A new modified form of the European psychosis called colonialism, which produced a new layer of European exploitation, replaced slavery in 1834 in the New World. The incisive analysis of Trinidadian African scholar Eric Williams identified that this period heralded the birth of the capitalist system by fueling the Industrial Revolution in Europe (15). From the perspective of this psychohistoriographic analysis, the capitalist system must be seen as a psychopathological construct, the material economic manifestation of the delusional greed of the colonizing European.

F. Treaty of Berlin: The Scramble for Africa—"Dem Tief We Lan" (Circa 1884)

By the end of the 19th century, the European nations were engaged in a frenzied scramble for Africa (16), as their attention was shifted from the exploitation of the New World to the underdevelopment of Africa in this period. In his book *How Europe Under-Developed Africa*, Guyanese African historian Walter Rodney (17) made clear the processes that were used by Europe to continue the ruthless rape of the African continent and the African people. Psychohistoriographic analysis has illustrated the cunning and Machiavellian strategies used by the European colonizer in the maintenance of the enslavement and exploitation process. As the development of the capitalist system ensured the sharpening of the class forces in Europe and around the rest of the world, this also formed the basis for the persistent poverty, described so eloquently by Jamaican African economist George Beckford (18), of the economic situation of African and Caribbean people.

G. The European Wars—"Fighting Over Our Treasures" (Circa 1914)

The scramble for Africa by European nations at the Treaty of Berlin in 1884 was the precursor of the two European wars, commonly referred to as "World Wars." These ferocious battles represented a struggle between the European nations over world hegemony. The contempt with which Europe simply divided up the African continent is a reflection of the lunacy with which Europe midwifed modern Africa—through the creation of boundaries that served their grandiose and delusional interests, in their frenzied quest for African land, labor, and raw materials. Magubane (19) points out how British Prime Minister Lord Salisbury, in a speech on May 6, 1898, divided the nations of the world into the living and the dying, with the relegation of African nations into the category of the dying nations. Magubane asks the question whether we can dismiss the callousness of the actions of the Europeans as characteristic of their time and of no interest to us in the present. This psychohistoriographic analysis provides an answer to the question, by forcing us to apply the thinking and actions of the time into a psychopathological continuum of the European delusion, which has existed for five centuries and is most certainly still alive at present.

H. White on White Racism—"Dem ah Kill Dem One Anoder"

In the sweep of history in the latter half of the millennium, certain critical historical events can be identified which at first glance might not fit easily into the psychohistoriographic analysis that has identified the European psychopathology. These events are the American Revolution in 1776, the French Revolution of 1795, and the Bolshevik Revolution of 1917. However, on the contrary, these events merely buttress the conclusion of the existence of the European psychosis, in that they underscore the reality that the delusion has existed and continues to exist, as evidenced by the hostility of one white ethnic group for another.

The early European settlers in America were themselves escaping from the racial and ethnic cleansing of their own kith and kin in Europe, who were attempting to perpetuate their tyranny across the Atlantic. The white French aristocracy treated the French peasants who stormed the Bastille with the same contempt and oppression that they meted out to their African slaves. The truth is revealed in the increased violent expression of the virulence of the European delusional system by the white American revolutionaries toward their own African slaves. Unlike the African slaves, however, the French peasants subsequently were absorbed into the French racial tapestry after the revolution. Liberty, equality, and fraternity were the watchwords of the French revolution, but only for white French people, not for their black African and Caribbean slaves.

The Soviet revolution contained within it similar expressions of the virulence of the European psychosis. Despite proletarian platitudes of comradeship with people of color, the harsh expression of racism by Soviet people to blacks at home and abroad has often been reported. Numerous examples of white-on-white racism insert themselves into the psychohistoriographic analysis, but receive the same analysis and treatment. The English attempt to subjugate the Irish, and more recently the Serb genocide against the ethnic Albanians, serve as other examples. In this regard, we must not forget the atrocities and the mental suffering of the Jewish Holocaust in Nazi Germany in the 20th century. This is another example of white-on-white racism within the context of the European delusional system. But as with the other examples of white-on-white racism, once the problem has been resolved with the oppressor, the victims of this type of racism become the perpetrators of an even more virulent form of racism against black people. The behavior of the Jewish State of Israel toward the Palestinian people in the latter half of the 20th century and the early 21st century illustrates this complicity with the European madness.

I. Independence from the Empire—"Gimmie Back Mi Lan" (Circa 1955)

Emancipation represented the first watershed defeat of the European psychosis and its retreat into its new form of colonialism. The independence period in the decades of the 1950s and 1960s represents the next major historical defeat of this psychopathology, the dissolution of the "empire," and the birth of the next phase, now known as neocolonialism and, subsequently, globalization. Crippling racism was experienced by the soldiers of color from India, Africa, the Caribbean, and America who fought for the West in the trenches against the Kaiser in the First European War. The racism that was meted out by their colonial masters acted as a catalyst for revolutionary anticolonial fervor on their return home. By the early 1930s, political discontent and rebellion was springing up all around the British, Spanish, and French Empires. By the end of the Second European War, the colonized people of the Caribbean, India, and Africa had pushed Europe against the wall and forced the political break-up of these Empires by the creation of politically independent nation-states.

Once again, the racist psychosis had been confronted and pushed against the wall by the struggles of black people around the world. Once again, the most virulent elements of the delusion were pushed back and encapsulated. Once again, the resultant compromise with Europe allowed the psychosis to survive in exchange for major political concessions to people of color. However, the fundamental mainstay of the psychopathological European social system, the economic control of the resources of their former colonies, remained intact. The European psychosis metamorphosed, and lived to reform itself again. But with each defeat, more of the psychosis was forced to encapsulate, while the struggle for survival of the remnants of the delusion became more desperate.

J. Defeat of Apartheid: The African Renaissance (Circa 1993)

The 30-year period from 1960 to 1990 saw the turbulent realignment of political and strategic forces around the world as the European psychosis was pushed back and forced to encapsulate further. The Civil Rights Movement in the United States forced the ruling center of the European psychosis to check its more virulent elements. The escalation of racial tension in the United Kingdom forced the "mother" of the European Psychosis to admit that institutional racism was alive and well in Britain. The recent McPherson Report (20), which looked into the death of African Caribbean teenager Stephen Lawrence, substantiates the numerous previous reports of racism in the police force in Britain. Most blacks living in Britain know, as a daily reality, that race is the basis of social barriers that are endemic in modern British society. The perception of many black people living in the United Kingdom (challenging the postmodern orthodoxy), is the presence of a pervasive racist conspiracy that riddles British society and makes daily living for most black people in Britain a living hell.

The stupendous victory of the African people against the Afrikaner Apartheid System in South Africa is seen by some as being nothing short of a miracle. The victory represented decades of struggle and courageous valor by the African masses in the face of the most vicious expression of the European psychosis witnessed on earth. The fact that this virulent form of the European psychopathology was allowed to flourish by the rest of the Western world reflects a paradox. Even in the face of significant encapsulation of the white delusions around the globe, evidenced by emancipation and the independence movement, bizarre, grandiose delusions and psychotic thoughts were allowed to flourish in a raw and unexpurgated form in apartheid South Africa, in many respects nurtured by the West. The victory over apartheid in 1993 represents the next major world historical victory against the European psychosis and has itself given birth to the fledgling epiphany of the African Renaissance.

Jamaican African visionary leader Marcus Mosiah Garvey articulated the concept of Pan-Africanism at the turn of the 20th century. His newspaper, *The Negro World*, was translated into 25 languages and, long before the telephone or the Internet, it was being read and studied by African people in every corner of the globe. In 1945, at the first Pan-African Conference, held in Manchester, England, the vision of that movement was given flesh by the African Founding Fathers. Ghanaian African Kwame Nkrumah, Kenyan African Jomo Kenyata, Trinidadian African George Padmore, American African William E. B. Dubois, and Peter Abrahams, a South African who was later exiled in Jamaica, were the major players. By 1963, the Organization of African Unity came into being at the Founding Conference held in Addis Ababa. Soon after that conference, HIM Emperor Haile Sellasie gave his famous address to the United Nations in California on February 28, 1968, which has been immortalized by the Bob Marley song, "War" (21):

> Until the philosophy which holds one race superior and
> another inferior is finally and permanently
> discredited and abandoned . . .
>
> everywhere is war
> mi sey war . . .

we Africans will fight we find it necessary
we know that we shall win, as we are confident in the
victory of good over evil

The relentless battle of people of color against delusional European racism in this period was undoubtedly the cause of the eventual defeat of the Afrikaner Apartheid system in South Africa. The recent declaration of the formation of the African Union in July 2002, fashioned on the European Union, represents the most recent advance of this encapsulation process. From the perspective of the psychohistoriographic analysis, this victory represents the latest in the escalating historical negation of the racist delusional system. As with the other watershed periods described, the victory was neither final nor complete, but represented a compromise formulation with the European delusion. The victory forced a further negation of the delusion, placing political power in the hands of the African masses, but leaving the ownership of the commanding heights of the economy in the hands of the whites.

It is simple for the seasoned observer, the insightful historian, the grounded psychologist to recognize the similar components of institutionalized racism, whether it exists in postcolonial Jamaica, the deep southern United States, in Stephen Lawrence's Britain, or in postapartheid South Africa. White people still own the commanding heights of the economy, and blacks are forced to scrape out a meager survival in a social reality that relegates them to an economic second class. Even in the countries where blacks are in the majority and are in political control of the society, the tangible elements of the racist delusional system still control the reality for black people.

From the perspective of this analysis, the insights gained have revealed that the birth of the capitalist economic system represented a psychopathological manifestation of the insane European social system. The surplus generated by the theft, exploitation, and slavery imposed by this lunacy has formed the material basis for the birth and growth of the capitalist economic system, and has left black people with a catch-22 situation. Without control of the commanding heights of the economy, black people are destined to eke out an existence in the ghettos of the canefields and the copper mines, in the inner cities and the townships.

The profound importance of the insight that the capitalist system is a psychopathological mushroom of European madness being imposed on the rest of the world will be of greatest importance in our consideration of the African Renaissance. The psychohistoriographic analysis predicts that the next watershed points in human history must confront this lunatic economic construction. In Thabo Mbeki's words, ". . . we are subjected to the strange situation that the process of the further reproduction of wealth by the countries of the North has led to poverty in the countries of the South" (22). Without the confrontation and defeat of this economic madness, there can be no African Renaissance, and the historic defeats of the past will simply have dashed the struggles of the African people at home and abroad against the treacherous reefs of European psychopathology. But the compelling and relentless defeats of the system provide a historic comfort that human life on this globe will not tolerate the continued existence of this lunacy.

IV. CONCLUSION: THE AFRICAN RENAISSANCE AND MENTAL HEALTH

Many will find the perception of racism in this account as a reduction to the level of psychopathology, and will consider this to be problematic. However, this is the essence of this analysis, and is the principal insight from the process of psychohistoriography. No doubt, this perception will challenge thinkers from Africa and elsewhere, and will at the very least be controversial. Few can deny however, that much of the time and resources of the world for the second half of the millennium have been devoted to the irrational European desire to own the world.

The greatest challenge to the mental pathology of European colonialism and enslavement has come from black popular revolt. Stuart Hall and his colleagues (23) have picked up the psychic challenge of the black revolt of the period, and begun to articulate the intellectual and philosophical challenge to postmodernism. The Western-dominated paradigm of postmodernism assumes the ability to explain all and to apply meaning to peoples of all cultures in a unitary way. Stuart Hall (24) and Catherine Hall (25) have posited the antithetical construct to postmodernism, which has become known as postcolonialism. Postcolonial theory describes how the processes of colonization and decolonization have been indelibly branded within the cultures of the colonizers as well as within those of the colonized, thus displacing the "story" of capitalist modernity from its European centering to its dispersed global peripheries, from peaceful evolution to imposed violence, redirecting the focus of the transition from feudalism to capitalism and replacing this with the formation of a world market controlled essentially by Europe.

Most importantly, Hall and his colleagues have constructed an intellectual and philosophical platform in Britain for black people to redefine issues of their own mental health. It is hard to comprehend how European society successfully renders people with black skins "invisible." Melba Wilson (26) argues that "In mental health terms, the invisibility engendered by the image, when combined with the overall tendency to portray people with mental health problems outside the bounds of normality compound the disadvantage experienced by black people in both the mental health and criminal justice systems." The stereotypical images of black men as violent rapists, black people as lazy and unproductive, and black families as unstable and pathological are clearly rooted in the experience of racism.

At a recent conference on Pan-African mental health held in Dakar, Senegal in April of 2000, a call was made for the establishment of a Pan-African Association of Mental Health Professionals. Such an association would certainly facilitate a blueprint for mental health in the African Diaspora. I suggest that the blueprint should include the following elements:

- A vehicle for African Unity across the Diaspora
- Development of psychological processes designed for the negation of the effects of racism and colonization in people of color in the Diaspora
- The training of culturally sensitive mental health workers for every community of black people in the African Diaspora

- The creation of community based mental health services across the African Diaspora
- The deinstitutionalization of European colonial custodial mental hospitals in the African Diaspora
- The establishment of rehabilitation facilities across the Diaspora that place work as therapy and the use of art, dance, music, and drama as the vehicles for African mental health
- The use of evidence-based mental health methodologies for Africans at home and abroad

Perhaps the most important mental health imperative for African people in the world today is to find strategies for navigating capitalism, and the encapsulation of the European psychosis. African people have as much right as any ethnic group to be in all parts of the world and to claim ownership of the world community that we have helped to build by our labor and our blood. Once there are white Africans, there will certainly be black Europeans. Our navigation maps must include creating safe places where African people can be culturally safe and secure. We must restore the driving ambition of our people, which has tended to be erased by this pervasive delusional system. We have to continue our process of stepping out of being the underclass and being our own masters as we create economic wealth across the globe, which will teach us how to live with ourselves in a harmonious and unified way. This must be the focus and the vision for all black people—the unity of Africans at home and abroad.

REFERENCES

1. Foucault M. *The order of things: an archaeology of the human sciences.* New York: Random House, 1973.
2. Makgoba MW. Introduction. In: Makgoba MW, Shope T, Mazwai T, eds. *African Renaissance, Cape Town.* Cape Town: Mafube, 1999:xii.
3. Fanon F. *The wretched of the earth.* London: Penguin Books, 1967.
4. Hickling FW. Sociodrama in the rehabilitation of chronic mental illness. *Hosp Community Psych* 1989;40:402–406.
5. Manley M. *The politics of change.* London: Andre Deutsche, 1980.
6. Becker C. What is historiography? *Am Hist Rev* 1938;44:1–28.
7. Goveia EV. *A study of the historiography of the British West Indies at the end of the 19*th *century.* Mexico City: Instituto Panamericano de Geografio e Historia, 1958.
8. Brodber E. Oral sources and the creation of social history in the Caribbean. *Jamaica J* 1983;16:2–8.
9. Mills C. Race and class: conflicting or reconcilable paradigms. *Soc Econ Stud* 1987;36:69–108.
10. Las Casas B. *History of the Indies*, completed in 1559. Mexico City: Fondo de Cultura Economica, 1951.
11. Thornton R. *Rethinking Columbus: Rethinking Schools special edition.* Milwaukee: Rethinking Schools, 1991.
12. Patterson O. *The sociology of slavery.* Jamaica: Sangsters, 1973.
13. Hickling FW. The political misuse of psychiatry: an African Caribbean perspective. *J Am Acad Psych Law* 2002;30:112–119.
14. Halliday A. *A general view of the present state of lunatics and lunatic asylums in Great Britain, Ireland, and some other Kingdoms.* London: Thomas and George Underwood, 1828.
15. Williams E. *Capitalism and slavery.* London: Longmans, 1970.
16. Pakenham T. *The scramble for Africa.* London: Abacus, 1992.
17. Rodney W. *How Europe underdeveloped Africa.* London: Bogle L'Overture, 1972.

18. Beckford G. *Persistent poverty.* Oxford: Oxford University Press, 1972.
19. Magubane BM. The African Renaissance in historical perspective. In: Makgoba MW, Shope T, Mazwai T, eds. *African Renaissance, Cape Town.* Cape Town: Mafube, 1999:10–36.
20. McPherson W. *The Stephen Lawrence Report.* London: The Stationary Office Agencies, 1999.
21. Marley RN. *War.* London: Island Records, 1977.
22. Mbeki T. Foreword. In: Makgoba MW, Shope T, Mazwai T, eds. *African Renaissance, Cape Town.* Cape Town: Mafube, 1999:XVII.
23. Hall S. *Racism and reaction: five views of multi-racial Britain.* London: Commission for Racial Equality, 1978.
24. Hall S. When was 'the post-colonial'? Thinking at the limit. In: Chambers I, Curti L, eds. *The post-colonial question: common skies, divided horizons.* London: Routledge, 1996:242–260.
25. Hall C. Histories, empires and the post colonial moment. In: Chambers I, Curti L, eds. *The post-colonial question: common skies, divided horizons.* London: Routledge, 1996:65–77.
26. Wilson M. Expectations and experiences. In: Fernando S, Ndegwa D, Wilson M, eds. *Forensic psychiatry, race and culture.* London, New York: Routledge, 1998:179–201.

SECTION III

International Mental Health Policy

13

International Mental Health in the 21st Century

Gregory L. Fricchione

Division of International Psychiatry, Massachusetts General Hospital, Boston, Massachusetts 02114

I. INTRODUCTION

Recently there has been a new focus in the area of international health. To quote outgoing director general of the World Health Organization (WHO), Dr. Gro Brundtland, "not only how people are dying but how they are living becomes a key ingredient in any international health planning" (1). Part of the reason for this new focus was the development of an important research tool called the disability-adjusted life years (DALYs) measure. The DALY is a health gap measure extending the concept of potential years of life lost due to premature death to include equivalent years of healthy life lost due to disability. The DALY refers to the sum of years of life lost because of premature mortality in the population plus the years of life function lost because of disability for incident cases of the health condition in question. The DALY becomes an overall global burden of disease single unit of measure that can be applied to all regions of the world (2–4).

In addition to the health burden of mental illness, there are hidden and undefined burdens to consider (5). This "hidden burden" is reflected not in pathological findings but in social consequences that lead to unemployment, stigmatization, and human rights violations. The concept of "undefined burden" encompasses the negative impact that social and economic effects have on families, friends, and communities of those suffering with mental illness. Social capital and community development are potential casualties of mental illness–related disabilities.

In this chapter, we will look at why mental illness has become a big-ticket item in terms of the disease cost to the world. We will also look at why the importance of mental health to global health has become clearer in the public health community. Worldwide prevalences of mental disorders will be reviewed, with an in-depth look at the situation in one part of the developing world, Ethiopia. Attempts to provide primary care mental health services in the developing world will be examined, along with the need for international mental health research. Then, we will summarize the WHO Mental Health Global Action Program, an attempt to respond to the world's needs in this area. And finally, we will describe the new effort at the Massachusetts General Hospital to establish an International Division of Psychiatry to contribute to efforts to reduce the global burden of disease secondary to mental illnesses.

II. MENTAL ILLNESS: A BIG-TICKET ITEM?

Why is mental illness suddenly on the radar screen of policymakers in international public health? It turns out that mental illnesses confer extensive disability not only in rich countries, but also in middle-income and poor countries. Moreover, mental illnesses appear to be on the rise throughout the world. Twelve percent of all DALYs lost in 1998 were secondary to mental illnesses. This includes 23% of DALYs in rich countries and 11% in poor countries. Major depression is the fifth of the ten leading causes of the global burden of disease. Indeed, five of the ten leading causes of the global burden of disease are mental illnesses, with alcohol abuse, bipolar disorder, schizophrenia and obsessive-compulsive disorder following on the heels of major depressive disorder. In high-income countries, dementia is the third leading cause of neuropsychiatric burden. Moreover, mental illnesses are expected to rise to 15% of the global burden of disease by the year 2020. This would make them the second leading cause of global burden behind cardiovascular disorders.

The 2001 World Health Report found that a disabling mental illness afflicts up to 20% of children and adolescents (6). According to this report, suicide is the third leading cause of death among adolescents. In a 2002 report to WHO, Belfer (7) focused on the mental health needs of children and adolescents in developing countries. He stressed specific problems, such as the fact that 80% of war victims were children and women and that there were 21.5 million refugees in the world in 1999. It is clear that children's mental health should be a priority area (8). For more information about issues affecting children, see Belfer's chapter in this volume on international child mental health.

There are several reasons why mental illnesses have increased in importance on the global public health scene. The increase in life expectancy has led to an increase in the dementias. At the same time, societal breakdowns with frayed family and social bonds have led to less social support and, therefore, an increase in propensity to mental diseases. Civil wars and international unrest have increased the incidence of refugee trauma and subsequent posttraumatic stress disorder (PTSD), and the number of refugees has increased. Major shifts in societies toward technology and commercialization may have contributed to alienation and depression. Taken together, these factors can add up to a hostile environment for mental health.

III. THE PREVALENCE OF MENTAL DISORDERS

The Composite International Diagnostic Interview (CIDI) was designed in 1990. It was a compilation of the Diagnostic Interview Schedule adjusted for both the

TABLE 13-1. *Lifetime prevalences of DSM-III-R disorders in ICPE survey studies.*

	Brazil	Canada	Germany	Mexico	Holland	Turkey	United States
Anxiety disorders	17.4	21.3	9.8	5.6	20.1	7.4	25.0
Mood disorders	15.5	10.2	17.1	9.2	18.9	7.3	19.4
Substance disorders	16.1	19.7	21.5	9.6	18.7	0.0	28.2
All study disorders	36.3	37.5	38.4	20.2	40.9	12.2	48.6

Prevalences are expressed in percentages.
(Adapted from WHO International Consortium in Psychiatric Epidemiology. Cross-national comparisons of the prevalences and correlates of mental disorders. *Bull World Health Organ* 2000;78:413–426.)

International Classification of Diseases and the fourth edition of the *Diagnostic and Statistical Manual of Mental Disorders* (DSM-IV) nosologies and diagnostic criteria. The International Consortium in Psychiatric Epidemiology, having been formed in 1998 by the WHO to carry out cross-national comparative studies of the prevalences and correlates of mental diseases, had a chance to use this common interview throughout the world. In 1998, it reported on lifetime prevalences in seven regions of North America, Latin America, and Europe (9).

Prevalence estimates from the International Consortium data varied widely, ranging from a greater than 40% lifetime prevalence for any mental illness in the Netherlands and the United States to levels of 12% in Turkey and 20% in Mexico (see Table 13-1 for a summary of lifetime prevalence data). Mental disorders were found to be often chronic; this was most true for anxiety disorders. The studies also found that early onset of mental disorders was common. The median age of onset for anxiety disorders was 15 years, for mood disorders 26 years, and for substance use disorders 21 years old. Socioeconomic measures of disadvantage and poverty such as low income, poor education, unemployment, and unmarried status were all positively associated with mental disorders.

The International Consortium concluded that mental disorders are among the most burdensome of all classes of disease because of their high prevalence and chronicity, complicated by an early age of onset leading to serious impairment. They suggested that there was a great need for demonstration projects involving early outreach, prevention, and early intervention for people with mental disorders. They also stressed the need for quality-assurance programs to look into the widespread problem of inadequate treatment of mental disorders. A study conducted by deJong et al. (10) in 2001 looked more specifically at the prevalence of PTSD in postconflict societies . This study found PTSD in 37.4% of people exposed to war, conflict, or mass violence in Algeria, 28.4% in Cambodia, 17.8% in Gaza, and 15.8% in Ethiopia.

IV. MENTAL HEALTH IN THE DEVELOPING WORLD: THE EXAMPLE OF ETHIOPIA

Examining in more detail what is known about the mental health situation in one developing country may be instructive. Ethiopia is a country in eastern Africa with a population of 70 million in an area five times that of France. There are many manmade and natural disasters in Ethiopia including drought and famine, human immunodeficiency virus (HIV) infection (which has orphaned over a million children), internal displacement due to civil wars, and other stressors and traumas. There are only nine psychiatrists in the country. One hopeful development has been the start of a psychiatry residency program at the University of Addis Ababa. Amanuel Hospital, which is located there, is the only psychiatric hospital, with 360 inpatient beds. New cases of mental illness at Amanuel Hospital numbered 6,461 in 1997, and 13,303 new cases were seen at other centers around the country. In addition to the nine psychiatrists available in Ethiopia, there are 148 practicing psychiatric nurses. There is a university outpatient clinic at the University of Addis Ababa and another unit at the Armed Forces Hospital. There are 45 treatment centers in the country, with 37 of them outside of Addis Ababa, staffed by two psychiatric nurses each (11).

In rural Ethiopia, in the Butajira region, Alem and colleagues (12) found the prevalence of mental distress to be 17.4%. Mental distress is highest in women, the elderly, the illiterate, those with low incomes, those with smaller families, or persons who are widowed and divorced. Alcohol abuse is also seen in this group. A history of a suicide attempt was found in 332 out of 10,468 subjects (3.2%). Sixty-three percent of these distressed individuals were females with a history of mental problems, family conflict, poverty, or a loss experience. Males who attempted suicide were more likely to have had physical illness or alcoholism and to have made their attempt by hanging, poisoning, or the use of guns. Problem drinking was found in 3.7% and Khat use was found in 50%. In a study conducted by Awas et al. (12) in 1999, using the CIDI, major mental disorders had a lifetime prevalence of 31.8%. Of these, anxiety was found in 75.7%, mood disorders in 6.2%, dissociative disorders in 6.3%, somatoform disorders in 5.9%, and schizophrenia in 1.8%.

In comparison, in the United States Epidemiological Catchment Area study, the lifetime prevalence of major mental disorders was 29% to 38% (13). Major depressive disorder was in the range of 3.7% to 6.7%, whereas anxiety and somatoform disorders ranged from 10.4% to 25%. Schizophrenia was in the 1.0% to 1.9% range. Tadesse et al. (14), in 1999, found that the prevalence of child and adolescent disorders in the Ambo district in Ethiopia was 17.7%. This is comparable with the prevalence that Schaffer et al. found in the United States in 1996, which was 21% (15).

In the urban Addis Ababa region, Kebede et al. (16) reported in 1999 that mental distress was prevalent at 11.7% in their sample of 10,203 individuals. Mental distress was associated most with women, the elderly, lack of education, unemployment, and small family size. The prevalence of schizophrenia was 0.4% and that of schizo-affective disorder was 0.5%. The lifetime prevalence of affective disorders was 5%, whereas that of phobic anxiety was 4.8% and other anxiety was 2.7%. An underreporting in the urban areas of Ethiopia may have occurred secondary not only to the impact of stigma, but also to governmental pressures existent at the time of the surveys.

No discussion of mental health in Ethiopia would be complete without reference to the AIDS epidemic. The work of Sahlu et al. (17) in 1999 in Jharma reflects the severe epidemic that has occurred in Ethiopia. As of 1997, there were 2,600,000 cases of HIV infection in the country. This translates into the third largest population burden in the world. The overall adult prevalence of HIV infection in Addis is between 10% and 23%. No one has carried out a study of the psychiatric comorbidity associated with this epidemic in Ethiopia, but the prevalence of depression alone in other samples of HIV patients ranges from 11% to 35%.

The WHO's atlas of mental health resources reported in 2001 that there was no mental health policy, no national mental health program, no community care in mental health, no substance abuse policy, and no applicable mental health law in Ethiopia (18). There were also no child mental health programs and no geriatric mental health programs. Another obvious barrier was the low number of psychiatrists, psychiatric nurses, psychologists, neurologists, and social workers.

V. PRIMARY CARE MENTAL HEALTH SERVICES IN THE DEVELOPING WORLD

In 1974, the WHO Alma-Ata Conference established three priorities in mental health: chronic mental handicaps (including mental retardation, dementia, and addictions), epilepsy, and "functional" psychoses. Four hundred and fifty million people around the world suffer from mental disorders today. Nearly one third of the global burden of disease is due to the 25% lifetime prevalence of mental disorders. In 2001, the World Health Organization issued the World Health Report, which focused on mental health (6). It suggested the following solutions to the problems of world mental health:

1. Provide treatment in primary care
2. Make psychotropic medications available
3. Give care in the community
4. Educate the public
5. Involve communities, families, and consumers
6. Establish national policies and legislation
7. Develop human resources
8. Link with other sectors
9. Monitor community mental health
10. Support more research.

Before looking at the WHO Mental Health Global Action Program designed to put these solutions into effect, we will focus on the need to mainstream mental health care within the primary care medical system. In a recent report, summarizing past experience, Cohen (19) finds that for the common and severe mental disorders, the evidence for effective treatment in the developing world is only indirect. This is due to the lack of adequate research data from programs that the WHO has supported in the past. Cohen does find that epilepsy is effectively treated in primary care settings, and he acknowledges that integrating mental health into primary care is still the best option, despite a lack of research evidence to date. He proposes that new programs should prioritize local needs, focusing on depression, psychosis, epilepsy, and HIV-related conditions. He also suggests that sociocultural interventions must compliment the use of medications and psychotherapies. This means that medical model approaches to mental illnesses must occur within the cultural context in which service provision is taking place.

In seeking to maximize compliance and acceptance, there is a choice of models to review. The WHO Collaborative Study on Strategies for Extending Mental Health Care trained health care workers to recognize and manage a limited number of conditions under the occasional supervision of a mental health specialist. In the Botswana Model, psychiatric nurses in primary care clinics supervise health care workers and are ultimately responsible for patient care under the periodic supervision of a consulting psychiatrist. The training of health care workers varies greatly in the developing world, and it is not known which mode is more effective in terms of patient outcomes. It must be a priority to study the best ways to train health care workers in mental health modalities. For example, should there be an emphasis on improving diagnostic sensitivity or specificity or on treatment methods? Programs should focus on the needs and wishes of communities they are expected to serve, not a "one size fits all" approach. One limitation of the few previous studies is that only public mental health and primary care approaches have been studied. Private practice models must also be studied in the developing world, because they are now providing much of the mental health care.

Intervention data are most important in assessing the service models. Demonstration projects with rigorous evaluation and outcomes methodology offering different site-appropriate mental health service models should be prioritized. In 1979, in Tanzania, there were two psychiatrists, five medical officers, and 40 mental health nurses. In 1980, the WHO/Denmark primary care/mental health integration plan was put into effect in Tanzania (19). It was designed to train health care workers in two pilot regions and to implement mental health services there. Early evaluations showed that of the 4,615 patients that were seen, 3.9% received a psychiatric diagnosis: 31.7% had anxiety, 14.4% had psychosis, 13.9% had epilepsy, 9.4% had substance abuse disorders, 2.8% had depression, 0.6% had mental retardation, and 17.2% had other conditions. The diagnostic accuracy was not determined. However, prevalence estimates were low compared with elsewhere in Africa, and most patients seemed to present with somatic complaints. Nevertheless, psychosis and epilepsy rates were higher than expected. Treatment was given to 396 patients (8.6%), whereas only 180 patients (3.9%) had received a psychiatric diagnosis. Most of those who were treated received medication, whereas only 13 patients received psychotherapy. Phenobarbital was given to 225 patients, whereas epilepsy was diagnosed in only 25 patients. Ninety-seven received antipsychotic medications, whereas only 45 presented with psychotic complaints. The program was also plagued by the poor availability of medications. Nevertheless, despite the shortcomings noted earlier, a decrease was noted in the number of admissions to the three regional psychiatric units in 1983. No follow-up studies were done.

In Botswana in 1977, there was overcrowding both in hospitals and jails, leading to a WHO Technical Assistance Campaign (19). In 1980, a psychiatric nurses program was begun with assignment to six psychiatric catchment areas. A service network of all primary care facilities was created in each region. The main strategy employed health care workers who reminded patients that the nurses would be visiting during regular rounding to these facilities. The nurses would see patients along with the facility staff to help the health care workers in their training and enable them to know the case so they could help maintain treatment. Health care workers were not expected to be self-sufficient. The specialist nurse was ultimately responsible while the health care worker provided routine ongoing care. Unfortunately, there was no funding for outcomes research.

In 1982, 80% of hospitals, health centers, and clinics were included in the Botswana program, with two thirds visited monthly and one third every 2 months by a nurse. The one psychiatrist made regular rounds in the catchment areas for consultations on difficult cases. The demand for psychiatric inpatient stays dropped by 75%. Outpatient department appointments at the mental hospital at Lobatse also decreased. This program continued into the mid-1990s, but now is somewhat overwhelmed by the AIDS epidemic.

VI. THE ETHIOPIAN PUBLIC HEALTH TRAINING INITIATIVE

In 1997, the Carter Center and the Ethiopian government established the Ethiopian Public Health Training Initiative, which emerged from discussion between former US President Jimmy Carter and Ethiopian Prime Minister Meles Zenawi. The Ethiopian Public Health Training Initiative has two major objectives: to strengthen the teaching capacities of the public health colleges in Ethiopia through education of their teaching staff, and to collaborate with Ethiopians in developing curriculum materials specifically created to meet the learning needs of the health center team personnel.

The first workshop took place in 1997 and focused on developing plans for the first 4 years of what was to be a 10- to 12-year project. Seven workshops were held over 3 years at the Nazareth, Gondar, Dilla, and Jimma campuses. Modules to educate public health care workers have been produced on such topics as malaria, diarrhea and dehydration, pneumonia, measles, HIV/AIDS, syphilis, tuberculosis, trachoma, ascariasis, protein energy malnutrition, intestinal roundworms, breastfeeding and weaning practices, immunization, acute febrile illnesses, anemia, and family planning. In May 2002, the Ethiopian Council approved a program to establish a mental health module to be used to help train health care workers in Ethiopia. This module will likely focus on common mental illnesses and conditions and on the severe illnesses and conditions selected by the WHO Global Action Program.

A technical committee is hard at work designing the mental health training module. The hope is that this training module will be used in the five public health colleges in Ethiopia to help educate health care workers in mental health management. These health care workers will work in the 35 units that are staffed by two psychiatric nurses each. These units are visited on a routine basis by the ten psychiatrists of the country, who supervise the psychiatric nurses and the health care workers on the difficult cases. Interaction with primary care takes place at the unit level, because patients present themselves at these health units seeking general care. Psychiatric nurses and health care workers are therefore charged with educating primary care physicians, nurses, and health care workers about mental health. It will be important to build in outcome studies on the Ethiopian experience. As underscored in the next section, there are many needs in international mental health research.

VII. INTERNATIONAL MENTAL HEALTH RESEARCH IN THE DEVELOPING WORLD

Kleinman and Han (20) recently pointed out that research is essential to improve the health of populations, to address the global burden of disease, to organize and fund appropriate systems of care, to prove outcomes, and to reduce disability. They suggested that intervention studies should be carried out on the economic and social contexts of mental illness. Ethnographic studies on how stigma emerges out of moral norms and perceived threats to what is most at stake for local communities must also be done and should be multidisciplinary. These studies would include the perspectives of anthropology, epidemiology, and psychiatry. The authors recommend a population laboratory approach, wherein a detailed database collection could be made on approximately 100,000 people, complete with epidemiological surveillance, pertinent clinical research, sociological surveys, and anthropological ethnographies. In these laboratories, demonstration projects in different cultural contexts using comparable diagnostic criteria, a treatment-process focus, and blinded assessment of outcomes could be achieved. This is much needed as a strategy for generalizing intervention programs.

Especially needed are gender studies looking at the effects of poverty, refugee status, and exposure to violence and infectious disease on the mental health of women and the production of depression. Special focus might be placed on postpartum depression, given its potential public health implications and intergenerational effects. Some studies should also focus on men and the effects of alcoholism and violence. Attention should also be paid to HIV/AIDS and multiple-drug–resistant tuberculosis. Issues of compliance, depression, and course of illness are of special importance in these epidemics. Political violence and refugee trauma resulting in "invisible wounds," in the words of Mollica (21), are important areas for research around the world. As stated earlier, there are over 21 million refugees, and 80% of them are women and children. Mental health problems in some refugee groups (including the Rwanda and Burundi camps) are as high as 50% (10,22).

Suicide should be another area of special interest, especially in certain countries such as China, where it is greatly underreported yet still a major public health crisis. Kleinman and Han (20) note that in some areas of the world, suicide is underreported by as much as 100%. They also advocate for mental health services research looking at primary care models, including both public and private sectors. They stress that the recognition and treatment of common mental disorders through integration of mental health services into primary care is obligatory. It will require high-level training, best-practices research, and global ethical norms. The development of international collaborative centers for research is suggested as a way to achieve these goals. These collaborative centers should be multidisciplinary, as stated earlier. Throughout all efforts in mental health research in the developing world, local area prioritization of the topical areas of interest for research should be a common approach.

Given the dimension of the burden of disease secondary to mental illnesses around the world, a renewed interest in the possibility of promoting mental health and preventing mental illnesses has emerged. In December 2000, the Inaugural World Conference on the Promotion of Mental Health and the Prevention of Mental and Behavioral Disorders: The Coming Together of Science, Policy, and Programs Across Cultures was held at the Carter Center in Atlanta, Georgia (23). A strategy for worldwide action to promote mental health and prevent mental and behavioral disorders emerged. At this conference, considerable progress was recognized in several areas: randomized controlled trials, time series studies, and quasi-experimental community trials have demonstrated the significant success of programs in reducing important risk factors and problem behaviors (23). For example, child abuse, preterm deliveries, low birth weight, and insecure attachments can be decreased through interventions made during the prenatal, infant, and toddler years.

In addition, aggressive behavior and violence can be decreased through parent training, good behavior–focused interventions in elementary schools, and comprehensive mental health promotion programs in primary and middle schools. The initiation of smoking in 14-year-olds can be lowered through interventions during early elementary school. By the same token, drug use in 12th graders can be decreased through life-skills training during the middle school years. Adolescent unprotected sexual encounters can be reduced through behavioral-skills training during high school. Teenage pregnancies can be reduced and negative marital communication styles and divorce can be decreased through education and skills training in young couples.

Research results have thus clearly shown that elements of mental health can be improved and protective factors can be enhanced. Home visitation and parent education can lead to a healthy start in life, healthier behavior in pregnant women, and better child–parent attachment. School-based curricula can maintain improvement of school climate, with secondary effects on self-esteem, life skills, and prosocial behavior. Professionals can learn stress-management skills, thus reducing their risk for occupational stress. Social support systems can foster emotional well-being. Research trials have also revealed that the onset of some specific mental disorders can be prevented, at least in the short term, through cognitive behavioral approaches. Such findings have been reported for major depression in adolescents at high risk, for generalized anxiety disorder in children ages 7 to 14 years who are anxious, and for posttraumatic stress disorders in victims of motorcycle and industrial accidents. These early studies are promising and suggest that research in prevention and promotion programs should become more of a priority (23).

VIII. THE WHO MENTAL HEALTH GLOBAL ACTION PROGRAM

Despite the presence of many barriers—including low priority, centralization of services in large institutions, lack of awareness among health care workers and policymakers, poor service organization and financing, poor quality assurance, lack of psychotropic medication availability, and stigma—the WHO in 2001 defined a Mental Health Global Action Program to address many of the needs outlined earlier in this chapter. Through its Project Atlas, WHO collected information from 185 countries, covering 99.3% of the world's population. This analysis showed that 41% of countries did not have a mental health policy as of 2001. Twenty-five percent of countries had no legislation on mental health. Twenty-eight percent had no separate budget for mental health, and of those countries that did, 36% allocated less than 1% of their health budget to mental health. Thirty-seven percent of countries did not have community mental health care facilities, and more than 25% did not have access to basic psychiatric medications at the primary care level. More than 27% of countries did not have a system for collecting or reporting mental health information. Most of the beds for mental health care are still in separated mental hospitals and, strikingly, 70% of the world's population had access to less than 1 psychiatrist per 100,000 people.

The goal of the Mental Health Global Action Program initiative is to support WHO member states in the enhancement of their capacity to reduce the stigma and burden of mental disorders. As mentioned earlier, the initiative focuses on the burden of six conditions: depression, schizophrenia, substance use disorders and dependence, dementia, epilepsy, and suicide. Four core strategies are to be used. Information concerning the magnitude, burden, determinants, and treatment of mental disorders is to be disseminated to enhance awareness. It is hoped that information dissemination will lead to advocacy against stigma and discrimination and provide for better policy decisions. The formulation and implementation of integrated policy and services is the hoped-for result of improved information and advocacy. In turn, it is hoped that integrated policy and services will generate more advocacy and even better decisions. Along the way, research capacity is expected to drive these relationships. A broad-based "university" for research in mental health is envisioned, making use of the worldwide network of WHO collaborating centers and mental health experts to set up local and regional fellowships in mental health research and evaluation. This will lead to promotion of local research capacity, contributing to the development of culturally relevant mental health information. In the final analysis, this will increase WHO's ability to understand and respond to changing trends in priority areas of inquiry.

IX. CONCLUSION

The need for enhancing international mental health has developed a new urgency now that the burden of disease secondary to mental illnesses around the world has been recognized as a public health crisis. What information we do have about the epidemiology and burden of mental illnesses needs to be disseminated. This information then needs to build a groundswell of support for developing mental health policy and legislation in countries around the world where they do not presently exist. With the coming of policy improvements, there is hope that service and resource development may receive higher priority. However, in order for services and resources to be used efficiently and effectively, better research in outcomes and demonstration projects are an absolute must. Innovative clinical research of the kind that recently showed positive effects of using group interpersonal therapy for depression in rural Uganda can be done in the developing world (24). This is particularly important in studying the integration of mental health services into the primary care infrastructures that exist in the developing countries. Models such as the one being built in Ethiopia that use a layered caregiving approach with colocation of primary care services and mental health services at the health unit level with healthcare workers seeing patients together are promising, but will need to be studied vis-à-vis the outcomes. The supervision of health care workers by psychiatric nurses and the supervision of psychiatric nurses and health care workers by visiting psychiatrists makes most efficient use of the resources presently available. Colocation with education of primary care physicians and nurses would be a natural extension at the local level.

Here in the Department of Psychiatry at Massachusetts General Hospital (MGH), a Division of International Psychiatry has been set up so that we can do our part to help meet the challenge of global mental health care. MGH should serve as a source of relevant expertise and assistance to developing nations, fostering clinical care and research relevant to local needs and conditions. The division will join and pursue efforts that not only offer assistance, but also emphasize what we can learn from colleagues abroad about how mental illnesses appear, are treated, and are managed by systems of care in other contexts and cultures. Together with these colleagues, we may be better able to address widely applicable and important questions in mental health policy, prevention, and treatment. We envision that the division will be a site for research, education, and collaboration in action-oriented programs with others as we pursue what can be learned and accomplished in a bidirectional way.

We feel that the best way to realize our goals in international education, clinical care, service improvement, and research is to develop an international psychiatry research and training center here under the auspices of the new International Division of Psychiatry. We hope this center can help revolutionize the development and apportionment of state-of-the-art psychiatry, adapted for use in areas of the world with scarce resources. Such an enterprise could contribute to the development of mental health policies, mental health service resources, mental health research, and the implementation of services in an empathic and evidence-based fashion in the developing world. Indeed, an evaluation of intervention programs is perhaps the most important requirement for future research in developing countries. As we have seen in Kleinman and Han's report (20), the development of international collaborative centers based in developing countries can bring together researchers from different regions to compare and learn new research techniques. The MGH Division of International Psychiatry will offer to collaborate with international centers abroad in an effort to establish what may constitute best practices in overseas locations and areas of need.

REFERENCES

1. Brundtland GH. Mental health in the 21st century. *Bull World Health Organ* 2000;78:411.
2. Murray CJL, Lopez AD, eds. *The global burden of disease: a comprehensive assessment of mortality and disability from diseases, injuries and risk factors in 1990 and projected to 2020. Global Burden of Disease and Injury Series, vol. 1.* Cambridge, MA: Harvard School of Public Health on behalf of the World Health Organization and the World Bank, 1996.
3. Murray CJL, Lopez AD, eds. *Global health statistics. Global Burden of Disease and Injuries Series, vol. 2.* Cambridge, MA: Harvard School of Public Health on behalf of the World Health Organization and the World Bank, 1996.
4. Murray CJL, Lopez AD. Alternative projections of mortality and disability by cause 1990–2020: Global burden of disease study. *Lancet* 1997;349:1498–1504.
5. Weiss MG, Isaac M, Parkar SR, et al. Global, national, and local approaches to mental health: examples from India. *Trop Med Int Health* 2001;1:4–23.
6. World Health Organization. *The World Health Report 2001. Mental health: new understanding, new hope.* Geneva: World Health Organization, 2001.
7. Belfer ML. International child and adolescent mental health review. In: Lewis M, ed. *Child and adolescent psychiatry: a comprehensive textbook.* 3rd ed. Philadelphia, PA: Lippincott Williams & Wilkins, 2002:1352–1360.
8. World Health Organization. *Caring for children and adolescents with mental disorders. Setting WHO directions.* Geneva: World Health Organization, 2003.
9. WHO International Consortium in Psychiatric Epidemiology. Cross national comparisons of the prevalences and correlates of mental disorders. *Bull World Health Organ* 2000;78:413–426.
10. deJong J, Komproe I, VanOmmeren N, et al. Lifetime events and post traumatic stress disorder in four post conflict settings. *JAMA* 2001;286:555–562.
11. Alem A. State of mental health in Ethiopia. Presented at the Ethiopia Public Health Training Initiative, 7th Curriculum Development and Staff Strengthening Workshop, May 13–18, 2002. Dilla College, Dilla, Ethiopia.
12. Awas M, Kebede D, Alem A. Major mental disorders in Butajira, southern Ethiopia. *Acta Psychiatr Scand Suppl* 1999;397:56–64.
13. Narrow WE, Regier DA, Rae DS, et al. Use of services by persons with mental and addictive disorders. Findings from the National Institute of Mental Health Epidemiologic Catchment Area Program. *Arch Gen Psychiatry* 1993;50:95–107.
14. Tadesse B, Kebede D, Tegegne T, et al. Childhood behavioural disorders in Ambo district, western Ethiopia. I. Prevalence estimates. *Acta Psychiatr Scand Suppl* 1999;397:92–97.
15. Shaffer D, Fisher P, Dulcan MK, et al. The NIMH Diagnostic Interview Schedule for Children Version 2.3 (DISC-2.3): description, acceptability, prevalence rates, and performance in the MECA Study (Methods for the Epidemiology of Child and Adolescent Mental Disorders Study). *J Am Acad Child Adolesc Psychiatry* 1996;35:865–877.
16. Kebede D, Alem A, Rashid E. The prevalence and socio-demographic correlates of mental distress in Addis Ababa, Ethiopia. *Acta Psychiatr Scand Suppl* 1999;397:5–10.
17. Sahlu T, Kassa E, Agonafer T, et al. Sexual behaviours, perception of risk of HIV infection, and factors associated with attending HIV post-test counselling in Ethiopia. *AIDS* 1999;13:1263–1272.
18. World Health Organization. *Atlas of mental health resources in the world 2001.* Geneva: World Health Organization, 2001.

19. Cohen A. *The effectiveness of mental health services in primary care: the view from the developing world. Nations for Mental Health.* Geneva: World Health Organization, 2001.
20. Kleinman A, Han C. *Global mental health: research that matters for the developing world.* Geneva: World Health Organization, 2002.
21. Mollica RF. Invisible wounds. *Sci Am* 2000;282:54–57.
22. deJong JP, Scholte WF, Koeter MW, et al. The prevalence of mental health problems in Rwandan and Burundese refugee camps. *Acta Psychiatr Scand* 2000;102:171–177.
23. Mrazek PJ, Hosman CMH, eds. *Toward a strategy for worldwide action to promote mental health and prevent mental and behavioral disorders.* Alexandria, VA: World Federation for Mental Health, 2002.
24. Bolton P, Bass J, Neugbauer R, et al. Group interpersonal psychotherapy for depression in rural Uganda, an RCT. *JAMA* 2003;289:3117–3124

14

International Child Mental Health

Myron L. Belfer

*Department of Social Medicine, Harvard Medical School, and Boston Children's Hospital, Boston, Massachusetts 02115 and Senior Adviser, Child and Adolescent Mental Health, World Health Organization, Geneva, Switzerland**

I. INTRODUCTION

International child mental health is no longer an esoteric topic of concern only for those interested in policy, research, or humanitarian aid. The understanding of child mental health from an international perspective is of relevance to clinicians and researchers throughout the world because of transnational migration, immigration, exposure to violence, and exploitation. Clinicians and researchers must be aware of what is known about cultural factors in the presentation and course of illness, cultural issues affecting diagnosis and treatment, and important issues for cross-cultural research. This chapter will provide a review of (a) humanitarian issues related to child mental health with a discussion of the implications of the United Nations Convention on the Rights of the Child, (b) the implications of cultural and societal issues for the assessment of children and understanding the epidemiology of child psychopathology, and (c) the implications of work with diverse populations of children for the development of clinical services and research.

II. CONTEXTUAL AND HUMANITARIAN ISSUES IN THE DEVELOPING WORLD

International child and adolescent mental health is intimately connected to the often compromised place of children in society, an understanding of diverse behavioral styles that are bound inextricably to cultural beliefs both historical and current, the ability and willingness to identify psychopathology, and the priority placed on the

*Opinions expressed in this chapter do not represent the policy or positions of the World Health Organization.

use of scarce resources for the care of those with mental illness in developing countries. With unprecedented migration and immigration of children from foreign countries into established alien societies, there is an urgent need on the part of child clinicians to understand more about the cultural dimensions and implications of the mental health problems they are encountering in clinical practice and research. Western concepts of illness, care, and the place of children in society are not universally accepted and may be inappropriate in many cultures.

Contemporary crises, such as children affected by war and the orphaning of children as a result of the HIV/AIDS epidemic, have heightened the awareness of many societies of the mental health needs of children. Thus, we are seeing an opportunity to bring about an improvement in the policies related to child mental health, to develop rational and modern treatment for child disorders, and to reduce the stigma associated with seeking care. To enhance the understanding of child and adolescent mental health in an international context, among those for whom child mental health is still not a priority issue, there is the need to foster an appreciation of a developmental perspective, to link child mental health with reducing overall psychiatric morbidity, and to create initiatives that counter the stigma associated with mental illness. Great challenges remain in the development of systems of care, and the training of professionals and other caregivers in the approaches to caring for the mentally ill child and adolescent. It is a challenge to child and adolescent clinicians and allied professionals to be active participants in understanding the nature of the problems being faced and to become part of the solution (1).

The overall health and well being of children is an international concern. Over 179 countries have ratified the 1989 United Nations Convention on the Rights of the Child (2). It commits countries to "ensure that all children have the right to develop physically and mentally to their full potential, to express their opinions freely, and to be protected against all forms of abuse and exploitation." Unfortunately, ratification of the treaty is no guarantee that the rights of children will be protected. The almost universal absence of national child and adolescent mental health policy has limited the development of coordinated efforts to enhance care because of a lack of accountability, programmatic guidance, priority setting, and funding (3).

It is simplistic to state, but meaningful to understand, that what may appear pathological in one country or society may be deemed normative or adaptive in another. Although it may be helpful to have a consensus about a frame of reference regarding psychopathological conditions, the observer must keep an open mind in attributing cause to behaviors, interpreting responses to events, or judging parental/familial interactions with children. The complexity of understanding children and adolescents embraces anthropological, social, psychological, political, and human rights dimensions. In trying to integrate knowledge gained in non-Western cultures, it is important to appreciate the distinction between emotional and behavioral problems, as often reported (4,5) from countries in the developing world, and mental disorders as commonly understood in the fourth edition of the *Diagnostic and Statistical Manual of*

Mental Disorders (DSM-IV) or the tenth revision of the *International Statistical Classification of Diseases* (ICD-10).

In developing countries, the impact of technology is differentially affecting parts of society. On the one hand, technological advance offers an unprecedented opportunity to the educated, but on the other, it accelerates inequality among the less educated. Urbanization combines with the technology revolution to further challenge accustomed ways, which may stress individuals and families (6). Children and adolescents, as students or as part of a family, experience new stresses that either convey advantage or disadvantage depending on access, intelligence, and resources. In response to these changes in society, resilience-building programs in schools, along with primary care health programs in communities, form what is recognized as the backbone of international child and adolescent mental health programming. The application of sophisticated tertiary care, even if deemed appropriate, is too often unavailable. However, the desired goal of prevention remains elusive as the political will fails to match the public rhetoric.

Child and adolescent psychiatrists are a rare commodity in developing countries. Other trained child mental health professionals vary in number and distribution in developing countries. The mode of practice often differs from that in more developed countries using primary care health providers, family and nonfamilial community members, traditional healers, and religious leaders. Pediatricians are also in relatively short supply, and thus the primary care provider with varying levels of training has become central to the provision of services. It is also of importance to note that the competencies of the child and adolescent mental health clinician must fit the needs of the society in which they exist. For example, epilepsy and mental retardation clearly fall within the expected clinical competencies of child and adolescent psychiatrists in developing countries, but are not expected competencies of child and adolescent psychiatrists in developed countries. When child psychiatry is a very scarce resource there may only be the opportunity for a consultative role, limited diagnostic capability, and an inability to be part of or stimulate discussion of national policy. At the same time, child and adolescent psychiatrists brought into developing countries may play a vital role in educating other professionals in medicine, psychology, education, social work, nursing, and the volunteer community. There is a clear need for increasing trained personnel to work in the primary care sector, but such training has lagged.

Significant gains have been made in raising consciousness about the mental health of children and adolescents. The importance now attributed to mental disorders and mental health, in general, is reflected in the World Health Organization (WHO) focus on mental health in its 2001 World Health Report (7) and in the mental health focus for World Health Day in 2001. In addition, the World Bank now considers mental health among its priority areas of concern. Recent analyses of the burden of disease give added weight to the arguments for considering child and adolescent mental disorders as a priority for policy development and research on longitudinal risk for morbidity and mortality. By bringing attention to the "burden" of mental illness (8) as measured in disability-adjusted life years (DALYs), it is possible to

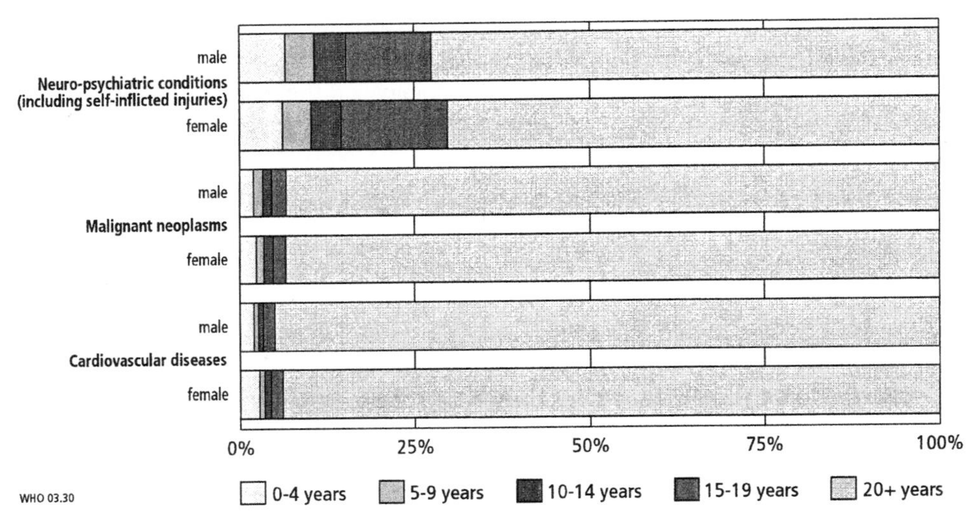

FIG. 14-1. World: Disability-adjusted life years (DALYs) in 2000 attributable to selected causes, by age and sex. (Reprinted from World Health Organization, Department of Mental Health and Substance Abuse. *Caring for children and adolescents with mental disorders: setting WHO directions.* Geneva: World Health Organization, 2003:3.)

have a more standardized assessment of the burden of disease measured in terms of lost opportunity, diminished function, and the cost of treatment and rehabilitation. Although the concept of DALYs has some inadequacies, it has achieved a supportive response from policymakers. From the child mental health perspective, DALYs have limitations in that they do not quantify negative or positive effects of behaviors but only address outcomes, and fail to adequately factor in associated costs related to child and adolescent mental disorders. As a result, the importance of behaviors that start during childhood and adolescence but result in disease and death only later in life may be underestimated by this approach.

The data reflected in Figure 14-1 (9) detail the burden of disease among noncommunicable disorders. Neuropsychiatric conditions and self-inflicted injuries represent a disproportionately large share of the burden of disease in younger people and a significant proportion of the overall burden.

Malnutrition

Malnutrition impacts the developing brain and may lead not only to delayed cognitive development, but also to more subtle behavioral manifestations including attentional problems and learning disabilities (10–12). Some studies suggest that the behavior disorders associated with malnutrition are secondary to impaired maternal capacities and not due to the malnutrition itself, because there is conflicting evidence that malnutrition does not contribute to behavioral disturbance later in life (13,14). Clearly, in the international context, the impact of malnutrition, whether on the child or on the mother, needs to be considered.

Conflict and Violence

The global problem of displacement from family, home, community, and country is of enormous importance to understanding the mental health of child populations. Displacement from war resulted in approximately 21.5 million refugees in 1999. An additional 30 million, 80% of whom are children and women, are displaced internally. In trying to appreciate the magnitude of the impact on the mental health of children and adolescents one needs to consider the importance of "place" in healthy development as described by Fullilove (15). Further, Sampson and colleagues (16), in their study of inner city Chicago, have specifically addressed the importance of the community as a mediator of the impact of violence on children and adolescents. The concept of "collective efficacy" in communities, as operationalized in the Chicago study, must now be seen as an important variable when assessing the impact imposed by poverty and displacement during or after ethnic conflicts and other traumatic events (16).

In developing countries, the notion of "place" and community are of equal or greater importance to that observed in domestic studies. The disruption of traditional communities by war, famine, and natural disaster leaves children and adolescents in vulnerable situations that impact mental health. Internal displacement due to war and famine leads to the break up of families, months and years of uncertainty, disruption of education, and morbidity from physical illness. Forced emigration and loss of parents and relatives in war often means abandonment or orphaning of children and adolescents. On the one hand, these stressors may serve to demonstrate the enormous resiliency of youth, but they often lead to depression, suicide, and a range of stress responses (17). Regardless of whether one focuses on pathological outcomes or observed resilience, gaining attention for a consideration of the mental health of these impacted individuals is a challenge in the context of life-threatening conditions.

A priority concern of those working in international child and adolescent mental health is often the acute and continuing tragedies that involve youth in armed conflict or the consequences of conflict. Eighty percent of the victims of war are children and women (18). The result of armed conflict is often displacement, which creates for large numbers of children and adolescents psychological consequences as severe as the more high profile concerns with posttraumatic stress disorder (PTSD) and short-term consequences; those with experience in frontline work in war-affected areas believe that longer-term consequences and depression deserve as much attention.

In the turmoil of some developing countries, children are now being forced to become "child soldiers," and other others are drawn into the conflict by being exploited for sexual purposes or labor. These horrific experiences place an as yet not fully understood burden on the psychological development of the child either as victim or perpetrator. To what extent does resiliency allow for future healthy development? Is permanent scarring evident and, if so, in what ways—disturbed interpersonal relationships, distorted defenses, heightened aggression, reduced empathy, and self-destructive behavior (17)? Many of the affected people are finding their way to the West or other parts of the world as asylum seekers, through resettlement programs or immigration. Once in these new settings, many of these young people are finding their way into the mental health or juvenile justice systems. Understanding the experience of these children and the consequences for their psychological development is essential to the provision of appropriate and effective clinical services.

In addition to the research already noted, there is a large body of internationally focused data from conflict areas where displacement from homes, families, communities, and countries has been part of the life experience of children. Representing this body of work, Zivic (19), in a study of Croatian children during war, found significantly higher depressive and phobic symptoms in displaced refugee children than in local children in stable social conditions. These displaced children were faced with exposure to war and violence, and may have seen family members murdered. Less often but even more horrific, some children have been forced into being the murderers of their family or conscripted to serve as child soldiers. Others find themselves either displaced to other countries or internally displaced and left to fend for themselves. Street children engage in survival tactics that include criminal activity and prostitution. In an effort to find a context for survival, the formation of youth gangs is increasingly evident, especially in societies where there is a lapse in government organization and control. More often than not, the children are the victims rather than the perpetrators.

HIV/AIDS

In sub-Saharan Africa, Russia, and parts of Asia, AIDS is now a pandemic. Special attention needs to be given to the consequences of AIDS for children and youth. The impact on children and adolescents is evident. Sexual exploitation has led to a high incidence of youth infection, with the inevitable outcome of death due to lack of available treatment. Parental disease has resulted in fetal transmission, and parental death from AIDS has led to a burgeoning population of AIDS orphans. An estimated 1.5 million children under the age of 15 years are living with HIV/AIDS (20). Over a quarter of the youth population in sub-Saharan Africa is infected. Among the ten most affected countries, all in sub-Saharan Africa, approximately 6,000,000 children under the age of 15 years have lost their mother or both parents to AIDS. For those infected but struggling with the illness, there is the prospect of having to adjust to declining physical and mental functioning and often living isolated lives. Thus, the mental health consequences of AIDS as a chronic and pervasive illness must be considered. There is the obvious concern with the direct effect of AIDS on the youth who have manifestations of neuropsychological dysfunction, including dementia, depression, and other disorders that go largely untreated. Then there are the children and adolescents living as orphans in stigmatized environments, vulnerable as the result of the loss of a parent or parents. They may be disenfranchised, with their depression going unrecognized. Others must assume the role of parent for younger children, leading to circumscribed opportunities for self-development. Research has yet to fully assess the mental health impact on this generation of youth, and adequate data to predict the future impact on societies remain elusive.

The mental health consequences of AIDS are well documented in US studies and are presumed to be similar in the international arena (21). In developing countries, it is more likely that recognition of the neuropsychological consequences will be overshadowed by the totality of the devastation. This lack of recognition of depression, dementing illness, and other consequences of HIV infection may contribute to the continuing spread of the epidemic. As documented by Carlson and Earls (22), whether through social policy, as evidenced in the Leagane children of Romania, or as the consequence of the pandemic of AIDS, the rearing of children in orphanages or in other situations that deprive children of appropriate stimulation and nurturance has potentially long-lasting consequences for societies.

III. CULTURE AND PSYCHOPATHOLOGY IN CHILDREN

A. Epidemiology

Determining the epidemiology of childhood mental disorders in Western society is a challenge. Internationally, the ability to determine the precise magnitude of mental disorders is even more complex. Reporting systems are inadequate, the definition or recognition of disorders varies or has variable interpretations, and the cultural component of what constitutes a disorder is only now being more fully appreciated by epidemiologists and researchers. Of significance in developing countries is that any measure of mental disorder takes place against a background of child and adolescent mortality and morbidity that may obscure the importance of associated child psychiatric morbidity and co-occurring disorders. This, among several other factors, contributes to the inaccuracy of data in developing countries. Thus, in studying the epidemiology of psychiatric disorders in children and adolescents in developing countries, it is important to define not only the prevalence and incidence of the disorders, but also the associated impairment and burden of disease as measured in the cost to society of lost productivity, cost of care, and lost human potential. There is no single study or consistent set of independent studies on the epidemiology of child and adolescent disorders conducted in the past 20 years that can be identified as definitive or relevant across societies. Those studies performed 20 years ago reflect the deficiencies noted earlier and certainly do not reflect the current realities of the countries from which the data were reported (23,24).

When faced with the realities in developing countries, as noted, there is the danger of becoming a diagnostic nihilist in attempting to understand mental disorders in youth. Yet, with all the caveats noted, responsible investigators have clearly identified disordered mental functioning that meets defined criteria (25), albeit not the same criteria. There is clear evidence that what would generally be called depression, psychosis, and mania can be defined and treated. The problem arises when one considers the context for the presentation of child and adolescent mental disorders. Is a hallucination during a ritual a disturbance in need of treatment? If the hallucination persists, should it be treated? What diagnostic label is appropriate?

Until there is adequate and accurate reporting, it cannot be assumed that the current state of child and adolescent mental health in the developing world is substantially different from that in the developed world, or that one can be overly optimistic based on ignorance of what represents impairment associated with mental disorders in developing countries. This sense is supported by the finding of WHO studies of primary care clinicians that a significant proportion of patients seeking care had mental disorders, and that their communities were aware of the problem (26). It is important to bear in mind the study of Giel and Van Lujik (4) who found, counter to prevailing belief, that mental disorders were diagnosed more frequently than infectious diseases in the health centers in Africa that they studied. Most countries today have access to appropriate epidemiological study guidelines, and it will be a matter of setting a national priority and allocating resources to ascertain the data in developing countries. The recent delineation of "cultural epidemiology," combining classical epidemiology with the information derived from cultural anthropological study, offers a unifying approach that may advance the understanding of child and adolescent disorders as seen in developing countries and inform our understanding in clinical settings worldwide (27).

Fayyad et al. (28) summarized the significant international epidemiological studies, and concluded that the range and rates of psychiatric symptomatology in children in the developing countries are similar to those in the developed world. There appeared to be universal risk factors correlated with manifest psychopathology, including parental separation and divorce, psychological deprivation, and culture-specific factors such as polygamy.

Recently Tadesse et al. (29) reported a prevalence of childhood behavioral disorder of 17.7% in Ethiopia. The behavioral disorders were more frequent in boys than in girls. These latter data were gathered with a version of the Reporting Questionnaire for Children developed by the WHO (29,30). Studies by Hackett et al. (31) in India and Bird et al. (32) in Puerto Rico found an excess of males with externalizing disorders. The findings support the Western view of a male predisposition to externalizing disorders. Thabet and Vostanis (33) reported a pattern of anxiety symptoms and disorders among children living in the Gaza Strip comparable to that found in previous epidemiological research in Western societies. There were high rates of anxiety disorders and school-related mental health problems. Further, Thabet and Vostanis found the same prevalence rate (21%) of anxiety-related disorders as did Kashani and Orvashel (34) in the United States. Importantly, Thabet and Vostanis state that their findings did not support the commonly held belief that, in non-Western societies, anxiety and other mental health symptoms are predominantly expressed through somatizing symptoms. Again, expressing what was once thought a controversial view, citing Nikapota (5), they state that child mental health symptoms do not differ significantly across cultures, and that culture-specific mental health disorders are rare. These views of comparability with Western epidemiological data are at odds with older studies, and may reflect new social and economic realities.

What of the disorders that are now occupying considerable attention in developed countries such as attention-deficit/hyperactivity disorder (ADHD), autism, and anorexia nervosa? In the case of eating disorders, there is clear evidence that the incidence may be affected by Western influences (35). There is little doubt that these disorders are seen, but what resources need to be invested in the treatment of these disorders in countries that have little access to the medications or programs that might be indicated? The diagnosis and treatment of these disorders highlights both a weakness and strength of having an international perspective. The recognition and labeling of disorders come as a result of improved international communication. However, the process of assessment is most complex, taking into account cultural concepts of what is normal or abnormal, and how parents perceive the presence or absence of a diagnosable disorder (24).

Increasingly, it is the pharmaceutical industry that provides the local education of providers in countries throughout the world. The attendant focus on particular disorders of interest to the pharmaceutical industry may distort the presentation of children and adolescents for treatment in clinics and lead to misconceptions about the incidence and prevalence of disorders. There may be an indirect incentive for the overdiagnosis of disorders such as ADHD or anxiety. The ability to evaluate the impact of these practices is quite variable throughout the world.

B. Cultural Influences on the Assessment of Psychopathology

Understanding the culture and context of any individual is crucial to the provision of care and the accurate diagnosis of disorder. For example, Murthy (36) reports that studies have found that suicide rates among immigrants are more closely aligned to the rates in the country of origin than to the rates in the country of adoption. The methods of suicide are those used traditionally in the culture of origin. As an example, suicide by burning was nearly ten times more common in females from the Indian subcontinent than in the overall female population in England and Wales (36,37). Canino et al. (38) also documented and advocated for the recognition of the persistence of relevant culture-bound syndromes in evaluating children in a US domestic context. In a particularly relevant study for international work, van Ommeren et al. (39) report on the context for the explanation of an apparently mysterious medical illness in Bhutanese adolescents. The manifestation of the mysterious illness clearly related to beliefs present in the local culture that were used for symptom attribution, even though from a research perspective more traditional concepts of loss and childhood trauma were statistical predictors of the illness. As reported by van Ommeren et al. (39), the fear of possession and the associated fear of dying led to high anxiety and somatoform anxiety symptoms that were interpreted as direct evidence of being possessed and dying. The latter led to a compounding of presenting physical symptoms. This confirms an earlier observation by Castillo (40) in South Asia of the type of reciprocal relationships noted by van Ommeren et al., wherein the experience of trauma may be one of the risk factors for spirit possession.

Although understanding the cultural surround associated with perceived psychopathology is of great concern, there is the need to balance this concern with the obvious danger of attributing to a culture the symptoms representing treatable mental illness. Nikapota (41) underscores the importance of determining "culture-appropriate" criteria to permit consistency in diagnosis. For example, in India, de-emphasis on the expression of thoughts and emotions in children, when identified by clinicians as representing a degree of pathology, could explain the greater preponderance of reported neurotic, psychosomatic, and somatization disorders (42). Thus, culture can influence the definition of normalcy or disorder. Malhotra and Chaturvedi (43) clearly articulate this perspective, stating that culture "proscribes the values and ideals for the behavior of individuals; determines the threshold of acceptance of pathology; and provides guidelines for the handling of pathology and its correction."

Mathews et al. (44) report on the influence of culture in the diagnosis and perception of Tourette's syndrome in children in Costa Rica. In this instance, important to the cross-cultural understanding of disorders in children and adolescents is the observation that although the phenomenology of a disorder may be similar across cultures, there may be a differential impact on perceived impairment. In the Mathews et al. (44) study, the degree of impairment associated with comorbid attentional and obsessive compulsive symptoms was less than that observed in other reported populations. The authors attribute this difference in perceived impairment to the fact that needs and expectations differ in differing cultures. For example, expulsion from school in an agrarian culture has less impact that it does in an urban setting. A culturally relevant perception in Costa Rica is that tics are thought of as a "bad habit" and not as a physical problem. Thus, the individual may be subject to discipline but not necessarily brought for other types of care outside the home. A general point made by Mathews et al. (44) is that where cultural forces affect disease definition, close scrutiny of symptom expression and possible adjustment of phenotype definition may be important. The authors observe that in many parts of Latin America, tics, including those associated with Tourette's syndrome, are still seen as being psychogenic rather than of physical origin and are treated with psychotherapy or behavior modification. Perhaps the willingness to accept the physical etiology of tic disorders is related to the level of impairment associated with a disorder in a cultural context. Such observations enhance the understanding of the contribution of culture to assessment.

To gain more standardized data for epidemiological and services planning, there is now great interest in the development of assessment tools that incorporate the diversity of cultural parameters. Beyond the now common strategy of translation and back translation, investigators are pursuing the development of more specific culturally relevant assessment instruments. These newer instruments are being added to the more commonly available, usually Western-developed, instruments for the assessment of depression, anxiety, PTSD, stress, and quality of life. It remains for there to be a sufficient body of cross-cultural research, with the use of modern standards for instrument design and validation, for the field of cross-cultural child and adolescent psychiatric research to have a full array of useful instruments to complement clinical interviewing and provide valid cross-cultural data for comparison.

A prime example of an instrument that has been widely translated and back translated is Achenbach's Children's Behavior Checklist (CBCL), including the Teacher's Report Form (TRF) and the Youth Self Report (YSR). This instrument finds wide acceptance in studies assessing children's adaptive behavior and psychopathology (45). There is a broader literature on comparing the factor structures of children's emotional and behavioral problems in different countries (46–48). In the view of many, the researcher is not on firm ground extrapolating from an essentially symptom-related assessment to a formal diagnosis meeting accepted standards. A general caution is that there needs to be standardization of any instrument for the culture in which it is used (49). A more accommodating view is offered by Slobodskaya (50), who argues that if the internal consistencies of syndrome scales, such as in the CBCL, are "sufficient," the scores could also be used for direct cross-cultural comparisons. Among Slobodsykaya's findings is the observation that cultures may have a "high cultural threshold" for recognizing emotional and behavioral problems and, as in the findings from Russia, this may result in increased reports of somatization. In the final analysis it must be borne in mind that the CBCL, which is very useful for a variety of assessment purposes, does not provide diagnoses that meet DSM-IV or ICD-10 criteria, and for most clinical purposes requires supplementation with more detailed assessment or with clinical interviews.

Posttraumatic Stress Disorder

The impact of the exposure of children to natural disasters and the trauma of war and other forms of violence is an area of both clinical concern and research. The literature reflects differing views of the impact of these traumas on children in terms of vulnerability, specific impact, and long-term consequences. Some believe that the diagnostic label of PTSD is often unwarranted and that the major pathological outcome is depression that goes unrecognized. Others advocate for placing the emphasis on the resilience of children and not on the outcomes leading to PTSD in the relatively small number of affected individuals (51). Earlier studies tend to place the emphasis on the diagnosis of PTSD and later studies on the potential resilience of affected individuals and the evidence for depression as a longer-term outcome. The child and adolescent literature reflects these conflicting views (52–55). The resiliency of children over the long term seems to be a consistent dominant finding, but individual investigators identify depression, externalizing behaviors, and PTSD as evidence of specific consequences (56). Laor et al. (56), in a developmental study of Israeli children exposed to Scud missile attacks, found higher externalizing and stress symptoms in displaced children than in those able to maintain family and community connections. Children in these circumstances may find themselves without the protection and support of parents at critical junctures in their lives. Children are forced to act in more mature ways far earlier than normal development would dictate or allow. Thus, it may be the combination of contextual factors along with the presence or absence of a diathesis that leads to the manifestation of mental disorder.

Further, according to Sack et al. (57), diagnostic status does not relate to functional status. Sack et al. (52) not only showed persistence of PTSD, but also demonstrated that there was sometimes a delayed onset of symptoms. In their study, there was a persistence of the PTSD diagnosis in youth over time, but they appeared able to function well. Studies of Kuwaiti children exposed to the threat of violence (58), and those from Iran (59), show the persistence of PTSD but with varying levels of functional impairment. Nader et al. (60) reported moderate to severe PTSD in 70% of Kuwaiti children after the Gulf War, but with less evident residual functional impairment than might have been expected. Terr (61) demonstrated persistent effects on children from traumas with lasting functional deficits. Ahmad (62) reported that 25% of displaced Kurdish children evidenced PTSD, and Weine et al. (55) found similar rates in Bosnian adolescents who had moved to the United States during the war. Hussain et al. (63), reporting on the impact of the siege of Sarajevo, noted that it was not the exposure to sniper fire, but rather the loss of a family member and deprivation of food, water, and shelter, that had a severe adverse impact on the children. The clinical manifestation of the trauma was avoidance and re-experiencing symptoms. The studies of Ahmad (62), Weine(55) and Husain(63) all support the importance of understanding the context in which a diagnosis of PTSD is made. This has significant implications for the mode of treatment and possible course of illness.

Attention Deficit Hyperactivity/Hyperkinetic Disorder

Attention deficit hyperactivity/hyperkinetic disorder is now reported worldwide. Regardless of the societal context, this disorder is reported with a remarkably high frequency, often from a country baseline of only a few years before when the diagnosis was not made at all. Prevalence studies of ADHD comparable to those in the West have been reported for populations in China, Brazil, India, Nigeria, and the United Arab Emirates (28). In the current era, the problem of accurate diagnosis is one that needs to be emphasized. The popularization of the diagnosis through the media and pharmaceutical advertising campaigns in both developed and developing countries, and the association made with poor school performance, delinquent behavior, and substance abuse, whether warranted or not, has led parents, teachers, and administrators to devote considerable attention and resources to the disorder. In some developing counties, the marketing of remedies to treat ADHD are aggressive and promise spurious outcomes, such as increased happiness and academic success in standard educational examinations.

Depression and Suicide

The diagnosis of depression is made in an increasingly sophisticated manner, but this is not the case in resource-poor areas. Western concepts of bipolar disorder are of interest in relation to children and adolescents, but unfortunately the Western reports too often lead to too rapid and/or inappropriate diagnoses in settings where the technical expertise does not exist to make such complex diagnoses. Meanwhile, on the positive side, there is increasing recognition in all parts of the world that children can be depressed and that the disorder merits treatment.

Suicide in youth is a pervasive world mental health problem. In Western cultures, suicide is presumed to be overwhelmingly associated with mental disorder. Elsewhere in the world, it is often very difficult to tease out the mental disorder associated with the suicidal act. The social, familial, and acute environmental factors may often overshadow or negate the presence of any causal mental disorder. The worldwide research data linking suicide with defined mental disorders, including depression, must be viewed with an understanding that the overall findings of causal linkage are based on relatively few studies using currently acceptable diagnostic criteria. Fleischmann et al. (64) surveyed the English-language scientific literature on completed suicide in young people worldwide and found that the literature, in the aggregate, reports on only 785 cases where depression was defined to meet DSM-IV (or III/III-R) or ICD-10 criteria. Thus, respect should be accorded for the views coming from developing countries about causal links to other than mental disorders. Studies of suicide in the West have focused on risk factors associated with cognitive distortions, substance use, and familial factors (65), and these are certainly of great relevance in an international context.

In trying to assess the high rates of suicide in some developing countries, it appears that the balance in determining suicidal risk may rest with environmental stressors and the perception of "no way out." Exceedingly high educational or performance expectations for children and youth may be a potent determinant of suicidal acts in the absence of a defined mental disorder (66). It should be noted that the traditional protective effect of religion in certain cultures seems not to operate among the younger generation (28), and suicide to assuage guilt, shame, or humiliation may be condoned in certain cultures. From this perspective, in India and other developing countries, the focus of the suicidal individual is not on achieving some exalted goal, but rather on being able to have enough of a dowry to be married, to not be isolated because of rape, or to be successful in passing a school advancement examination. It seems more apparent that suicide is viewed by those without demonstrable mental disorder as a solution to social and personal dilemmas, as noted previously, that bring with them thwarted expectations for a happy or successful life. This alteration in emphasis is important when considering intervention strategies, and when training workers to triage and treat suicidal children and adolescents.

In India, suicide rates have been steadily rising. Psychiatrists believe this is due in part to the accelerating pace of social and economic change. A consistent finding in India is that the dominant risk factor is a combination of social and economic issues. Farmers in debt take pesticide and ostracized women immolate themselves (67).

Case Illustration

In India, four sisters aged 16 to 24 years committed suicide by hanging after an evening during which they bought sweet cakes and samosas and played word games.

The context was that they were part of a once prosperous family in which the father died of tuberculosis due to lack of medical treatment. Now they were periodically without sufficient food, but with a mother too proud to ask for help. This family was socially isolated due to parental marriage across religious lines and had suffered an unexpected financial downturn due to a road-widening project that took their once fertile land.

In Hong Kong, amidst the impressive high-rise buildings and fancy stores, there reside families barely able to subsist. In this context of economic hardship, due in part to massive economic adjustment in the Far East, there is the phenomenon of family suicide. Chan (68) reported that families would come together and in a well-planned manner, seal themselves inside their small apartments, and light a charcoal heater. In a relatively brief time, the members of the family are asphyxiated. This has become an acceptable form of suicide in that the bodies remain intact and have an attractive appearance due to the monoxide poisoning. To the extent that it has been possible to determine the psychological state of the family before the suicides, there has not been the report of major psychiatric disturbance.

Substance Abuse

Substance abuse in children and adolescents is a worldwide problem (69). In developing countries, the problem is of no less importance than in Western countries and exacts a tremendous toll in terms of morbidity and mortality. The use of psychoactive substances not defined as drugs of abuse, such as khat, inhalants, and alcohol, are accessed by youth regardless of economic circumstance or religious prohibition (70). In Egypt, patterns of drug use are as follows: First-time use of any drug including tobacco is reported at age 14 years, with progression to the use of alcohol and cannabis by age 17 years and the use of synthetic hypnosedatives by age 18 years (71). There is progression to the use of opioids and/or cocaine by age 20 years. Most users are polysubstance abusers (71). Ahmad and Hasani (72) found that 30.23% of their sample of Iranian high school students reported using substances one or more times during their lives. Of those who reported use, 25.4% reported cigarette use, 9.6% alcohol use, 3.5% opium, and 2.8% hashish, with lesser percentages for marijuana, heroin, LSD, cocaine, and morphine. Current use as opposed to lifetime use was 13.86% with a proportional use of the substances noted above. Substance use was significantly higher among males than females (72). Khat is used extensively in East Africa and the Middle East. In Somalia, Ethiopia, and Kenya, khat is used at all levels of society from about age 10 years (73). Khat may induce a mild euphoria and excitement that can progress to hypomania. In youth, khat use, especially if combined with the use of other psychoactive substances, may lead to psychosis. In Nigeria, heroin is now cheaply available and the pattern of use has shifted from use in affluent minority communities to marginalized young and unemployed males (70,74).

Solvent and inhalant use is disproportionately prevalent in poor economies. In South America, inhalant use is dominant among youth affected by psychoactive substances. In Sao Paolo, Brazil, up to 25% of children age 9 to 18 years abuse solvents (75). In the Sudan, gasoline is the inhalant of choice; in Mexico, Brazil, and elsewhere in Latin America, paint thinner, plastic cement, shoe dye, and industrial glue are often used. Solvent use is also found among the aboriginal groups in Australia and on Canadian Indian reservations (76). In Mexico, 3 of every 1,000 people between the ages of 14 and 24 years use inhalants on a regular basis (77). These figures do not include two high-risk groups, the homeless population, and those younger than 14 years, where inhalation is much greater. Several community studies carried out in different parts of Mexico show that starting ages are as young as 5 or 6 years (77). In conflict-impacted countries, it is now common to see youth using inhalants as they take up life on the streets. Recent data suggest that the percentage of young people using inhalants decreases as age increases and other substances such as alcohol and marijuana are substituted. Child soldiers are routinely offered and use drugs and/or alcohol in the course of their combat or aggression.

Mental Retardation and Epilepsy

Mental retardation and epilepsy are major disorders that often dominate the services of child mental health and pediatric professionals in developing countries. The prevalence rates of mental retardation in developing countries were estimated over a decade ago to be in the range of 8 to 12 per 1,000 for children aged 3 to 10 years (78–80). Mental retardation and epilepsy are the most common mental disorders in India (43,81). The rate of serious mental retardation in some developing countries may reach 16.2 per 1,000 population (82), significantly higher than the rate in the West, which is 4% to 8% (83). Cerebral palsy and postnatal etiologies of retardation are much more common in transitional societies than in developed countries.

Untreated epilepsy limits the potential for any individual to participate in society. Unfortunately, although the cost of medication is relatively small, access to care is often limited. The care of the mentally retarded varies widely in developing countries. In some, special effort is made to provide for productive lives with meaningful vocational education, especially in agrarian economies. All too often, the moderately and severely retarded are housed in minimal care institutions where illness and premature death are common.

IV. SERVICE DELIVERY IN THE DEVELOPING WORLD

Service Gaps

The notion of an ideal continuum of care for children remains a dream in all but the wealthiest and most enlightened areas of the world. In developing countries, services tend to reflect low levels of spending, archaic forms of institution-based care left over from much earlier times, or fragmentation due to lack of collaboration, idiosyncratic program development, lack of funding, and lack of knowledge about appropriate modes of care for children and adolescents with mental disorders (84). However, these observations should not be assumed to be universal, because there are some excellent programs for children and adolescents with mental disorders in the developing world and, in particular, in low-income countries. Often, this reflects the priority or advocacy of particular individuals to obtain the resources needed for the programming rather than representing a national commitment to provide the particular services.

The Western concept of a continuum of care for the treatment of seriously emotionally disturbed children and adolescents will remain a hope in most of the developing world. The reshaping of institution-based care and the training or retraining of those used to older models of care requires resources that are beyond the reach of most nations. However, the encouragement of the development of innovative forms of intervention using traditional healers, religious communities, parents, and communities should be a priority.

To be avoided is the naïve and too-rapid introduction of Western concepts of managed care, privatization, and insurance that are not suitable in the developing world and tend to distort existing systems in ways that may erode basic services that are desperately needed as a safety net. These initiatives come in countries that have barely viable rudimentary systems of care for child mental health. Those promoting these "reforms" are often not familiar with or wish to ignore the negative outcomes that have led to a reduction in services to the most needy through the imposition of these fiscally driven efforts. Although managed care and health services research has had the beneficial impact of stimulating the development of some innovative systems of care, unfortunately the investment needed to foster these systems of care does not exist in the developing countries.

Of particular concern in areas that are "postconflict" or where natural disasters have occurred is the role of nongovernmental organizations (NGOs). These NGOs are often rapid responders to crises. However, when they arrive in the impacted areas, there is often little regulation of their delivery of services. This can lead to duplication of services, poor needs assessment, and the delivery of services not appropriate to the target population. In some instances, the situation of the community can be made worse by the raising of expectations for services that then cease when the money flow to the NGO ceases at the end of the crisis, or when the emergence of a crisis in some other locale diverts the attention of the NGO. That NGO services are often delivered in the absence of a plan for sustainability is a major problem in the delivery of care in developing countries and those impacted by conflict.

Training for Service Delivery

Short-term, focused training in specific areas related to diagnosis or intervention, often sponsored by NGOs, can provide a level of specialized care that may have an impact. However, these programs often do little to help develop a system of care or provide basic education that lays the groundwork for more comprehensive mental health care. The development of models of care in developing or resource-poor countries that utilize parents, teachers, pediatricians, and others can be informed by the findings from studies in developed countries, but also must incorporate the knowledge and creative capacities of the local individuals. Of special interest is the need to validate indigenous methods of care and models that are not dependent on specialists. This approach will allow new programs to avoid the pitfalls seen with the development of highly touted, but ineffective, programs in developed countries that are sometimes viewed with inflated expectations.

The prospect for the future of child mental health practice in developing countries is tied to economic growth, health literacy, and reduction of stigma. The creative efforts to develop programs to reach children and adolescents in developing countries need to be supported. Child and adolescent psychiatry will remain a scarce resource to be utilized in ways that will not have a duplicative impact. This means that the training of volunteers and peers, the support of family intervention programming, and the use of community-based early intervention need to be the focus of attention. In some countries, the lack of child mental health personnel has stimulated some remarkable efforts to train individuals from diverse backgrounds to be effective in identifying—and intervening to ameliorate—child mental health problems. Kapur and Cariapa (85), who developed an impressive school consultation program in Bangalore, India, demonstrated that the training of teachers as counselors in India was effective. In Alexandria, Egypt, child counselors have also been trained to develop culturally accepted sophisticated interventions in schools (86).

Program Illustration

In Alexandria, the Department of Community Medicine has supported the development of a cadre of school counselors. These counselors come from the ranks of volunteers, social workers, and psychologists. Without prior child mental health training, the workers are provided with course work on common child mental health problems and then supervised in field placements. The counselors work with parents around children identified by both the school and parents as having some type of behavioral problem. They also serve as contact points for the school, parents, or pediatricians to bring children with more severe behavioral disturbance to the attention of the few fully trained mental health professionals.

Much emphasis is placed on mental health training for primary care practitioners, but the reality for child-focused practitioners is that training in child mental health has lagged. It must be borne in mind that without appropriate training, primary practitioners have been shown to have a poor record of recognizing mental disorders. The challenge is even greater in reference to child and adolescent disorders than that with adult psychiatric disorders. Giel (87) reported in his study in developing countries that primary care practitioners identified only 10% to 20% of the disorders that his group were able to diagnose. The WHO has devoted considerable effort to the development and distribution of training manuals to aid primary care practitioners in the recognition of mental disorders (41,88,89). More recently child mental health training modules have been incorporated in the WHO's widely used Integrated Management of Childhood Illness program.

An example of a primary care, comprehensive program comes from India, where the anganwadi system has developed to provide basic nutrition and educational support in villages. This is both an appropriate preventive intervention and a way to assess youngsters presenting with disorders (90). The anganwadi system focuses on providing essential services to very young children. Like HeadStart, the program provides nutrition, basic education, socialization, and a venue for more specialized intervention for children perceived to be at risk or in need of additional services (91). There must be a concern in the development of these indigenous systems of care that not too much dependence is placed on family structure and support at a time when urbanization and industrialization is eroding the traditional family structure. Both the extended and new nuclear family face mounting challenges leading to a vulnerability for both the adults and their children.

Prevention and Mental Health Promotion versus Services

It would appear that prevention is the way to approach the problem of reducing the toll of mental illness in developing countries. However, mental health initiatives in developing countries are often dependent on outside sponsorship. Such sponsorship, whether in the form of grants from donor countries or foundations, most often requires evidence-based intervention with a definable outcome. The field of prevention in both developed and developing countries offers little support for evidence-based programming for the prevention of child and adolescent mental disorders. Compounding this problem is the investment needed to adapt promising prevention programs for implementation in developing countries. For any program to go to scale, there is the need for broad political and community support. Unfortunately, there is often a lack of political will to support prevention programming. The need for a long-term perspective beyond the election cycle in most countries, and the lack of short-term outcomes, often does not fit with political agendas in developed or developing countries. With an increased emphasis on mental health and mental disorders in the World Bank and WHO, there is some cause for optimism that additional financial and programmatic resources may facilitate the implementation of prevention programming.

Currently, Life Skills Education, as promoted by the WHO over decades, is the backbone of prevention programming in many developing countries (92). Life skills training provides, in the context of the school curriculum, a program to enhance psychosocial competencies. The training focuses on basic skills such as decision making and problem solving, creative and critical thinking, communication and other interpersonal skills, self-awareness and empathic skills, and coping with stress and emotions. The aim is to promote mental well-being and enable children to take more responsibility for their lives and feel more effective (98). The program is now part of a larger Health Promoting Schools initiative supported by the WHO (93).

Systemic Issues

Throughout the world it is rare to see child mental health incorporated in national health policy. In many countries, developed or developing, no coherent health policy exists that would provide a framework for program development. In countries that do have a systematic health policy, it is rare that child mental health rises to a prominent position. Until child mental health becomes integrated into health policy, stable budgetary support for child and adolescent mental health programs will not be realized.

Advocacy for child and adolescent mental health is evident throughout the world, but competition with other interests often forces the issue off the policy agenda. When there are crises that involve children, such as the child soldiers in the Sudan, or female genital mutilation, the issue of child mental health for a time gains the spotlight. Unfortunately, the advocacy and concern diminishes with time and rarely finds a sustaining constituency.

Professional NGOs play an important role in promoting child mental health, disseminating information, providing a forum for professional exchange, and advocating for specific causes. The constituency bases of these organizations differ, but they generally have broad representation and provide an opportunity for interested individuals to learn more about specific topics or develop ideas in a context of knowledgeable individuals. Many of the NGOs have affiliated regional organizations that permit ongoing local involvement. The following are some of the more established international NGOs that represent professional groups: International Association for Child and Adolescent Psychiatry and Allied Professions, World Association for Infant Mental Health, International Association for Adolescent Psychiatry, the World Federation for Mental Health, and the World Psychiatric Association.

V. RESEARCH TRENDS

Mohler (94) has described in detail the current state of cross-cultural research, and further refines the understanding of what it means to incorporate a cultural perspective into research. He states that the past limitations of cross-cultural research methods in child mental health reflect the complexity of the concept of culture and the difficulty of testing its direct and indirect multiple level effects on child development. As discussed earlier, Weisz et al. (95) note that although some data suggest a more universal presence of identifiable syndromes, the cross-cultural validity of syndromes in child psychopathology are far from having been investigated in depth. The Child Behavior Checklist, which is the most widely used instrument, has been tested and used in multiple cultures, but even with the CBCL, validation studies have been limited (95).

Earls and Eisenberg (96) highlighted three areas for enhanced research activity in relation to child and adolescent mental health. The first is research to understand how changes in contemporary society are reflected in the prevalence and incidence of mental disorders. The second is research to enhance the understanding of how different childrearing methods impact normal and deviant behavioral and emotional development. The third area of interest involves research on the design and delivery of mental health services.

In a further refinement of one of these interest areas, Earls (97) described how compulsory schooling leads to the need to better understand the impact of learning disorders. The appropriate diagnosis and remediation of these disorders is a first-order priority in countries where technological advance places a premium on knowledge acquisition and use. As yet, research in this area has not been implemented in developing countries, but the pressure to implement such studies is mounting. As AIDS among adults impacts the educational infrastructure and the family context that supports education, another researchable dimension of education would be the consideration of how effective alternatives to traditional educational models, especially in impacted countries, should be developed.

Childrearing practices represent an area of cross-cultural research that has broad implications both in developing and developed countries. Research into the understanding of the differential impact of childrearing methods should be an area of collaborative inquiry between those interested in mental health and those concerned with the role of women and the family in evolving societies. It is not evident that any one method of childrearing is superior to another. It may be that developing and developed societies can learn from one another about the optimal methods for child rearing in the face of the evolution of individual societies. Experience in developed countries with the effects of urbanization, industrialization, the changing roles of women, and increased survivorship of children may form the basis for translation into programs for developing countries. However, the healthy development of youngsters growing up in adversity in developing countries may provide information on how to enhance understanding and develop new interventions for "at risk" children in developed countries. An example of a high-visibility topic where developing and developed countries could engage in collaborative research is the finding from a recent epidemiological study in Sweden that raised new concerns about the risk status of children growing up in single-parent homes (98). This phenomenon, for a host of reasons, is worldwide. Continuing research is needed to define critical factors and possible remedial or preventive interventions to ameliorate postulated consequences of growing up in a single-parent household.

Munir and Earls (99) have articulated a set of ethical parameters for research that must be considered when conducting research among the children and adolescents of developing countries. To apply a different standard, using the difficulty of implementing protocols as justification, would violate the support of a rights framework so essential for progress to be made on behalf of children in developing countries. There can be no exploitation of the situation of children in developing countries for the sake of implementing research.

The issues related to the development of mental health services are addressed elsewhere in this chapter. The diversity of cultures, the acceptance of change, and the continuing availability of resources for program implementation are issues that need to be confronted in international health services research. The development of pilot programs that are not sustainable does not promote infrastructure development, but does promote a cynicism that erodes the potential for the success of future efforts.

The uncritical adoption of Western models that incorporate unproven, controversial, or rejected concepts, including those of managed care, a variety of insurance schemes, and tertiary care, is a trend that needs review and study. Services research will clearly advance the cause of child and adolescent mental health if it can incorporate protocols to obtain economic data about the burden of disease and the effectiveness of programs for the care of child and adolescent mental disorders.

VI. CONCLUSION

Knowledge of child and adolescent mental health problems throughout the world is an important part of the education of all child and adolescent clinicians. The perspective gained from appreciating the stresses on children and adolescents in parts of the world embroiled in conflict and the nature of the responses offers the opportunity to learn more about the resilience of children and adolescents and about what we must do to develop more effective intervention programs. With vast immigration and migration, the likelihood that a clinician in a developed country, or any country serving as a haven for refugees, will see a child, adolescent, or family from a different culture has been significantly increased. To have the appropriate cross-cultural literacy and sensitivity to recognize the potential for cultural differences in presentation, acceptance of a diagnosis, and intervention is an essential.

The dearth of trained child and adolescent professionals in developing countries challenges us to find the most effective means for inculcating knowledge and providing meaningful services. It is unrealistic to assume that any effort will meet the needs for child and adolescent psychiatry as determined by conventional planning assumptions. As services evolve in developed countries, there is probably much that can be learned from the way in which less developed countries have found the means to support families and individuals to be relatively self-sufficient, even when impacted by mental disorders.

Given the enormity of the challenge to extend child mental health in a meaningful manner globally, the establishment of regional centers of excellence should be considered. These centers would incorporate resource libraries, have access to consultants, support training, and in some instances provide clinical diagnostic functions. Ultimately, the goal is to establish a sufficient cadre of child mental health professionals trained to an acceptable standard with the capacity to relate in a culturally appropriate manner to the mental disorder of children and adolescents, and to be able to support the healthy development of children and adolescents.

REFERENCES

1. Sugar JA, Kleinman A, Eisenberg L. Psychiatric morbidity in developing countries and American psychiatry's role in international health. *Hosp Commun Psychiatry* 1992;43:355–360
2. United Nations Convention on the Rights of the Child, UN General Assembly, November 20, 1989.

3. Shatkin J, Belfer ML. The Global absence of child and adolescent mental health policy. *J Child Adolesc Ment Health*, 2004;9:104–108.
4. Giel R, Van Luijk JN. Psychiatric morbidity in a small Ethiopian town. *Br J Psychiatry 1*969;115: 149–162
5. Nikapota AD. Child psychiatry in developing countries: a review. *Br J Psychiatry* 1991;158:743–751
6. Rahim S, Cederblad M. Effects of rapid urbanization on child behavior and health in part of Khartoum, Sudan. *J Child Psychol Psychiatry* 1984;25:629–641
7. World Health Report 2001. *Mental health: new understanding, new hope.* Geneva, Switzerland: World Health Organization, 2001
8. Desjarlais R, Eisenberg L, Good B, et al., eds. *World mental health.* New York: Oxford University Press, 1995.
9. World Health Organization, Department of Non-communicable Disease and Mental Health, Department of Mental Health and Substance Dependence, 2003.
10. Chavez A, Martinez C. *Growing up in a developing community. A bio-ecologic study of the development of children of poor peasant families in Mexico.* Mexico: Institute of Nutrition of Central America and Panama, 1982.
11. Agarwal DK, Upadhyay SK, Agawal KN, et al. Anaemia and mental function in rural primary school children. *J Trop Paediatr* 1989;9:194–198.
12. Galler JR, Ramsey F, Solimano G, et al.. The influence of early malnutrition on subsequent behavioral development. *J Am Acad Child Adolesc Psychiatry* 1983;22:8–15.
13. Miranda CT, Turecki G, Mari JJ, et al. Mental health of mothers of malnourished children. *Int J Epidemiol* 1996;25:128–133.
14. Galler JR, Ramsey F. A follow-up study of the influence of early malnutrition on development: behavior at home and school. *J Am Acad Child Adolesc Psychiatry* 1989;28:254–261.
15. Fullilove MT. Psychiatric implications of displacement: contributions from the psychology of place. *Am J Psychiatry* 1996;153:1516–1523.
16. Sampson RJ, Raudenbush SW, Earls F. Neighborhoods and violent crime: a multi-level study of collective efficacy. *Science* 1997;277:918–924.
17. Belfer ML, ed. Cultural and societal influences in child and adolescent psychiatry. *Child Adolesc Psychiatr Clin North Am* 2001;10.
18. Lee I. Second international conference on wartime medical services. *Med War* 1991;7:120–128.
19. Zivic I. Emotional reactions of children to war stress in Croatia. *J Am Acad Child Adolesc Psychiatry* 1993;32:709–713.
20. UNICEF. *State of the world's children.* UNICEF, 2000.
21. Munir K, Belfer ML. HIV/AIDS in children and adolescents: US and global perspectives. In: Weiner JM, Dulcan MK, eds. *Textbook of child and adolescent psychiatry.* Washington, DC: American Psychiatric Press, 1993:869–890.
22. Carlson M, Earls F. Psychological and neuroendocrinological sequelae of early social deprivation in institutionalized children in Romania. *Ann N Y Acad Sci* 1997;807:419–428.
23. Odejide AO, Oyewunmi LK, Ohaeri JU. Psychiatry in Africa: an overview. *Am J Psychiatry* 1989; 146:708–715.
24. Hackett R, Hackett L. Child psychiatry across cultures. *Int Rev Psychiatry* 1999;11:225–235.
25. Tadesse B, Kebede D, Tegegne T, et al. Childhood behavioural disorders in Ambo district, western Ethiopia. I. Prevalence estimates. *Acta Psychiatr Scand Suppl* 1999;100:92–97
26. Harding TW, deArango MV, Balthazar J, et al. Mental disorders in primary health care: a study of frequency and diagnosis in four developing countries. *Psychol Med* 1980;10:231–241.
27. Weiss MG. Cultural epidemiology: an introduction and overview. *Anthropol Med* 2001;8:5–30.
28. Fayyad JA, Jahshan CS, Karam EG. Systems development of child mental health services in developing countries. *Child Adolesc Psychiatr Clin North Am* 2001;10:745–762.
29. Tadesse B, Kebede D, Tegegne T, et al. Childhood behavioural disorders in Ambo district, western Ethiopia. II. Validation of the RQC. *Acta Psychiatr Scand Suppl* 1999;100:98–101.
30. World Health Organization. *Child mental health and psychological development. Report of the World Health Organization Expert Committee.* Tech. Report Series 613. Geneva: World Health Organization, 1977.
31. Hackett RJ, Hackett L, Bhatka P. The prevalence and associations of psychiatric disorders in children in Kerala, South India. *J Child Psychol Psychiatry* 1999;40:801–809.
32. Bird HR, Gould MS, Yager T, et al. Risk factors for maladjustment in Puerto Rican children. *J Am Acad Child Adolesc Psychiatry* 1989;28:847–850.

33. Thabet AAM, Vostanis P. Social adversities and anxiety disorders in the Gaza Strip. *Arch Dis Child* 1998;78:439–442.
34. Kashani JH, Orvaschel H. A community study of anxiety in children and adolescents. *Am J Psychiatry* 1980;147:313–318.
35. Becker AE. *Body, self, and society: a view from Fiji.* Philadelphia: University of Pennsylvania Press, 1995.
36. Murthy RS. Approaches to suicide prevention in Asia and the Far East. In: Hawton K, Van Heeringen K, eds. *International handbook of suicide and attempted suicide.* London: John Wiley & Sons, 2000: 625–637.
37. Raleigh VS, Balarajan R. Suicide and self-burning among Indians and West Indians in England and Wales. *Br J Psychiatry* 1992;161:365–368.
38. Canino I, Chou JC-Y, Christman JJ, et al. Cross-cultural issues and treatments of psychiatric disorders. *Am J Psychiatry* 1991;148:543–544.
39. van Ommeren M, Sharma B, Komproe I, et al. Trauma and loss as determinants of medically unexplained epidemic illness in a Bhutanese refugee camp. *Psychol Med* 2001;31:1259–1267.
40. Castillo RJ. Spirit possession in South Asia, dissociation or hysteria? Part 2: case studies. *Cult Med Psychiatry* 1994;18:141–162.
41. Nikapota AD. *Recognition and management of children with functional complaints: a training package for the primary care physician.* New Delhi: WHO Regional Office for South-East Asia, 1993.
42. Malhotra S, Malhotra A, Varma VK, eds. *Child mental health in India.* New Delhi: MacMillan, 1992.
43. Malhotra S, Chaturvedi SK. Patterns of childhood psychiatric disorders in India. *Ind J Pediatr* 1984; 51:235–240.
44. Mathews CA, Amighetti LDH, Lowe TL, et al. Cultural influences on diagnosis and perception of Tourette Syndrome in Costa Rica. *J Am Acad Child Adolesc Psychiatry* 2001;40:456–463.
45. Crijnen MM, Achenbach TM, Verhulst FC. Comparison of problems reported by parents of children in 12 cultures: total problems, externalizing and internalizing. *J Am Acad Child Adolesc Psychiatry* 1997;36:1269–1277.
46. Auerbach JG, Lerner Y. Syndromes derived from the Child Behavior Checklist for clinically referred Israeli boys aged 6–11: a research note. *J Child Psychol Psychiatry* 1991;32:1017–1024.
47. Berg I, Fombonne E, McGuire R, et al. A cross cultural comparison of French and Dutch disturbed children using the Child Behaviour Checklist. *Eur J Child Adolesc Psychiatry* 1997;6:7–11.
48. Weisz JR, Sigman M, Weiss B, et al. Parent reports of behavioral and emotional problems among children in Kenya, Thailand and the United States. *Child Dev* 1993;64:98–109.
49. Roussos A, Karantanos G, Richardson C, et al. Achenbach's Child Behavior Checklist and Teachers' Report Form in a normative sample of Greek children 6–12 year old. *Eur J Child Adolesc Psychiatry* 1999;8:165–172.
50. Slobodskaya HR. Competence, emotional and behavioral problems in Russian adolescents. *Eur J Child Adolesc Psychiatry* 1999;8:173–180.
51. Stichick T. The psychosocial impact of armed conflict on children: Rethinking traditional paradigms in research and intervention. *Child Adolesc Psychiatr Clin North Am* 2001;10:797–814.
52. Sack WmH, Him C, Dickason D. Twelve-year follow-up of Khmer youth who suffered massive war trauma as children. *J Am Acad Child Adolesc Psychiatry* 1999;38:1173–1179.
53. Mollica RF, Poole C, Son L, et al. Effects of war trauma on Cambodian refugee adolescents' functional health and mental health status. *J Am Acad Child Adolesc Psychiatry* 1997:36:1098–1106.
54. Pynoos RS, Frederick C, Nader K, et al. Life threat and posttraumatic stress in school age children. *Arch Gen Psychiatry* 1987;44:1057–1063.
55. Weine SM, Vojvoda D, Becker DF, et al. PTSD symptoms in Bosnian refugees 1 year after resettlement in the United States. *Am J Psychiatry* 1998;155:562–564.
56. Laor N, Wolmer L, Mayes L, et al. Israeli pre-schoolers under Scud missile attacks: a developmental perspective on risk-modifying factors. *Arch Gen Psychiatry* 1996;53:416–423.
57. Sack WmH, Clark GN, Kinney R, et al. The Khmer Adolescent Project II: functional capacities in two generations of Cambodian refugees. *J Nerv Ment Dis* 1995;183:177–181.
58. Abdel-Khalek AM. A survey of fears associated with Iraqi aggression among Kuwaiti children and adolescents: a factorial study 5.7 years after the Gulf War. *Psychol Rep* 1997;81:247–255
59. Almquist K, Brandell-Forsberg M. Refugee children in Sweden: post-traumatic stress disorder in Iranian preschool children exposed to organized violence. *Child Abuse Neglect* 1997;21:351–366.

60. Nader K, Pynoos R, Fairbanks L, et al. A preliminary study of PTSD and grief among the children of Kuwait following the Gulf crisis. *Br J Clin Psychol* 1993;32:407–416.
61. Terr LC. Chowchilla revisited: the effects of psychic trauma four years after a school-bus kidnapping. *Am J Psychiatry* 1983;140:1543–1550.
62. Ahmad A. Symptoms of post-traumatic stress disorder among displaced Kurdish children in Iraq: victims of man-made disaster after the Gulf War. *Nordic J Psychiatry* 1992;46:314–319.
63. Hussain SA, Nair J, Holcomb WM, et al. Stress reactions of children and adolescents in war and siege conditions. *Am J Psychiatry* 1998;152:1718–1719.
64. Fleischmann A, Bertolote JM, Belfer ML, et al. Completed suicide and psychiatric diagnoses in young people: a review. *J Child Adolesc Ment Health* 2004 *(in press).*
65. Shaffer D. The epidemiology of teen suicide: an examination of risk factors. *J Clin Psychiatry* 1988; 49:36–41.
66. Bertolote J. Suicide prevention: what works? *World Psychiatry* 2004 *(in press).*
67. Dugge CW. A mirror for India: suicide of 4 sisters. *International Herald Tribune* April 25, 2000, p. 2.
68. Chan KPM, Hung SF, Yip PSF. Suicide in response to changing societies. *Child Adolesc Clin North Am* 2001;10:777–796.
69. Belfer ML, Heggenhoughen K. Substance abuse. In: Desjarlais R, Eisenberg L, Good B, Kleinman A, eds. *World mental health: problems and priorities in low-income countries.* New York: Oxford University Press, 1995:87–115.
70. Day G. Geographical, economic and political situation in West Africa: significance of drug trafficking and abuse. In: *Drug control in Africa.* Padova: ARFI, 1992:9–14.
71. El-Akabawi AS. Drug abuse in the Arab world: a country profile of Egypt. In: Okasha A, Maj M, eds. *Images in psychiatry: an Arab perspective.* Cairo: Scientific Book House, 2001:143–150.
72. Ahmad J, Hasani M. Prevalence of substance use among Iranian high school students. *Addict Behav* 2003;28:375–379.
73. Alem A, Kebede D, Kullgren G. The prevalence and socio-demographic correlates of khat chewing in Butajira, Ethiopia. *Acta Psychiatr Scand Suppl* 1999;100:84–91.
74. Asuni T, Pela OA. Drub abuse in Africa. *Bull Narc* 1986;38:55–60.
75. Carlini-Cottrim B, Carlini EA. The use of solvents and other drugs among children and adolescents from a low socioeconomic background: a study of Sao Paolo, Brazil. *Int J Addict* 1988;23:1145–1156.
76. Cameron FJ, Debelle GD. No more Pacific Island paradises. *Lancet* 1984;1:1238.
77. Cravioto P, Anchondo R-L, de la Rosa B, et al. Risk factors associated with inhalant use among Mexican juvenile delinquents. In: *Epidemiological trends in drug abuse.* Rockville, MD: NIDA, DHHS, 1992:472–477.
78. Narayanan HS. A study of the prevalence of mental retardation in Southern India. *Int J Ment Health* 1981;10:128–136.
79. Belmont L. *The international pilot study of severe childhood disability. Final report. Screening for severe mental retardation in developing countries.* Utrecht: Bishop Bekkers Institute, 1984.
80. Tao KT. Mentally retarded persons in the People's Republic of China: a review of epidemiological studies and services. *Am J Ment Retard* 1988;93:193–199.
81. Lal N, Sethi BB. Estimate of mental ill-health in children in an urban community. *Ind J Pediatr* 1977;44:55–64.
82. Stein Z, Durkin M, Belmont L. Serious mental retardation in developing countries: an epidemiological approach. *Ann N Y Acad Sci* 1986;42:8–21.
83. Eisenberg L. Children and youth. In: Desjarlais R, Eisenberg L, Good B, et al, eds. *World mental health.* New York: Oxford University Press, 1995:155–178.
84. World Health Organization, Department of Mental Health and Substance Dependence. *Caring for children and adolescents with mental disorders: setting WHO directions.* Geneva: World Health Organization 2003.
85. Kapur M, Cariapa I. Evaluation of an orientation course for teachers on emotional problems among school children. *Ind J Clin Psychol* 1980;7:103.
86. El-Din AS, Moustafa AT, Mohit AS, et al. A multisectoral approach to school mental health, Alexandria, Egypt, Part II. *Health Serv J East Mediterr Reg* 1993;7:34–40.
87. Giel R, de Arango MV, Climent CE, et al. Childhood mental disorders in primary health care: results of observations in four developing countries. *Pediatrics* 1981;68:677–683.
88. Graham P, Orley J. WHO and the mental health of children. *World Health Forum* 1998;19:268–272.

89. Graham P, Orley J. WHO's activities related to psychosocial aspects of health (including child and adolescent health and development). In: DeGirolamo G, Eisenberg L, Goldberg DP, et al., eds. *Promoting mental health internationally.* London: Gaskell, 1999:117–131.
90. Mathur GP, Mathur S, Singh YD, et al. Detection and prevention of childhood disability with the help of anganwadi workers. *Ind Pediatr* 1995;32:773–777.
91. Jazairy I, Alamgir M, Panuccio T. *The state of world rural poverty: an inquiry into its causes and consequences.* New York: International Fund for Agricultural Development, 1992.
92. World Health Organization. *Life Skills Education in Schools, Programme on Mental Health.* WHO/MNH/PSF/93.7A.Rev2. Geneva: World Health Organization, 1997.
93. World Health Organization. *Child Friendly Schools's Initiative.* MNH/PSF/1. Geneva: World Health Organization, 1997.
94. Mohler B. Cross-cultural issues in research on child mental health. *Child Adolesc Psychiatr Clin North Am* 2001;10:763–776.
95. Weisz JR, Eastman K. Cross-national research on child and adolescent psychopathology. In: Verhulst F, Kooot H, eds. *The epidemiology of child and adolescent psychopathology.* Oxford: Oxford University Press, 1995:442–465.
96. Earls F, Eisenberg L. International perspective in child psychiatry. In: Lewis M, ed. *Child and adolescent psychiatry: a comprehensive textbook.* Baltimore: Williams & Wilkins, 1991:1189–1196.
97. Earls F. Child psychiatry in an international context: with remarks on the current status of child psychiatry in China. In: Super CM, ed. *The role of culture in development disorder.* New York: Academic Press, 1987;235–248.
98. Weltoft GR, Hjern A, Haglund B, et al. Mortality, severe morbidity, and injury in children living with single parents in Sweden: a population-based study. *Lancet* 2003;361:289–295.
99. Munir K, Earls F. Ethical principles governing research in child and adolescent psychiatry. *J Am Acad Child Adolesc Psychiatry* 1992;31:408–414.

15

Mental Health in Areas of Conflict

*Barbara Lopes Cardozo and †Gregory L. Fricchione

**National Center for Environmental Health, International Emergency and Refugee Health Branch, Centers for Disease Control and Prevention, Atlanta, Georgia 30345; and †Department of Psychiatry, Massachusetts General Hospital, Boston, Massachusetts 02114*

I. INTRODUCTION

The mental health consequences of armed conflict did not receive much attention until the late 1980s. As circumstantial evidence mounted, researchers began to pay closer attention to what we now know is a serious problem afflicting people who are affected directly or indirectly by war. In addition to injury and physical illness, psychological health hazards result from conflict-induced trauma and stress. Refugees, internally displaced populations, and other victims of conflict are likely to suffer from high rates of depression, posttraumatic stress disorder (PTSD), other anxiety disorders, and other forms of mental distress.

By some estimates, the total number of people affected by violent conflict in a single year can exceed 500 million (1). Studies in specific conflict and postconflict areas suggest that a substantial number of these people suffer from symptoms of mental illness. The psychological damage from brutalizing experiences during war and conflict have been neglected in international humanitarian aid circles because mental health issues were traditionally not considered a priority, when compared to seemingly more pressing issues such as physical injuries and infectious diseases. The usually enormous logistical and operational tasks as well as issues regarding security make it more difficult to relate to the psychological issues involved, because it seems in the short run they have a higher priority (2). In recent years the effects of psychological trauma, both short and long term, on the recuperation and rebuilding of societies have been rapidly gaining attention. Although considerable evidence supports the importance of this aspect of health care, few proven strategies exist to address mental health issues during and after times of conflict.

The impact of war on mental health encompasses a wide range of disorders, from severe mental disorders to mild adjustment problems. Among the most common manifestations of the consequences of conflict are depression and PTSD, but many other symptoms are regularly found when studying war and postwar populations. Beyond the immediate impact of mental illness on people who experience it and on their families, is a social and economic cost. Mental illness exacts a cost in the health care system beyond the psychiatric realm. Psychological distress often manifests as physical symptoms, placing an additional burden on health facilities (3). In addition, the potential for economic growth and social development may erode in countries, towns, and villages that are home to large numbers of people suffering from psychological problems. Furthermore, evidence indicates that the untreated emotional consequences of violent conflict can leave a residue of anger, and hatred and a desire for revenge among its victims (4). These, in turn, could lead to the resurgence of conflict.

Given the magnitude of the problem and the seriousness of its consequences, it is important to develop an effective response. Until now, efforts to address mental health during and after war have been, at best, haphazard. For the most part, existing strategies have not become fully integrated in the public health and primary health care systems of affected countries. Beyond the unevenness and insufficiency of the current response, evidence-based knowledge is lacking about the most effective mental health strategies to address this problem.

In this chapter, we will examine how armed conflict impacts the mental health of hundreds of millions of people affected each year by war and warlike conditions. We will provide an overview of the existing research examining the extent of the problem across a variety of populations recovering from armed conflict. In addition, we will examine the consequences of not effectively addressing psychological damage. Finally, we will offer an action plan to decrease the burden of mental illness and break the cycle of violence.

II. THE BURDEN OF MENTAL ILLNESS IN AREAS OF CONFLICT

Hundreds of millions of people are currently affected by violent conflict and war (5,6). UNICEF reports that 10 million children across the globe have been psychologically traumatized (7). In 2002, approximately 40 million people were displaced worldwide (8); 15 million were refugees and 25 million were internally displaced persons (9). The International Federation of the Red Cross listed conflicts in 62 countries with over 7.5 million war-related deaths (10).

Even in situations where populations are not subjected to the trauma of war, the prevalence of mental illness is substantial. Mental disorders alone accounted for 11% of the global burden of disease in 1998 according to the World Health Report of 1999 (11). The Global Burden of Disease Study (12) concluded that psychiatric conditions made up five of the ten leading causes of disability worldwide. Like the 1999 World Health Organization report, this study did not focus on victims of war. Recent research demonstrated that the prevalence of mental illness is much higher among war-affected populations than among the general population (13–15). Given the high number of people affected by war and the lack of attention to mental health problems, hundreds of millions of people are probably experiencing mental illness as a result of armed conflict. For individuals suffering from mental disorders brought about by violent conflict, the end of war does not automatically bring an end to mental illness. This means that there is a cumulative effect on the number of people affected by conflict.

Military scientists were the first to report and study mental trauma among soldiers during wartime. Psychiatric casualties make up between 10% and 50% of all casualties resulting from prolonged battle (16). In World War I, psychological casualties exceeded physical casualties two to one. The British Army reported that 7% to 10% of officers suffered mental breakdowns (16). In World War II, 33% of all medical evacuations were psychiatric. In the Korean War, 6% of all evacuees had a psychiatric diagnosis (17).

PTSD was first described as a diagnostic entity in 1980, in the third edition of the *Diagnostic and Statistical Manual of Mental Disorders* (DSM-III). The criteria for PTSD were revised in the updated third edition (DSM-III-R) and fourth edition (DSM-IV) (18) and have recently been included in the tenth revision of the *International Classification of Diseases and Related Health Problems* (ICD-10). Before that time, the disorder was called "shell shock," "battle fatigue," "combat neurosis," and "soldier's heart," reflecting the fact that PTSD was originally related to traumatic events encountered by soldiers in combat situations. Among Vietnam veterans, the estimated PTSD prevalence varied from 4% to 30%, with estimates consistently higher in females than in males (16,19). The prevalence of PTSD was much higher in wounded soldiers than in soldiers exposed to combat but not wounded.

Several studies have provided evidence from a number of settings that underscore the severe mental health sequelae resulting from mass violence (13,20). Despite methodological challenges involved in determining the prevalence of mental illness across cultures and in areas of conflict, progress has been made over the last decade toward assessing psychological and social issues. Specifically, the lack of accurate population estimates and culturally validated screening instruments had to be overcome to make culturally valid mental health assessments (21,22).

Refugee population–based studies reveal high levels of depression and PTSD; each occurs at rates many times higher than the baseline found in nontraumatized populations. A study of Cambodians living on the Thailand–Cambodia border found that of 993 adults interviewed, more than 80% reported poor health, depression, and somatic complaints despite good access to health services; 67.9% and 37.2% had symptom scores that correlate with Western criteria for depression and PTSD, respectively (23,24). A recent study of Burmese refugees living in Thailand found that 41.8% met clinical criteria for depression; the PTSD prevalence was 4.6% (3). A study of Rwandan and Burundian refugees living in poor and insecure conditions in Tanzania during the Rwanda Refugee Crisis of 1994 found that the prevalence of serious mental health problems was 50%, corresponding to a General Health Questionnaire (GHQ-28) score of at least 14 (25).

A longitudinal study of Bosnian refugees revealed the serious disability associated with the mental health effects of mass violence. In the initial 1996 survey, 45% of the refugees studied met DSM-IV criteria for depression, PTSD, or both. Comorbidity of these two disorders was associated with a 25% prevalence of physical disability (26). Three years later, after the cessation of conflict, this refugee population evidenced unremitting psychiatric disability and premature death in the elderly (27). Other studies support the Bosnia data, suggesting that suffering continues long after the crisis has ended (28,29).

Studies of civilian populations affected by mass violence reveal results comparable to those found in refugee populations. Lopes Cardozo et al. (13) found a prevalence of nonspecific psychiatric morbidity of 43% and an estimated prevalence of PTSD symptoms of 17.1% in a study of Kosovar Albanians after the war. Another study among survivors of war or mass violence in postconflict settings in Algeria, Cambodia, Ethiopia, and Gaza found a high prevalence of PTSD in each setting: 37.4%, 28.4%, 15.8%, and 17.8%, respectively (30).

Violence is one of the most common sources of PTSD. Studies of Holocaust survivors reported that more than 85% of survivors suffered from PTSD 10 years after the trauma (31). Psychosis cases have been reported among survivors of Nazi concentration camps, and a marked increase in schizophrenia was described in prisoners of Japanese camps (17).

III. MENTAL HEALTH CONSEQUENCES OF PSYCHOLOGICAL TRAUMA: CYCLES OF VIOLENCE

In civilian populations, common events that cause psychological trauma during and after violent conflict and war are persecution, separation from family and friends, displacement, killings, violence, rape, torture, and destroyed homes and property. Everyone is affected somehow by such traumatic events, but not everyone develops a mental disorder as a result of the experiences. In fact, most people adapt and continue on with their lives (20). In a population that has undergone war or violent conflict, one can expect to find what is shown in the trauma pyramid model (see Fig. 15-1) (32). The pyramid describes the full range of psychosocial manifestations from physical and mental exhaustion at the base of the pyramid for the entire population to family problems in the middle. At the top of the pyramid, a small proportion exhibits serious mental illness.

The psychological wounds of war may continue for many years and may even have transgenerational effects. Feelings of hatred and revenge in a postwar civilian population in relation to psychiatric morbidity were described in a mental health survey in Kosovo (4). After the 1999 Kosovo war, many Kosovar Albanians expressed feelings of hatred and a desire to take revenge. In two surveys conducted in Kosovo, people with PTSD and nonspecific psychiatric morbidity were more likely to have feelings of hatred and a desire for revenge (4,13). Additionally, a dose–response effect appeared to exist between nonspecific psychiatric morbidity and these feelings. We cannot be certain whether feelings of hatred existed before

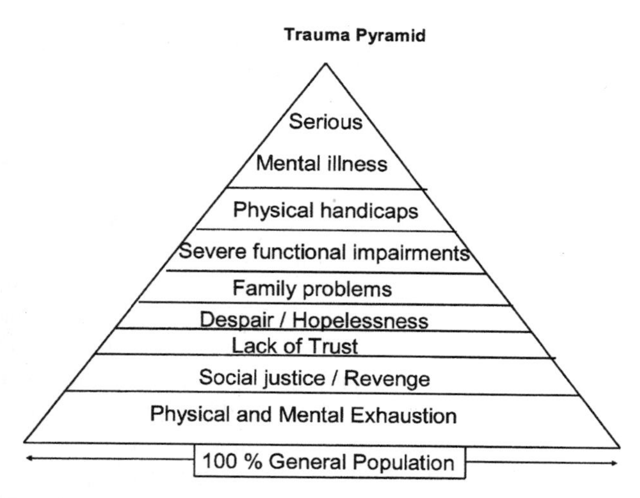

FIG. 15-1. The trauma pyramid. (Modified from Mollica RF. Invisible wounds. *Sci Am* 2000;282: 54–57.)

PTSD symptoms developed or vice versa, because this type of cross-sectional study cannot demonstrate a cause–effect relationship.

PTSD and other psychiatric morbidity may have developed during the war, when many people experienced multiple traumatic events. Such events also may have triggered feelings of hatred and wishes for revenge. However, anecdotal information and consideration of the historical events in Kosovo over the last 50 years suggest that feelings of hatred have existed for decades (4). Generational transmission of hatred also may occur when children are taught to hate and take revenge (33).

The association of anger with exposure to the stress of combat and, particularly, combat-related PTSD has been shown in a number of epidemiological studies (34). Individuals experiencing PTSD commonly present with anger (35). Addressing issues of anger as part of treatment for PTSD might be useful, as indicated by a study of former political prisoners, which showed an association between anger and posttraumatic stress reactions (36).

High rates of violence were found in a clinical study of Vietnam veterans in whom PTSD was diagnosed, again pointing to the likelihood that anger is a factor in PTSD (37). PTSD may, in fact, improve if feelings of hatred and anger are reduced, given that anger and hatred probably are associated. Conversely, effective treatment for PTSD and nonspecific psychiatric morbidity also may reduce feelings of hatred and revenge. If this were the case, successful treatment of PTSD might be beneficial in reducing continued cycles of violence. Future research efforts should focus on the hypothesis that mental illness caused by psychological trauma may contribute to perpetuation of the cycles of violence in war and conflict through feelings of hatred and a desire for revenge. Longitudinal studies and clinical research are necessary to test this hypothesis.

IV. MENTAL HEALTH ACTION PLAN FOR AREAS OF CONFLICT AND POSTCONFLICT AREAS

Given the high burden of mental illness in violent conflict, mental health assessments and programs should be integrated with humanitarian relief efforts. National and international support has increased for psychosocial and mental health programs in postconflict situations, such as in Rwanda, Bosnia, Kosovo, and East Timor. Early, rapid mental health and psychosocial assessments in complex emergencies and post-conflict situations can provide information about the mental health needs and resources of the communities concerned. Early interventions will not only improve the mental health status of those traumatized by war and conflict, but also will relieve suffering and reduce the burden on health facilities because persons suffering from psychological distress often present with physical complaints and do not receive proper care or attention for the underlying psychological problems.

The challenge of providing the needed attention to psychological problems after violent conflict has led the international humanitarian community to propose a wide range of psychosocial interventions. The term "psychosocial," however, has been the source of confusion and controversy. Psychosocial implies a dynamic relationship between psychological and social effects; that opens the field to a large variety of possible interventions, encompassing a multitude of approaches. As a result of the vagueness of this term, a debate has emerged in the field. Approaches to so-called psychosocial intervention include everything from social events, sports activities, and educational development to more medically focused efforts, such as psychiatric treatment and psychological debriefings. Many proponents of socially oriented interventions consider the focus on psychopathology counterproductive. Another view is that social and psychological/psychiatric interventions are complementary aspects of an effective mental health action plan. In an effort to resolve this controversy and provide some clarity, van Ommeren (38) has proposed separating the psychological/psychiatric interventions from social interventions and treating the two as distinct categories. Different phases of conflict and postconflict situations require distinct programs. The following psychological and psychiatric interventions have been proposed for the emergency phase of conflict and postconflict situations.

- Establishment of services through the primary health care system to address urgent psychiatric complaints
- Provision of essential psychotropic medications at health facilities
- Organization and establishment of outreach and nonintrusive psychological support, or "psychological first aid"

Some major nongovernmental organizations and United Nations Organizations focus on social interventions, directing their services towards vulnerable groups such as women, children, orphans, and the elderly. Others specialize in unique types of social intervention; the International Committee of the Red Cross, for example, is commonly involved in tracing and reuniting families.

Another important aspect of social intervention during the acute phase of a conflict is reassuring war-affected populations about what is a normal psychological reaction to their experience. Without this information, individual reactions may worsen among people experiencing not only the effects of trauma, but also anxiety and fear from poorly understood symptoms of psychological distress.

After the acute phase of a conflict, or during the transitional and reconsolidation phase, a different set of measures is needed. During this stage, the emphasis is on long-term planning. Survivors of war and conflict may suffer from mental health problems for years after the conflict, even into future generations. Many people continue to suffer after the international relief agencies pull out of the program. Brief programs (2 years or less) may not be suited for mental health programs in postconflict situations. Programs intended for longer duration should have well-developed plans that ensure both financial and administrative continuity.

The two principal reasons for establishing a long-range mental health program in a postconflict situation are

- To provide positive and supportive action to restore normal functioning among the affected population and in society as a whole
- To prevent the long-term medical and psychosocial consequences of mental illness among the affected population

The choice of mental health services depends on the needs and traditions of the people being served, but they should include some of the following elements:

- Enlist the support of the national and local authorities, by encouraging recognition of the importance of addressing mental health issues, and the perils of failing to do so
- Utilize the country's existing structures and resources to develop sustainable mental health programs
- Integrate mental health programs into the primary health care system. Many issues faced by an agency trying to provide mental health services already may have been resolved by the existing health care system
- Incorporate mental health services into other resources within the community to help rebuild the structure of individual, family, and communities, beyond health care
- Involve the affected community in decision-making from the beginning. Representatives of the community should be made equal partners in program planning and implementation to best serve the people in greatest need
- Train and supervise local primary health care (PHC) workers in basic mental health knowledge and skills
- Educate aid workers and community leaders in basic psychological skills
- Ensure continuation of medication for psychiatric patients
- Train and supervise community workers to assist PHC workers
- Collaborate with traditional healers, who are often the most accepted by the general population, and whose support may be indispensable to a successful and sustainable program

V. CONCLUSION

The psychological damage of exposure to violence, terror, torture, and rape during war and violent conflict traditionally have not been addressed or given priority in the arena of international humanitarian aid. The literature suggests that mental trauma and its psychological consequences are a concern for a substantial portion of war-affected populations and should be addressed as major public health problems in countries plagued by collective violence. A functioning society, whatever the culture, is based on a stable community with a sense of individual and collective responsibility. Restoring psychological equilibrium through culturally appropriate community-based programs is key to preventing future conflicts. Mental illness also can impede the economic development of a country. Only in recent years have international organizations recognized this fact (20).

Although a substantial body of research has now demonstrated that mental health is a serious problem among postconflict populations and has provided evidence about the magnitude of the problem, one crucial area of research in this area still is urgently needed. To date, conclusive evidence is lacking that point specifically to the types of interventions that provide measurable results. A number of programs are now in place, but not enough attention has been devoted to examining their effectiveness. Until this is done, activities aimed at easing the mental health consequences of violent conflict will be carried out on a porous foundation. Scientific research is imperative to maximize the benefits of interventions by offering evidence for which programs and activities should be replicated in the growing number of societies trying to rebuild after a period of conflict. Much research still is needed to delineate the problems and identify the appropriate strategies; specifically, research into the prevalence of the problems as well as into methods of prevention and treatment is necessary to alleviate the psychological suffering of entire populations affected by war and violent conflict.

REFERENCES

1. WHO/EHA/EHTP. Emergency Health training Programme for Africa. Available at: http://www.who.int/disasters/repo/5512.pdf. Accessed August 22, 2004.
2. Golaz A, Guha-Sapir D, Lopes Cardozo B, et al. Overview of mental health issues in populations affected by war and genocide. In: *Proceedings of Fifth World Congress on Psychiatric Emergencies in a Changing World.* Brussels: Elsevier, 1999.
3. Lopes Cardozo B, Talley L, Burton A, et al. Karenni refugees living in Thai–Burmese border camps: traumatic experiences, mental health outcomes, and social functioning. *Soc Sci Med* 2004;58: 2637–2644.
4. Lopes Cardozo B, Kaiser R, Gotway CA, et al. Mental health, social functioning, and feelings of hatred and revenge of Kosovar Albanians one year after the war in Kosovo. *J Traum Stress* 2003; 16:351–360.
5. Spiegel PB. HIV/AIDS among conflict-affected and displaced populations: dispelling the myth and taking action. UN High Commissioner for Refugees (UNHCR), January 2004. Available at: http://www.reliefweb.int/w/lib.nsf/LibHome?OpenForm&Start = 1&Count = 1000&ExpandView. Accessed April 21, 2004.
6. Mollica R, Mc Donald L. Project 1 billion. Health ministers of post-conflict nations act on mental health recovery. Available at: http://www.un.org/Pubs/chronicle/2003/issue4/0403p56.asp. Accessed April 21, 2004

7. UNICEF. *The state of the world's children.* Oxford: Oxford University Press, 1996.
8. United Nations High Commissioner for Refugees. 2002 statistics on asylum seekers refugees and others of concern to UNHCR. Geneva : UNHCR 2003. Available at: http://www.unhcr.ch/static/statistics_2002/asr02-dr2-Table4.pdf. Accessed April 21, 2004
9. Global IDP project. A global overview of internal displacement, 2003. http://www.idpproject.org/global_overview.htm. Accessed August 22, 2004.
10. International Federation of Red Cross. *The world disaster report.* Oxford: Oxford University Press, 1998.
11. World Health Organization. World health report 1999. Available at: http://www.whomsa.org/it/text4/01_whr99.html. Accessed April 21, 2004.
12. Murray CJL, Lopez AD, eds. *The global burden of disease: a comprehensive assessment of mortality and disability from diseases, injuries and risk factors in 1990 and projected to 2020.* Cambridge: Harvard University Press, 1996.
13. Lopes Cardozo B, Vergara A, Agani F, et al. Mental health, social functioning, and attitudes of Kosovar Albanians following the war in Kosovo. *JAMA* 2000;284:569–577.
14. Mollica RF, Donelan K, Tor S, et al. The effect of trauma and confinement on functional health and mental health status of Cambodians living in Thai-Cambodia border camps. *JAMA* 1993;270: 581–586.
15. Lopes Cardozo B, Bilukha OO, Gotway C, et al. Mental health, social functioning and disability in post-war Afghanistan, 2002. *JAMA* 2004;292:575–584.
16. Armfield F. Preventing post-traumatic stress disorder resulting from military operations. *Mil Med* 1994;159:739–746.
17. Beebe GW. Follow-up studies of World War II and Korean war prisoners. II. Morbidity, disability, and maladjustments. *Am J Epidemiol* 1975;101:400–422.
18. American Psychiatric Association, Task Force on DSM-IV. *Diagnostic and statistical manual of mental disorders.* 4th ed. Washington, DC: American Psychiatric Association, 1994.
19. Kulka RA, Schlenger WE, Fairbank JA. Contractual report of findings from the National Vietnam Veterans Readjustment Study. Durham, NC: Research Triangle Institute, 1988.
20. Mollica R. Invisible Wounds. *Sci Am* 2000,282:54–57.
21. Mollica RF, Caspi-Yavin Y, Bollini P, et al. The Harvard Trauma Questionnaire: validating a cross-cultural instrument for measuring torture, trauma, and posttraumatic stress disorder in Indochinese Refugees. *J Nerv Ment Dis* 1992;180:111–116.
22. Goldberg DP, Gater R, Sartorius N, et al. The validity of two versions of the General Health Questionnaire (GHQ) in the WHO study of mental illness in general health care. *Psychol Med* 1997;27: 191–197.
23. Mollica RF, Donelan K, Tor S, et al. The effect of trauma and confinement on functional health and mental health status of Cambodians living in Thai-Cambodia border camps. *JAMA* 1993;270: 581–586.
24. Mollica RF, Poole C, Tor S. Symptoms, functioning and health problems in a massively traumatized population: the legacy of the Cambodian tragedy. In: Dohrenwend, BP, ed. *Adversity, strength, and psychopathology.* New York: Oxford University Press, 1998.
25. De Jong JP, Scholte WF, Koeter MWJ, et al. The prevalence of mental health problems in Rwandan and Burundese refugee camps. *Acta Psychiatr Scand* 2000;102:171–177.
26. Mollica RF, McInnes K, Sarajlić N, et al. Disability associated with psychiatric comorbidity and health status in Bosnian refugees living in Croatia. *JAMA* 1999;282:433–439.
27. Mollica RF, Sarajlic N, Chernoff M, et al. Longitudinal study of psychiatric symptoms, disability, mortality and emigration among Bosnian refugees. *JAMA* 2001;286:546–554.
28. Bramsen I, van der Ploeg HM. Fifty years later: the long-term psychological adjustment of ageing World War II survivors. *Acta Psychiatr Scand* 1999;100:350–358.
29. Yehuda R, Schmeidler J, Wainberg M, et al. Vulnerability to posttraumatic stress disorder in adult offspring of Holocaust survivors. *Am J Psychiatry* 1998;155:1163–1171.
30. De Jong JTVM, Komproe IH, Van Ommeren M, et al. Lifetime events and posttraumatic stress disorder in 4 post conflict settings. *JAMA* 2001;286:555–562.
31. Frankl VE. *From death-camp to existentialism; a psychiatrist's path to a new therapy.* Boston: Beacon Press, 1959.
32. Psychosocial effects of complex emergencies. Symposium report. Program on forced Migration and Health, School of Public Health. Washington, DC: Columbia University, 1999. Available at: http://cpmcnet.columbia.edu/dept/sph/popfam/pubs/docs/sym_99.pdf Accessed April 21, 2004.

33. Post JM. Terrorist on trial: the context of political crime. *J Am Acad Psychiatry Law* 2000;28: 171–178.
34. Novaco RW, Chemtob CM. Anger and combat-related posttraumatic stress disorder. *J Trauma Stress* 2002;15:123–132.
35. Kaplan HI, Sadock BJ. *Comprehensive textbook of psychiatry VI.* 6th ed. Baltimore: Williams & Wilkins, 1995.
36. Schutzwohl M, Maercker A. Anger in former East German political prisoners: relationship to posttraumatic stress reactions and social support. *J Nerv Ment Dis* 2000;188:483–489.
37. McFall M, Fontana A, Raskind M, et al. Analysis of violent behavior in Vietnam combat veteran psychiatric inpatients with posttraumatic stress disorder. *J Traum Stress* 1999;12:501–517.
38. WHO Department of Mental Health and Substance Dependence. Mental health in emergencies: mental and social aspects of health of populations exposed to extreme stressors. Available at: http://www.who.int/disasters/repo/8656.pdf. Geneva: World Health Organization, 2003. Accessed April 21, 2004.

16

Important Considerations in Fostering Growth of a Research Culture in the Developing World

Anne E. Becker

Department of Psychiatry, Massachusetts General Hospital, and Department of Social Medicine, Harvard Medical School, Boston, Massachusetts 02114

I. INTRODUCTION

A number of considerations are relevant to the imperative for fostering a "research culture" in the developing world to support mental health research. First, conclusive data support the high impact of neuropsychiatric illness globally. Severity of mental illness has a direct bearing on disability across diverse cultural contexts, underscoring its devastating socioeconomic, if not personal, impact (1). For example, neuropsychiatric illness accounts for 26.4% of the disability-adjusted life years (DALYs) among 15- to 44-year-olds worldwide. Indeed, five of the ten leading causes of DALYs in this age range are mental illnesses or self-inflicted injuries (2,3). Moreover, poor countries such as many in the Western Pacific, Africa, and Latin America have a disproportionate burden of social problems (for instance, natural disasters, war, rapid social change, nutritional deficiencies, material poverty) that contribute to risk for mental illness at the same time as they lack critical resources to support adequate mental health services (4,5). Indeed, there is a tremendous need for research on etiology, prevention, and treatment for populations in many areas of the developing world to better understand the contributions of the local social, cultural, and economic contexts of mental illness as well as the most effective remedies and

---

Adapted from a Consultation on the Development of a Research Culture and Capacity for Mental Health in the Western Pacific Region for the World Health Organization Western Pacific Region, November 20–22, 2002, Manila, Philippines.

prevention strategies—whether they be in the realm of pharmacologic or health policy interventions. Thus, there is an especially critical need for epidemiologic and social science research in the developing world to address elevated rates of illness and barriers to effective care in these populations.

There is both a critical need for and a critical deficit of research-generated knowledge about locally relevant approaches to treatment and prevention of mental illness. The World Health Organization (WHO) has reported that 40% of countries surveyed are without a national mental health policy and 30% do not have programs to improve mental health (6). Although the World Health Report 2001 concludes that more research must be supported to address the deficits in mental health care (6), only 5% of global research funds are used for studying health in developing countries (7). The increasing gap between the burden of mental illness and the resources to address it has prompted the WHO to spearhead efforts to promote research on mental health and substance abuse in developing countries (8).

II. THE DOMINANT GLOBAL RESEARCH CULTURE AND ITS EFFECTS ON LOCAL RESEARCH CULTURES

The critical shortage of research-based knowledge undoubtedly stems from multiple local sources, such as fewer economic resources, a relative lack of training opportunities for basic science and clinical researchers, seemingly more exigent competing priorities (i.e., health care delivery), and local cultures that offer relatively less support for research activity. However, there are additional important contributions to this deficit from extralocal sources. Arguably, there is a "dominant global research culture" that elevates certain sources of research knowledge that are more readily generated in Western countries than in resource-poor countries. Specifically, this is evident in the gross underrepresentation of mental health research from the developing world in the major psychiatric journals. A recent study by Patel and Sumathipala (9) surveying six major psychiatric journals (three from Europe and three from the United States) best illustrates this point. They found that only 6% of the studies published in these high-impact journals emanates from regions of the world that comprise over 90% of the global population. Moreover, less than 1% of articles published in these journals described mental health interventions in the developing world. Finally, acceptance rates for papers were significantly lower for studies from outside Europe and the United States. The authors were concerned that these data are indicative of a possible editorial bias against publishing such papers as well as a low submission rate from psychiatric researchers in developing countries—both worrisome issues.

The dominant research culture in psychiatry includes research priorities that are deeply embedded in the cultural and economic context of medicine in Western Europe and North America. For example, a perusal of the table of contents from recent issues of the *American Journal of Psychiatry* will reveal not only the predilection for articles generated in the United States, but also for content that focuses on the genetics of mental illness, neuroimaging as it relates to mental illness, and psychopharmacologic therapies. Notwithstanding these important and exciting research horizons, the preponderance of "cutting edge" biotechnologic research often appears to supplant .equally important research on the social contexts of mental illness. Because sponsorship may strongly determine research agendas, "lower-tech" interventions and findings in poorer nations do not often capture research funding so necessary to address basic mental health needs.

In addition, the professional research culture of Western biomedicine has evolved so as to privilege certain ways of knowing (e.g., quantitatively based data) over others (e.g., qualitatively based data such as clinical narratives). There is arguably a reification of the relevance of certain findings based on statistical significance regardless of their clinical meaningfulness, at the same time as anecdotal or observational data are devalued. The popularization of evidence-based medicine (EBM) in the 1990s further eclipsed the value of qualitative data in contributing to the medical and psychiatric literature. Randomized clinical trials provide information relevant to groups but not necessarily applicable to individuals across diverse personal and social contexts (10,11). Indeed, as Williams and Garner (10) argue, the "EBM culture" supports an unfortunate "covert assertion that only factors that can be measured are recognised as important." In addition, Lowe (12) argues that in countries such as Fiji, EBM supports a kind of "cultural hegemony, in which the questions that are important to rich countries, and answers that are appropriate to them, are imposed upon less-developed countries." In other words, the validity of clinical recommendations stemming from EBM generated in other countries may be questionable in such settings. Lowe concludes that practitioners in the Fijian setting will continue to exercise judgment concerning the applicability of EBM based on clinical experience.

The EBM culture of Western biomedicine raises two relevant issues to developing a research culture in non-Western societies. The first concern is in the devaluation of research knowledge generated by clinical observation and descriptive studies that may indeed begin important research dialogues in developing countries. The other underscores the importance of generating research questions and answers in local environments and not accepting wholesale research findings generated in tightly controlled research contexts. As Hohmann and Shear (13) persuasively argue, complementary research generated within both academic and community settings is necessary in pushing forward the frontier of effective medicine and prevention. Inclusion criteria are often quite narrowly defined, procedures rigorously standardized (often beyond what is likely to be realistic in a clinical practice), and a main outcome measure chosen in initial randomized controlled trials to optimize signal-to-noise ratios and establish whether an intervention is generally effective in a highly controlled study sample and setting. In contrast, community-based research demonstrates feasibility, acceptability, relevance, and generalizability in context. Research should be designed to generate treatment protocols that will be sustainable in the context in which it they are carried out (14,15). Hohmann and Shear enumerate key considerations when adapting research knowledge generated in academic settings to community settings; these involve looking at the target population, community

TABLE 16-1. *Considerations in extrapolating conclusions reached in academic settings to commmunity settings.*

Target population
- Will those most likely to be affected be accessible to the research team?
- Will racial, ethnic, social, or cultural differences affect the prevalence or phenomenology of the illness?
- Are those at highest risk to be in treatment?
- Is there a high prevalence of comorbid illness?
- What local cultural factors will influence acceptability of treatment?

Community issues
- Are there already sanctioned sources of care of this problem?
- What resources are there to pay for the care?
- Is the treatment site setting generalizable?
- How is the site organized to accomodate patient flow, etc.?
- Are there local barriers to implementation, such as time or cost?

Outcomes assessment
- What are the most salient outcomes for the target population?

(Adapted from Hohmann AA, Shear KM. Community-based intervention research: Coping with the "noise" of real life in study design. *The American Journal of Psychiatry;*159:201–207 (2002). Copyright 2002, the American Psychiatric Association; http://ajp.psychiatryonline.org/. Reprinted with permission.)

issues, and outcomes assessments, and are synopsized in Table 16-1. Indeed, the imperative nature of testing the relevance of imported EBM underscores the necessity of developing and implementing local research agendas in the developing world. The knowledge base generated in such research will not only guide treatment approaches locally, but also will contribute to vital understandings of etiology and risk factors for psychiatric illness in other contexts. Moreover, such efforts can ultimately contribute substantively to a local research culture (16).

III. STRATEGIES IN THE DEVELOPMENT OF A RESEARCH CULTURE

The development of a research culture often focuses on early to midcareer health professionals in the form of career development opportunities and research fellowships. Whereas such programs are laudable and necessary, a broader, multitiered approach is optimal, given the professional, social, and political contexts in which research opportunities, agendas, and resources are invariably embedded. In particular, in order for local research programs to be sustainable, policymakers must be persuaded to "buy-in" to (a) the local burden of mental illness, (b) the desirability and feasibility of conducting research to advance preventive and therapeutic efforts for mental illness, and (c) the need for support of local research and researchers in addressing these problems. Policymakers will need to be provided with epidemiologic and economic data about the impact of mental illness as well as be informed in language they understand about what can be done (5). Not only health professionals, but also individuals with mental illness and their families can be mobilized to advocate for better funding of mental health research. In addition, the lay public has to "buy-in" to the importance of research. Their potential participation as research subjects makes it imperative that they understand what is at stake for them in the successful advancement of the local research agenda. Indeed, research on research will be essential to promoting a research environment most conducive to popular acceptance.

Effective development of a research culture in developing societies may involve very complicated local strategies about addressing the stigmatization of mental illness. It will also be based on a foundation of public trust reinforced through infinite attention to the ethical and responsible conduct of research. This will include not only compliance with universal standards of ethical behavior (17), but also attention to local ethical exigencies (e.g., using care to ensure that participation is truly voluntary and not informally coerced by local authority). The local media can be used for public service announcements, and they can be involved in embedding prosocial messages in programming; examples in the United States include the successful campaign to promote the concept of a "designated driver" to reduce alcohol-related motor vehicle fatalities, and television dramas that raise public awareness of eating disorders and available treatment. Finally, the pharmaceutical industry can also play a positive role in disseminating information about mental illness to the lay public and policymakers (as well as in training local clinician researchers). However, a major caveat to pharmaceutical industry participation is to ensure that their financial agenda does not undermine building a research culture that will seek to find the best local solutions to prevention and therapy of mental illness—solutions that are not necessarily primarily pharmacologic. Innovative, cross-disciplinary approaches that include medical scientists, education specialists, and medical anthropologists and that possibly import skills and cooperation from the advertising, news, and entertainment industries will be key in developing a local backdrop against which a successful professional research culture can develop.

IV. LESSONS FROM OTHER RESEARCH AND PROFESSIONAL CULTURES: A LONG WAY TO GO

Medical anthropologic research has demonstrated the complexities of professional medical cultures in the United States. Whether young clinicians will follow a research career is not determined only by personal interest in scientific research and social interest in providing means, opportunities, and inducements for clinical and basic science researchers. Moreover, the ways in which personal interest in research develops cannot be extricated from the social environment that provides incentives or disincentives for this career trajectory. For example, the high cost of medical education and the evolving managed health care environment in the United States have had an adverse impact both on students' choice of medicine as a career (18) and on their decision to pursue research as a primary career outlet. Attempts to counter this trend are evidenced in financial aid programs and special federal financial inducements for individuals pursuing medical research careers (e.g., the National Institutes of Health Federal Loan Repayment Program, which requires a commitment to conduct qualified research activities for a minimum of 2 years). Strong institutional pressures associate career advancement in medicine with producing numerous high-quality publications on original research. The "publish or perish" mandate of American research culture contributes to an ethos of associating prestige and position with scientific productivity, even in the absence of financial rewards. Indeed, American humor observes that battles over academic research territory are fierce because "there is so little [financially, that is] at stake."

It is also essential to note that the socialization of medical students during their premedical and medical education contributes to the development of a research culture that associates prestige with publication and acquisition of research skills. Medical training represents a time at which students are taught the language and perspectives of clinical and research medicine. A major transformation occurs in the way patients and illnesses are constructed, and in ways of knowing about illness (19). In other words, the importance of early socialization of values, conduct, and motivating forces in laying a foundation for future interest in pursuing research cannot be overstated. Such an environment that fosters the early socialization of health care professionals to value research in developing countries will include a tradition of high-quality research locally that creates an established local career path that will attract new trainees (16).

Targeted efforts to promote a research culture among trainees in medicine and nursing in the United States have identified certain barriers to entry into research careers among health professionals that include inadequacy of protected time, lack of opportunities to acquire research methods, and lack of funding (20,21). It appears that certain characteristics are associated with more successful participation by trainees in research. These include program director support, protected time, faculty involvement, a didactic curriculum (e.g., a journal club), professional support and guidance, and opportunities for presenting research (22,23). Additional characteristics of successful research environments include starting early, an integrated curriculum, having required projects, defining research broadly, fostering clinically applied research and EBM, promoting visibility of research (e.g., having a bulletin board to describe projects and opportunities), and having a research committee (22). As useful as it is to draw from the American experience of principles of developing a robust research culture, it is essential to remember that just as research agendas need to be developed locally, local institutions and policymakers will know best how to provide means, opportunity, and motivation, and enhance the perceived value of research. Local input will thus be essential to creating a culture that supports productive research.

It is perhaps instructive to examine attempts to involve women and underrepresented minorities in research culture in a setting with an abundance of resources in order to illustrate the powerful cultural forces that require attention in developing a research culture anywhere, especially in resource-poor settings without a culture that supports and values scientific research. For example, the Department of Psychiatry at the Massachusetts General Hospital (MGH) is a setting that has a thriving research culture as well as infrastructure, personnel, and abundant funding that promotes an environment in which clinicians are steered toward research opportunities and careers. Having expanded annual research expenditures from 7 to 20 million dollars in just 8 years, the MGH Department of Psychiatry has an established track record of developing independently funded clinical research programs. In addition, there are well-conceived, concerted institution-wide efforts to promote career development for women, such as an Office for Women's Careers, seminars on conducting research, free statistical consultation on research, networking and mentoring opportunities, and intramural funding to support time and expenses for research. Despite such valiant efforts to promote opportunities for women in academic medicine and research at MGH, the proportion of women who have attained senior faculty positions remains unacceptably low (e.g., 11.8% are full professors and only 15.3% are associate professors) as compared with the nearly 1:1 gender ratio in the lowest academic rank of instructor (24). Indeed, this gender inequity reflects the national (US) trend; it is, however, disheartening to see the insurmountability of barriers to women's participation in medical research careers even in the setting of a firm institutional commitment and an abundance of resources that are designed to nurture a research culture for women. Notwithstanding the promise such a focused interventional program offers, it is an illustration that certainly is humbling in the face of what we have not yet succeeded in accomplishing. This illustration also reminds us of the challenges of fostering opportunities for scientists with diverse skills, perspectives, and backgrounds in developing a research culture anywhere.

V. MECHANISMS FOR DEVELOPMENT OF RESEARCH CAPACITY: COMMON FEATURES

Key advances to developing mental health research capacity in developing countries have included the development of assessment tools that standardize assessment across cultural contexts (25), the development of consortia to facilitate cross-national research, such as the International Consortium in Psychiatric Epidemiology (26), the development of principles that define responsible conduct of psychiatric research across diverse cultural settings (17), and the nurturing of institutional collaboration that promotes research. Collaborative relationships ideally develop sustainable research capacity by well-conceived exchange programs and joint ventures that ensure that research can continue in the developing country site. Past models of training small numbers of clinician researchers raised concerns about sustainability and "brain drain" from sites in developing areas (27,28). However, thoughtful international exchange and collaborative programs to promote research in the developing world show promise. For example, "twinning" programs that establish a formal link between institutions from academic leaders and those in developing nations can result in sustained collaboration that includes promoting mutually useful and local research priorities in addition to health services (28). Moreover, training programs that specifically build in a component of sustained cross-institutional collaboration may provide a productive means of facilitating the rich exchange and leveraging of intellectual resources that can result from international collaboration. Illustrations of two such programs for Chinese and Southeast Asian junior and midcareer scholars have been developed in the Department of Social Medicine at Harvard Medical School.

The Freeman Foundation Chinese and Southeast Asian Fellowship and Exchange Program at Harvard Medical School has the broad mission of advancing communication and improving relations between Chinese and Southeast Asians and Americans. Its fellowship, student exchange, and faculty exchange programs were developed to provide research training to fellows and promote cross-institutional research collaborations. The program's explicit goal, therefore, is to actively facilitate teaching, dialogue, collaboration, and cultural exchange among participating fellows, students, and faculty in a mutually enriching way. In creating opportunities for Asian fellows to study medical anthropological theory and methods in the United States, and for Harvard students to travel and do research in Asia, the program has facilitated the development of several strong institutional relationships between Harvard and Asian universities, and has promoted an exchange of Asian and American perspectives.

Since 1996, the Freeman Fellowship Program has brought numerous scholars from China and Southeast Asia to Harvard to study health and social science research theory and methods. Faculty exchange (i.e., Harvard faculty making visits to the Chinese and Southeast Asian participating institutions) has been a key complement to the Fellowship Program. These visits have sustained the collaborative research relationships that were primed during the fellowship years, and have helped to develop a "critical mass" of researchers that will continue to promote, in each of these institutions, a thriving research culture in medical anthropologic research. This program has resulted in collaborative research that is presently ongoing at Gadjah Mada University in Yogyakarta, the Shanghai Mental Health Center, the Department of Social Medicine, Shanghai Medical University, Department of Psychological Medicine of the Zhongshan Hospital, and the Chinese University of Hong Kong. It has also resulted in a number of coauthored, scientific papers on mental health research in Indonesia and China. We feel that several key elements have resulted in the success of developing a social science research culture. First, the curriculum not only includes didactic seminars to provide a foundation of theory and research methods, but it also includes both a journal club and a writing seminar. The former introduces visiting scholars to the local research culture of reading scientific journals critically and deconstructing their assumptions; the latter develops writing skills. Both of these skill sets help fellows to effectively present research findings in English-language journals, thereby enhancing visibility of their research. In addition, formal mentorship is arranged (and it is expected that this will result in an enduring collaborative research relationship) and opportunities to present work are actively sought within the local Harvard community.

A similar second program for Chinese and Indonesian psychiatrists was developed and initiated in 2001 with funding from an International Clinical, Operational and Health Services Research and Training Award (ICOHRTA) of the Fogarty International Center. This program was developed to address the lack of psychiatrists with

TABLE 16-2. *Goals of the Harvard-CUHK ICOHRTA program.*

1. To provide fellows with basic competency in research design, and to build their competency in research methods to the level needed to conduct a selected research project.
2. To provide fellows with basic competency in the culture and mental health services paradigm.
3. To provide fellows with basic understanding of the relevance of the culture and mental health services approach to five priority mental health conditions: i.) depression and anxiety disorders; ii.) suicide; iii.) psychoses; iv.) substance abuse; v.) eating disorders.
4. To support fellows in developing specialized competency in relation to one of these priority conditions.
5. To provide fellows with the opportunity to design and carry out a research project, in collaboration with and under the supervision of faculty members from both the Department of Social Medicine and the CUHK.

systematic research training in China and Indonesia. Over a period of 5 years, the program will support 11 fellows who will participate in research training at both Harvard and the collaborating center, The Chinese University of Hong Kong (CUHK). The development of research projects that will be carried out in the home country is the primary goal. One innovative feature of this program is that fellows' research projects are funded upon their return to their home institutions. This funded research continues with supervision from faculty mentors at both Harvard and the CUHK. Ultimately, the goal of this program is to train a cadre of researchers in China and Indonesia in a set of research competencies that will ultimately reduce the burden of mental illness in these regions. The specific goals of the program are outlined in Table 16-2.

For these and similar programs to contribute substantively to local research culture in the Western Pacific, care must be taken to support local research agendas (29), to undertake research that will develop sustainable and realistic interventions for the local community (14), to establish and observe ethical guidelines about not enticing researchers from less-developed countries to ones with greater economic opportunities, and to choose collaborative research agendas (30,31). A set of guidelines for collaborative research based on the collective experience of WHO-coordinated study has been suggested by Dr. Norman Sartorius, past president of the World Psychiatric Association and former director of the Division of Mental Health, WHO, and is summarized in Table 16-3.

There have been other such fellowships organized by the WHO and the World Psychiatric Association that have contributed to the development of health researchers in developing countries (32). The development of such efforts will ultimately be enhanced by the continued relocation of training activities to the developing world (33).

VI. IMPORTANT CONSIDERATIONS IN THE DEVELOPMENT OF LOCAL AND GLOBAL RESEARCH CULTURES

A key consideration to developing a research culture in areas of the developing world is to ensure that a local "emic" perspective is consistently applied in setting

TABLE 16-3. *Guidelines concerning ethical aspects of scientific collaboration.*

1. Research problems must be recognized and defined jointly.
2. Solutions to the problems must have clear relevance to all participants.
3. Collaboration should do no harm to any party.
4. Collaboration should provide a structure for continued joint activity.
5. Collaboration should not exhaust the resources of any participant.
6. Investigators should work, write, and present work on an equal-status basis.
7. Data should be used in scientific publications and to promote collaboration and understanding among participant institutions and countries.
8. Rules of the strictest ethical review committee should apply to the entire collaborative network.
9. Organization of collaboration should be agreed upon by all and respect culture-specific requirements and methods of working.
10. Collaboration arrangements (e.g., with respect to use of data, authorship) should be discussed and agreed upon before work proceeds.

(Adapted from Sartorius N. Experience from the mental health programme of the World Health Organization. *Acta Psychiatr Scand Suppl,* 1988;344:72–74, with permission.)

local research priorities. In the developing Pacific Island countries, for example, research infrastructure has been historically poor and most health research has been both initiated and funded externally (29). To reduce the burden of mental illness in the Western Pacific, however, research colonialism (i.e., research in a developing country for the sole benefit of the outside institution or population conducting the research) must certainly be avoided, and so must "armchair" and "ivory tower" perspectives yield to perspectives that encompass local points of view in the development of research agendas in which the host culture's benefit is a priority. Mental illnesses are best understood and addressed from "emic" (insider) as well as "etic" (external) perspectives.

As crucial as it is to support the development of local research cultures, these cultures are inextricably located in a larger, global cultural context that exerts strong influence on them. Indeed, development of research culture locally should not consist of merely patterning it after Western research culture, but in being innovative in contributing to the development of more globally relevant research agenda. Just as the global research culture stimulates local ideas and research activity, the converse should be equally true, so that these collaborative partners enrich each other. Reducing the burden of mental illness globally will require promotion of a research agenda that is broadly inclusive of both social science and natural science perspectives. Ethnographic and qualitative research methods will need to be integrated more effectively into study design to infuse cross-cultural epidemiologic data with local relevance and to provide essential data on phenomenologic variations in mental illness, local explanatory models, social risk factors, and social course across diverse contexts. In addition, there is a need to foster a global research culture that is respectful of the strengths that developing countries bring to scientific progress.

VII. CONCLUSION

In summary, the development of local research cultures will enhance the visibility and voice of developing nations in developing and promoting local research agendas and in contributing to the global research agenda of reducing the burden of mental illness. Local research cultures can best be developed by an incorporation of the "emic" perspective on how research may be promoted and valued locally and by borrowing from the experience of successful programs to develop research culture. The success in the development of local research cultures will also include work toward moderating the hegemony of Western research methods and agendas to broaden the scope of research as well as to capitalize on the strengths of diverse research environments. Nations with a well-developed research infrastructure and culture need to seek creative new ways to share data and research software with developing countries. Mechanisms for creating international registries and databases and for developing reservoirs of methodologic support should be encouraged. Fellowship and exchange programs that allow for sustained research collaborations across institutions should continue to be encouraged and developed. Journals should be called upon to promote the visibility of work from developing nations. Any loss in intellectual potential represents a loss for the worldwide scientific community, and all of us share the responsibility to promote research in developing nations (34). Finally, leading research centers must be helped to appreciate the relevance of promoting research activity in diverse contexts to their own research agenda as well as be encouraged to meet their responsibilities in contributing to local research cultures. These changes will ultimately best advance our global capacity to develop and implement mental health preventive and treatment strategies across diverse contexts and to reduce the substantial global burden of mental illness.

REFERENCES

1. Ormel J, VonKorff M, Bedirham U, et al. Common mental disorders and disability across cultures: results from the WHO Collaborative Study on Psychological Problems in General Health Care. *JAMA* 1994;272:1741–1748.
2. Murray CJL, Lopez AD, eds. *Global burden of disease.* Cambridge: Harvard School of Public Health on Behalf of the World Health Organization, 1996.
3. Becker AE, Kleinman A. Anthropology and psychiatry. In: Sadock BJ, Sadock VA, eds. *Kaplan & Sadock's comprehensive textbook of psychiatry.* 7th ed. Philadelphia: Lippincott Williams & Wilkins, 2000:463–476.
4. Desjarlais R, Eisenberg L, Good B, et al. *World mental health: problems and priorities in low-income countries.* Oxford: Oxford University Press, 1995.
5. Sartorius N, Emsley RA. Psychiatry and technological advances: implications for developing countries. *Lancet* 2000;356:2090–2092.
6. Brundtland GH. Mental health: new understanding, new hope. *JAMA* 2001;286:2391
7. Mari JDJ, Lozano JM, Duley L. Erasing the global divide in health research: collaboration provides answers relevant to developing and developed countries. *BMJ* 1997;314:390.
8. World Health Organization. *Research for change.* Geneva: WHO, 2002.
9. Patel V, Sumathipala A. International representation in psychiatric literature: survey of six leading journals. *Br J Psychiatry* 2001;178:406–409.
10. Williams DD, Garner J. The case against 'the evidence': a different perspective on evidence-based medicine. *Br J Psychiatry* 2002;180:8–12.

11. Sackett DL, Rosenberg WMC, Gray JAM, et al. Evidence based medicine: what it is and what it isn't: It's about integrating individual clinical expertise and the best external evidence. *BMJ* 1996; 312:71–72.
12. Lowe M. Evidence-based medicine-the view from Fiji. *Lancet* 2000;356:1105–1107.
13. Hohmann AA, Shear KM. Community-based intervention research: coping with the "noise" of real life in study design. *Am J Psychiatry* 2002;159:201–207.
14. Garner P, Torres TT, Alonso P. Trial design in developing countries. *BMJ* 1994;309:825–826.
15. Bonair A, Rosenfield P, Tengvald K. Medical technologies in developing countries: issues of technology development, transfer, diffusion and use. *Soc Sci Med* 1989;28:779–781.
16. Sartorius N. Scientific work in third world countries. *Acta Psychiatr Scand* 1998;98:345–347.
17. Sartorius N. Ethics and the societies of the world. In: Okasha A, Arboleda-Florez J, Sartorius N, eds. *Ethics, culture, and psychiatry: international perspectives.* Washington, DC: American Psychiatric Press, 2000:3–14.
18. American Association of Medical Colleges. Available at: http://www.aamc.org/newsroom/pressrel/2002/021030.htm. Accessed November 18, 2002.
19. Good BJ. *Medicine, rationality, and experience: an anthropological perspective.* Cambridge: Cambridge University Press, 1994.
20. Temte JL, Hunter PH, Beasley JW. Factors associated with research interest and activity during family practice residency. *Fam Med* 1994:26:93–97.
21. Polk GC. Building a nursing research culture. *J Psychosoc Nurs* 1989;27:24–27.
22. DeHaven MJ, Wilson GR, O'Connor-Kettlestrings P. Creating a research culture: what we can learn from residencies that are successful in research. *Educ Res Methods* 1998;30:501–507.
23. Crow S, Rogers J, Larcombe K. Developing a research culture in education and practice. *Nurs Stand* 1997;12:34–35.
24. Partners Office for Women's Careers at MGH. *Partners Office for Women's Careers at MGH Winter Newsletter.* Boston: Massachusetts General Hospital, 2002:2.
25. Sartorius N, Janca A. Psychiatric assessment instruments developed by the World Health Organization. *Soc Psychiatry Psychiatr Epidemiol* 1996;31:55–69.
26. Kessler RC. The World Health Organization International Consortium in Psychiatric Epidemiology (ICPE). Initial work and future directions—the NAPE Lecture 1998. *Acta Psychiatr Scand* 1999; 99:2–9.
27. Pang T, Lansang MA, Haines A. Brain drain and health professionals: a global problem needs global solutions. *BMJ* 2002;324:499–500.
28. MacDonagh R, Jiddawi M, Parry V. Twinning: the future for sustainable collaboration. *BJU Int* 2002; 89:13–17
29. Finau SA. Health research in the Pacific: in search of a reality. *N Z Med J* 1995;108:16–19.
30. Bundred PE, Levitt C. Medical migration: who are the real losers? *Lancet* 2000;356:245–246.
31. Sartorius N. Experience from the mental health programme of the World Health Organization. *Acta Psychiatr Scand Suppl* 1988;344:71–74.
32. Sartorius N. Activities of the World Psychiatric Association in the period 1996–1999. *Curr Opin Psychiatry* 1999;12:i–iii.
33. Eddleston M. Encouraging high-quality clinical research in the tropics. *Lancet* 1999;353:1190.
34. Cuevas-Sosa A. Scientific and research culture in Mexico. *Lancet* 1999;354:685.

17

Project 1 Billion

A Global Model for the Mental Health Recovery of Postconflict Societies

[*]Laura S. McDonald, [*]Robina Bhasin, and [*,†]Richard F. Mollica

[*]*Harvard Program in Refugee Trauma, Cambridge, Massachusetts 02139; and*
[†]*Department of Psychiatry, Harvard Medical School, Boston, Massachusetts 02114*

I. INTRODUCTION: GLOBALIZATION AND HEALTH

We live in a world today where state boundaries have become less significant through the process of globalization. Industrialized countries can no longer afford to consider health problems beyond our borders irrelevant to international policymaking. The trends of globalization—defined as "the process of increasing economic, political, and social interdependence and global integration that takes place as capital, traded goods, persons, concepts, images, ideas, and values diffuse across state boundaries"(1)—have made health care and health outcomes of populations worldwide a primary focus of consideration in policymaking and action. This concern for the health of populations far beyond national borders is embedded in our view of health as a core human right; as expressed in the 1950 United Nations Declaration of Human Rights (Art. 25), "Everyone has the right to a standard of living adequate for the health and well-being of himself and his family, including food, clothing, housing and medical care and necessary social services"(2,3).

Despite landmark advances in science and technology, inequities in research and access to care characterize international public health. Heightened cooperation among researchers, institutions, and health practitioners has led to important findings and efficacious treatment for several illnesses; yet, tragically, a number of preventable diseases such as malaria and tuberculosis continue to take the lives of millions of people worldwide (4,5). Global health indicators continue to decline, while disparities in health outcomes and access to care between industrialized and developing countries continue to grow. The United Nations Development Programme (UNDP) reported in 2003 that in 21 countries, a larger portion of people were going hungry than in 1990; in 14 countries, more children were dying before age 5 years. Further, the Human Development Index (HDI), a measurement of healthy life expectancy, education, and standard of living, declined in 21 countries in the 1990s, compared to decreases in only four countries in the decade prior (6). This trend, according to UNDP Administrator Mark Malloch-Brown, "signifies an urgent call for action to address health and education as well as income levels in these countries" (7).

Despite these harrowing realities, only 10% of the $70 billion allocated on an annual basis to health research and development worldwide is directed toward 90% of the world's health problems, a phenomenon referred to as the "10/90 gap." This serious misallocation of resources translates to devastating outcomes for a majority of the world's populations, negatively affecting the health, social and economic well-being, and long-term economic and social development of the countries in which they live. Current trends of globalization, coupled with the growing negative impact of mass violence, should incite policymakers, organizations, and scientific and health communities to focus on addressing related causes and outcomes, which are affecting millions of individuals worldwide.

II. GLOBALIZATION AND MASS VIOLENCE

Mass violence has taken a devastating toll on the health of populations worldwide in recent decades. Since 1980, more than 60 countries have experienced significant periods of conflict, affecting up to 1 billion persons (8). According to the World Bank, 80% of the world's 20 poorest countries have had major conflicts in the past 15 years (9). In the 11-year period from 1990 to 2000, there were 56 different major armed conflicts in 44 locations (10). Since World War II, the majority of conflicts have taken place in Africa, Asia, and the Middle East, and have been increasingly characterized by devastating consequences for civilian populations, who are often specifically targeted for violence. The Carnegie Commission notes that, "in some wars today, 90% of those killed in conflict are noncombatants, compared with less than 15% when the century began" (11). Every country in sub-Saharan Africa has either been affected by mass violence directly or borders on a devastated country, thereby having to deal with large influxes of refugees and/or political instability. Conflicts in Sudan and the Democratic Republic of Congo (DRC) have taken an unimaginable toll. The conflict in Sudan has resulted in 2.0 million deaths, creating the world's largest internally displaced population (IDP) of more than 4 million (12). Approximately 3.3 million people have died as a result of war-related causes in the DRC, with the highest war death toll documented worldwide in the last half of the 20th century (13).

The 20th century was marked by massive population movements resulting from forced displacement. The US Committee for Refugees estimates that in 2000 there were over 35 million refugees and IDPs worldwide (14). According to Human Rights

Watch, Asia hosts 45% of all refugees, followed by Africa (30%), Europe (19%), and North America (5%) (15). These figures translate into 1 in every 300 persons worldwide having been forced to flee persecution, violence, and war (16). When this article was under preparation, a humanitarian crisis was taking hold in the Darfur region of Sudan, where an estimated 2.2 million people are fleeing from forced displacement and regional conflict. This crisis, if it continues unabated without immediate provision of humanitarian assistance and a political resolution, will take a serious toll in human lives, individual and community well-being, and regional security.

The refugee experience is characterized by both the direct and indirect experience of violence (17–20). Refugees are often exposed to violence, sexual assault, torture, incarceration, and the threat of injury and death (21). A recent report published by the US Committee for Refugees underscores the harrowing realities faced by refugees, as "more than seven million refugees have been confined to refugee camps, segregated settlements or otherwise deprived of their rights for ten years or more" (22). Serious human rights violations often occur during conflict and displacement. A recent study by Amowitz et al. (23) found that among survivors of the conflict in Sierra Leone, 94% of 991 households randomly surveyed reported among their members at least one serious abuse during the previous 10 years of conflict; multiple types of violations occurred, including abductions, beatings, killings, rape and other forms of sexual violence, capturing for 24 or more hours, torture, forced labor, gunshot wounds, serious injuries, and amputations.

The impact of conflict and violence on children is staggering. According to a 1996 United Nations Children's Fund (UNICEF) report, 2 million children died and 4 to 5 million were seriously injured as a result of conflict during the decade prior (24). Studies from several countries report that children's most pervasive fear is of violent death (25). Several hundreds of thousands of children have been used as child soldiers in recent and current conflicts (26). A recent study of former Ugandan child soldiers reveals the extent of trauma these children experience at a very young age (27). Forced to perpetrate serious crimes against their families and communities, they are deprived of the opportunity for healthy development, seriously jeopardizing the possibility of a healthy adult life. A recent Human Rights Watch report (28) reveals the harrowing impact of conflict in Uganda on innocent civilian populations:

> The brunt of the war is borne by the civilian population, in terms of homes destroyed, goods stolen, children abducted and brutalized, family members killed and raped, all of which has reduced the more than one million Acholi inhabitants of northern Uganda to a state of destitution and despair.

In addition, in recent years, a significant increase in international terrorist activity has resulted in the loss of thousands of lives. Most significantly, the attacks of September 11, 2001, in the United States and in Madrid, Spain, in March 2004 have taken thousands of lives and have had a serious negative impact (29–32). Although precise figures are unknown, preliminary reports also reveal that many innocent civilians in both Afghanistan and Iraq have lost their lives as a result of activity in which they had no involvement (33,34).

III. MENTAL HEALTH CONSEQUENCES OF MASS VIOLENCE WORLDWIDE

Recent scientific studies have revealed the enormous mental health impact of mass violence on the health status and functioning of traumatized populations. As reviewed in more detail by Lopes Cardozo and Fricchione in this volume, scientific studies of war-affected refugee and civilian populations reveal rates of posttraumatic stress disorder (PTSD) and depression several times greater than baseline prevalence (35–39). Disability and suffering can continue long after the crisis has ended (40–44). A recent longitudinal study of Bosnian refugees revealed for the first time the serious disability associated with the mental health effects of mass violence. Comorbidity for depression and PTSD was associated with high rates of physical disability (25%) in this population (45). Even after the conflict had ended, these refugees experienced unremitting psychiatric disability, and there was premature death of the elderly (46).

A number of studies also reveal significant increases in PTSD, depression, and anxiety among children following the experience of mass violence (47,48). Studies have found high prevalences of PTSD and depression among children who have experienced conflict (49,50). Nader et al. (51) found in a study of Kuwaiti children following the Gulf war that over 70% presented with moderate to severe posttraumatic stress reactions. Studies undertaken after the attacks of September 11, 2001, reveal associated serious negative mental health outcomes in adults and children (52–54). Negative mental health sequelae resulting from terrorism have also been demonstrated in other settings (55–58).

The incidence of psychological distress and growing mental health problems worldwide has been acknowledged extensively in scientific and policy-based literature. The World Health Organization (WHO) estimates that approximately 450 million people suffer from some form of mental or brain disorder, including alcohol and substance abuse disorders (59). The landmark Global Burden of Disease (GBD) study (60), using the measurement of disability-adjusted life years (DALYS), has shed critical light on the prevalence of mental health problems worldwide by accounting for years lived with a disability. Psychiatric conditions accounted for five of the ten leading causes of disability worldwide. The study found that depression ranked as the fourth leading cause of disease burden in 1990. It is estimated that by 2020, the GBD attributable to mental and brain disorders will rise to 15%, and depression will move to rank as the second leading cause of disease burden by 2020. Further, this study predicts that the GBD caused by war will rank seventh in 2020. Because few postconflict or conflict-affected countries were included in this study, it has been estimated that the aforementioned statistics are likely to be two to four times greater in these countries than in those of nontraumatized populations.

The psychological wounds of conflict must be a key component of postconflict recovery and a truly sustainable rehabilitation. Organizations attempting to work within this context have expressed understanding of the importance of healing psychological injuries or "invisible wounds" (61) within the postconflict environment.

In a recent paper, for example, the World Bank argued that "failure to address mental health and psychosocial disorders in populations that have experienced mass violence and trauma caused by conflict will impede efforts to enhance social capital, promote human development and reduce poverty" (62). The growing scientific evidence documenting the serious negative health and mental health sequelae of mass violence, combined with the widely accepted view of health as a basic and inviolable human right, should propel health practitioners, policymakers, and scientific experts to seek ways to address the mental health consequences of mass violence. Furthermore, the forces of globalization should make developing a strong, appropriate, and evidence-based response to these devastating health outcomes a primary concern of industrialized and developing countries alike.

IV. EVIDENCE-BASED MENTAL HEALTH INTERVENTIONS

In recent years, there has been a revolution in the development of an evidence base for mental health interventions (42,63). The development of scientifically valid approaches to mental health recovery provides the justification and foundation for mental health assistance using a culturally appropriate and evidence-based action plan. Scientific studies reveal the capacity of indigenous primary health care systems (64–68), traditional healers (69–71), and nongovernmental organizations (NGOs) and international organizations (IOs) (72–75) to address the serious suffering and disability associated with mass violence. Further, although there are limited studies on the long-term effectiveness of training approaches, existing studies show that with modest training, primary health care providers can effectively identify and address mental health outcomes in a postconflict society (76); focusing on the primary health care setting has been widely acknowledged by scientific and health authorities as well as institutions as an effective way to foster healing (77,78).

The field of cross-cultural psychiatry has emphasized issues important in developing and designing culturally appropriate and effective treatments for depression, PTSD, and anxiety (79,80). The efficacy of a number of intervention techniques, including psychotropic drugs, cognitive behavior therapy (CBT) (81), and individual and group therapy (82), has been demonstrated in various settings. CBT has been shown to be efficacious in treating cases of PTSD that have failed to respond to supportive counseling (83,84). Talking therapy has also demonstrated efficacy in a number of contexts (85).

Although some studies have demonstrated the positive impact of eye-movement desensitization and reprocessing (EMDR), there is still debate surrounding the efficacy of this treatment (86–90). Studies on the effectiveness of debriefing in the conflict context have led to assertions that routine debriefing may not be as effective as initially considered and may lead to adverse consequences (91). The efficacy of art therapy, an approach to healing frequently supported by IOs and NGOs, has not yet been scientifically proven as an effective healing intervention (92). Evidence on the efficacy of psychiatric treatments for disorders prevalent in postconflict societies is increasing—and should continue to grow.

V. SOCIETAL RECOVERY: LINKAGES TO ECONOMIC DEVELOPMENT, SOCIAL CAPITAL, AND HUMAN RIGHTS

A growing trend of postconflict recovery efforts is the acknowledgment that health and mental health outcomes, services, and recovery can no longer be conceptualized as separate from other domains of postconflict recovery and growth. Intervention efficacy is resolutely contingent on a broad consideration of the existing social, economic, and political context. Science is beginning to reveal complex and interdirectional linkages between mental health outcomes and economic development, social capital, and human rights. As Figure 17-1 illustrates, each of these domains and corresponding contextual features warrants critical consideration in the design, development, and implementation of a mental health action plan for postconflict societies.

Positive correlations have been revealed between poverty, unemployment, substance dependence, and poor mental health outcomes (78,93–95). Poverty is likely to exacerbate the onset and severity of mental disorders. There is growing evidence that health can seriously impact economic outcomes (96). Although there exist little data on the specific impact of depression on economic behavior in the postconflict environment, high levels of hopelessness and despair affecting more than 40% of citizens living in local towns and villages is likely having a negative impact on social and economic development (61). A study in 2001 of individuals seeking care at primary health care centers in Bosnia found that almost 40% were suffering from serious depression and related disability. A recent unpublished study by Kapetanovic

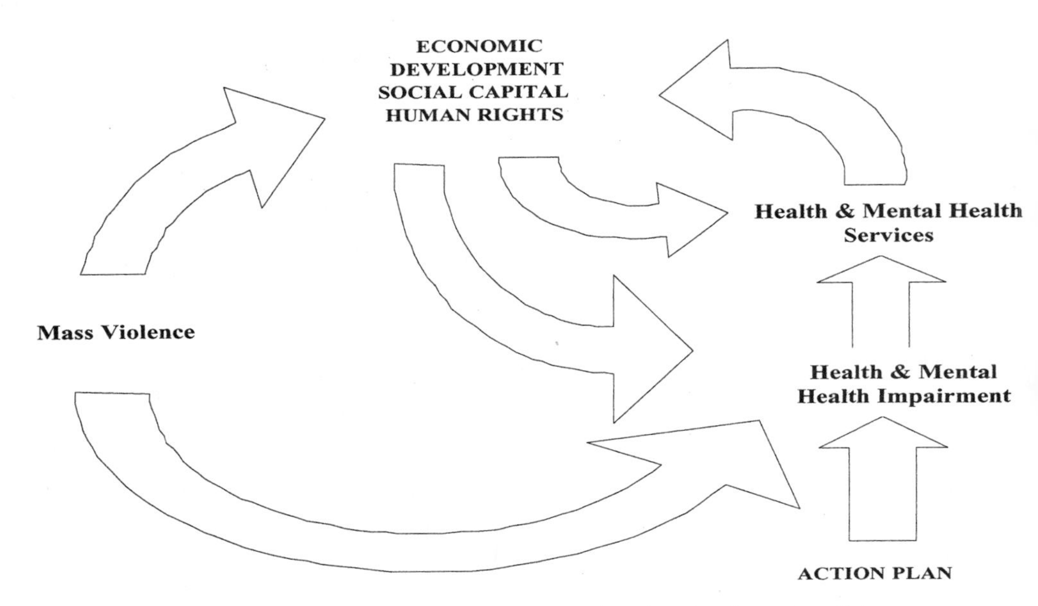

FIG. 17-1. Conceptual framework for a mental health action plan for postconflict recovery.

(97) of individuals seeking care at primary health care centers in Bosnia found that almost 40% were suffering from serious depression and related disability according to the criteria of the fourth edition of the *Diagnostic and Statistical Manual of Mental Disorders* (DSM-IV). One year later, major depression was diagnosed in 24% using a culturally validated algorithm based on DSM- IV. Findings such as this highlight the probability that the toll on economic productivity is significant.

Although related studies in conflict-affected societies are limited, the impact of mental illness on the labor market, measured in terms of job performance and productivity, has been well established in industrialized countries (see Geballe [98]). The economic costs of mental illness among traumatized civilian populations are measured in a number of ways, including days of work lost, job performance quality, and ability to plan for economic activities. In the United States, depression is associated with the highest rate of work-related disability. For example, the total annual cost in the United States due to depression in 1990 was estimated at $43.7 billion, owing to reduced productivity (55%), treatment costs (28%), and suicide-related mortality costs (17%). Those with depression have been found to be 27 times more likely to miss work, with 44% of those with depression reporting having missed at least 1 day of work in 3 months, compared with 2% of the general population (98). Research on PTSD has indicated that people with PTSD work an average of 3.6 days a month less than nontraumatized co-workers, resulting in an annual productivity loss of $3 billion per year (99,100).

Although the impact of mental health on economic productivity is likely to be significant, opportunities for self-agency and productivity have demonstrated positive impact on individuals' health and mental health. Findings from subsequent analysis of a study of Cambodian refugees living in a refugee camp on the Thai-Cambodia border suggest that employment and the opportunity to practice altruistic behavior can have a positive impact on individuals' mental and physical health (101). Moreover, although survivors may participate to some degree in "normal" daily activities in the aftermath of conflict, we have little information as to the impact of the experience of these individuals, despite their demonstrated resiliency, on themselves and their offspring.

The role of social capital has also been increasingly recognized as a key component of a healthy society, and must be given significant consideration in the postconflict recovery phase. The World Bank acknowledges its interdependent linkages in asserting that social cohesion—social capital—is "critical for poverty alleviation and sustainable human and economic development" (102). Positive social capital is characterized by functioning social networks that improve a collective approach to problem solving; it can be demonstrated through, for example, community engagement and efficacy, informal social support networks, norms of trust and reciprocity, and trust in various institutions (103). Violent conflict significantly damages social capital, leaving vengefulness, hatred, and mistrust in its wake. The restoration of social capital, therefore, must be the cornerstone of mental health recovery activities. Its restoration is critical in preventing the reemergence of conflict and in ensuring the health of the society in the short and long term (104).

Respect and concern for human rights issues within the postconflict setting must be factored into the mental health recovery of a society as well. It has been argued that, conceptually, conflicts do not "end" at a specific point in time, but rather occur on a continuum; simply because a conflict has officially ended or has been suspended as a result of a political peace agreement or ceasefire does not necessarily mean that widespread human rights violations are not being inflicted by both civilians and armed authorities within the postconflict setting. Indeed, some reports do reveal human rights violations continuing after a conflict's official end (105,106).

Further, the human rights community recognizes the survivor's understandable desire for justice, and possibly vengeance and restitution. A number of countries, including Bosnia, Sierra Leone, and Cambodia, have opted to hold international tribunals in order to bring justice to survivors of conflict and those who have lost loved ones. The delay of this process and, in turn, of justice, could be perceived as an obstacle to the societal respect for human rights, constituting arguably a lower-scale violation of human rights. In the case of Cambodia, for example, whose many citizens await a tribunal for a conflict that officially ended many years ago, it has been asserted that "without truth, justice and reparations, victims and their communities will feel that the new order has failed them" (107).

Given the serious devastating mental health consequences of mass violence, as well as the foreseeable impact of these outcomes on all domains of life, efforts to address these outcomes, with consideration for broader contextual issues as discussed earlier, should be central to postconflict recovery. The World Bank, a leading international development organization, has acknowledged the importance of mental health and of supporting the social and economic process of recovery to achieve a successful rehabilitation of postconflict societies (62,104). The World Bank has noted that although most of its intervention in the reconstruction phase after conflict has focused on "rebuilding infrastructure, . . .capacity is also needed to promote economic adjustment and recovery, to address social sector needs, and to build institutional capacity. . . . Two overall objectives for Bank intervention are. . .to facilitate the transition to sustainable peace after hostilities cease and to support economic and social development" (108). Significant continued research on each of these areas within postconflict settings will play a critical role in further developing efficacious recovery methods.

VI. BARRIERS IN THE CURRENT APPROACH TO HEALING

Despite the development of evidence-based practices in addressing the mental health impact of mass violence and the growing realization that good governance on these issues is critical, these two issues have remained largely disconnected in terms of policy and approaches to addressing the mental health wounds resulting from mass violence. In the aftermath of conflict, the management of local authorities is frequently ineffective and disorganized. National health authorities, responsible for playing a key role in the recovery process, do not possess adequate human and financial resources for massive recovery efforts to be effectively undertaken. Furthermore, they lack both an international mandate for assistance and knowledge of best practices—each necessary for the creation of sustainable and effective mental health systems and activities.

Further, the efforts of IOs and NGOs, largely funded by international donors, have been criticized for disregarding, overlooking, or underutilizing the available and indigenous healing resources (109). There exists little information as to how community structures are incorporated into international efforts (110). An approach to individual and collective recovery in the postconflict phase that is not founded on knowledge, experience, and the participation of the indigenous healing system is likely to result in (i) underutilization of services resulting from stigmatization and perceived treatment inefficacy, (ii) limited sustainability due to high dependence on vacillating donor funding cycles, and (iii) suboptimal resource allocation as a result of redundancy and the likelihood of limited sustainability of interventions following the departure of external organizations. This characteristic disconnect of NGO/IO intervention from existing indigenous systems and approaches impedes these organizations' capacity to gauge and respond effectively to existing needs at the local, national, and regional levels, while simultaneously depleting important indigenous structures (111).

Laying the foundation for uninformed efforts detached from local and national input is the lack of organization in the design and delivery of mental health assistance. This is widely acknowledged as a deficit of postconflict intervention in science- and policy-related literature (42,112). Further, despite advances in research on the treatment of psychological distress and mental illness among refugees and IDPs and related outcomes, few studies have been undertaken in the emergency and postconflict context. Although there is significant discussion surrounding the ethical issues of such research, building up the evidence base through randomized clinical trials and epidemiological studies in a wide variety of contexts is critical in ensuring efficacious assistance and resource allocation. The continued absence of this research base from the specific context will limit the provision of optimal care. Indeed, the absence of a viable mental health recovery action plan, based on culturally effective and evidence-based practices, severely limits the provision of effective mental health services to populations in need.

VII. THE MISSING LINK: A MENTAL HEALTH ACTION PLAN

The greatest barrier to effective mental health recovery in postconflict societies is the absence of an action plan that could guide policy, programs, and services. A mental health action plan based on state-of-the-art scientific evidence is critically needed, and would represent a landmark step in remedying the inherent flaws of the existing approach to mental health recovery efforts in the postconflict environment. Several features are essential to the success of an action plan in the short and long term. The plan must be (i) culturally valid and able to be customized for various settings and regions, (ii) equipped to utilize local resources and maximize involvement of the local indigenous healing system (including primary care practitioners, traditional healers and local NGOs, among others), (iii) financially feasible given current and anticipated resource constraints, and (iv) focused on recovery in a broad sense, including not only patient care, but also employment, economic development, reconstruction of civil society, and reconciliation.

For such an action plan to be developed and implemented, a partnership within this structure must be fostered among mental health practitioners (medical doctors, clinical psychologists, and social workers), the Ministers of Health, and related national health authorities. Each partner has something critical to offer. The Ministers of Health within postconflict societies are already charged with the responsibility for ensuring the society's well-being and are most aware of the in-country postconflict realities. In addition to familiarity with the culture, social structure, and operating mechanisms within the society, they are aware of existing financial and human resources and related constraints. At the same time, they often lack the scientific tools to create and realize such policy, programs, and services.

Mental health practitioners can play an essential role in meeting these barriers and limitations to forge an effective approach to recovery. Equipped with resources and scientific expertise derived from the rapidly growing evidence base, these individuals can provide guidance and consultation to national health leaders and policymakers. This partnership is critical, as mental health practitioners from abroad frequently have limited, if any, understanding of the field-level realities and key contextual issues that characterize the postconflict setting.

The successful design and applicability of a mental health action plan is contingent on a cohesive and balanced partnership of cooperative exchange between medical practitioners and policymakers. Together, they can ensure the timely provision of effective healing services based on resource availabilities, field-level constraints, and contextual issues characterizing the postconflict setting. Indeed, this new conceptualization of roles and strong partnerships in developing and promoting the mental health recovery process should be a focal point for an action plan on mental health recovery. New efforts founded on evidence-based practices, contextual realities, and national ownership and leadership can lead to the provision of effective and sustainable care to millions of suffering individuals.

VIII. PROJECT 1 BILLION: A COLLABORATIVE SCIENTIFIC INITIATIVE

A. The Genesis of Project 1 Billion

The Harvard Program in Refugee Trauma (HPRT) for more than two decades has worked with more than 10,000 survivors of mass violence worldwide and has collaborated with numerous governments in several postconflict societies, including Cambodia, Bosnia, and East Timor, to create mental health services programs. Through varied field-level and research activities, HPRT noted systemic limitations characterizing most postconflict societies. To gain field-level insight into the experiences of national health authorities and perceived barriers to developing and sustaining viable mental health services, HPRT convened a meeting of Ministry of Health officials from conflict-affected societies in Asia, Africa, Europe, and Latin America. This meeting, held in Sarajevo in 2002 and attended by scholars, scientists, policy makers and donors, provided important guidance in developing viable approaches to mental health recovery in the postconflict context (113).

The participants agreed that the next steps needed to ensure the mental health recovery of postconflict societies would be to (i) develop a framework for creating and financing culturally effective and sustainable mental health policies, (ii) determine science-based clinical and socioeconomic strategies that would be able to achieve significant positive results for mental health, (iii) prepare policy recommendations to be disseminated by the conference participants, (iv) convene a meeting of 45 Ministries of Health (MOH) from conflict-affected nations and international agencies, and (v) disseminate and implement the program through on-site technical assistance to a number of postconflict countries. This initiative, called Project 1 Billion—referring to the one billion persons who are affected by violence today—was believed to have the potential to lead to the formulation of new ideas and practices and, ultimately, to a global mental health agenda with significant bilateral and multilateral support.

B. Components of a Mental Health Action Plan

The primary objective of Project 1 Billion is to develop a global action plan for mental health recovery in postconflict societies, working collaboratively with national health authorities and guidance from Ministers of Health (113). Scientific research and guidance from mental health experts from a number of countries and cultural contexts have enabled us to develop a draft mental health action plan (see Appendix), and we are currently in the process of compiling a *Book of Best Practices* that can be used by MOH, policymakers, organizations, and donors. Both the *Book of Best Practices* and the action plan focus on six key areas: policy and legislation; financing mechanisms; service design and provision; training and education; role of organizations; and linkage of care to human rights, social capital and economic development (see Fig. 17-2). The long-term viability of an action plan requires consideration and action in each of these domains.

Our understanding that these six domains must be the cornerstone of any action plan grew out of the meeting in Sarajevo. Below we will discuss existing limitations in each area, as well as the opportunities that exist if an action plan is able to address each area effectively, and each domain's specific role in the viability of a mental health action plan for recovery.

1. *Policy and legislation.* To maximize resources in a broken system, policy is crucial. During the acute phase of conflict, the society's existing structures and facilities are completely destroyed and human survival is the most urgent priority. In the postconflict phase, governance and accountability are key. Within this context lies a critical juncture of opportunity for reconstruction of structures and system-wide healing approaches, incorporating up-to-date medical advances.

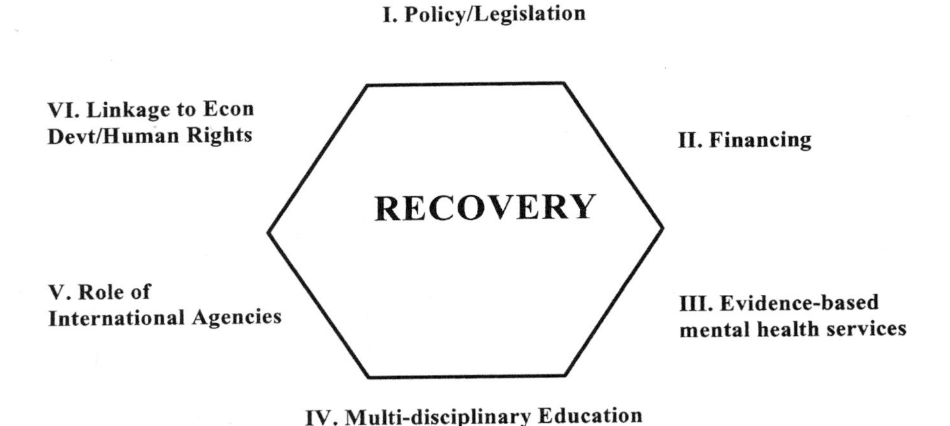

FIG. 17-2. Framework for mental health recovery.

Such an approach (which likely retains components of prior approaches and perceptions) can foster increased solidarity between actors and provide opportunities for the creation of a new level of excellence in service design and provision. Within this realm, long-term dependency on external sources can be avoided. Policy formulation is an essential step toward the development and acceptance of legislation.

In addition to guaranteeing intervention sustainability, and doing their part to ensure that health policy adheres to the action plan, national health ministries are well placed to work closely with allied ministries to ensure the proper and most effective implementation of the action plan. For example, ministries of education, labor, and economic development can assess and ensure access to mental health care within their respective domains, and can secure followthrough in the provision of science-based interventions and the dissemination of mental health–related public health information to the general public.

2. *Financing mechanisms.* The current approach to mental health recovery in postconflict rehabilitation, characterized by a profound disconnect between the indigenous community and international agencies, results in the establishment of parallel services that lead to the marginalization of the indigenous healing system. Further, there exist to date no clear guidelines for countries to follow in order to secure long-term funding. No central or recognized authority exists to plan and control finances in mental health care. Financial mechanisms that can ensure the sustainability of mental health services in the long term must be an essential feature of postconflict recovery efforts. The MOH should collaborate with donors and international and national organizations to create these financing mechanisms. This step will prevent the characteristic development of parallel systems of health care that ultimately become largely responsible for the collapse of the health care system when the recovery process is considered finished and the international

community withdraws its support. A fiscally healthy mental health system increases the confidence and long-term effectiveness of the entire indigenous healing community and ensures accountability.

3. Science-based mental health services. Science-based, culturally competent mental health services must be implemented to ensure the recovery of traumatized persons. State-of-the-art evidence-based best practices must be adapted for the local cultural context and evaluated for effectiveness. Institutions; human, financial, and material resources; and scientific literature should be harnessed to strengthen scientific research. Mental health training can build local capacities in many sectors of societies, especially those that have direct contact with mental health problems on a daily basis (i.e., primary care providers, school teachers and counselors, clergy, and traditional healers) (42).
4. *Multidisciplinary education.* To build and maintain culturally valid and cost-effective services, a standardized program for continuing mental health education must be established. The educational approach should be multidisciplinary and multisectoral to meet the needs of all practitioners and institutions that play a role in the implementation of mental health services, and evaluation mechanisms should be established to ensure their effectiveness. This approach teaches health professionals and healers scientific clinical skills and cultural competence. Providing new skills and promoting attitudes and behaviors that contribute to the healing of individuals, families, communities, and nations also creates the opportunity to break up cycles of violence. This program also teaches about the deleterious effects of trauma and fosters partnership between local and international agents, to facilitate exchange of knowledge and expertise. It is necessary to be aware, however, that conflict tends to occur and evolve unpredictably, and could lead to misplaced intentions and or interventions, as well as negative ideological, cultural, or religious attitudes and misunderstandings.
5. *Role of international agencies.* The lack of coordination among international efforts to address the mental health impact of war is a salient feature of the emergency and postconflict environment. Its absence in complex emergencies is considered by many to be a serious barrier to the provision of effective care to populations in need. Initiatives such as the Sphere Project (114), a collaborative effort of 228 NGOs, which includes minimum standards in disaster response for essential public health services, provide some guidance as to how coordination of efforts can be effectively undertaken. Coordinated assistance should be the cornerstone of any relief and/or development intervention in the conflict and postconflict phases.

The presence of additional human, financial, and technical resources creates the opportunity to not only "rebuild" but also to create more optimal services and infrastructure, as long as it is coordinated and collaboration exists among the international agents involved, the MOH, and indigenous capacities. Confusion about ownership that results from this lack of coordination threatens local capacity and permits the presence of hidden and conditional agendas linked to the provision of services.

6. *Linkages to economic development and human rights.* The linkage of mental health recovery to human rights and economic development is essential. Mental health services cannot function effectively in a society where human rights violations are common and opportunities for economic development are extremely limited, as evidenced by high rates of unemployment and poverty. Furthermore, the effectiveness of mental health interventions is likely to be undermined in a society characterized by blatant disregard for human rights. At the same time, good mental health is likely to play a key role in reducing hatred and feelings of revenge, fostering the development and promotion of social capital, reconciliation, and the reconstruction of civil society. During the postconflict recovery phase, mental health programs should be provided with consideration for and directly or indirectly linked to development and human rights activities.

To maintain and foster cooperation in these areas, and to ensure that each is taken into critical consideration during the course of program development and implementation, MOH should establish programs with other national ministries, including those of social welfare, labor, and education. These ministries can play a key role in promoting major aspects of the country's mental health activities, including, for example, ensuring activities that will foster economic production and development, such as education and vocational training programs. Monitoring and evaluation mechanisms to determine the impact of mental health on economic and social development should also be established in the initial phase to provide insight into both the determinants and degree of program success.

C. Implementation and Dissemination

The aforementioned action plan will be presented to Ministers of Health and technical advisers of approximately 45 postconflict countries at a meeting scheduled for December 3–4, 2004. At this meeting, an action plan devised on the basis of the previously outlined objectives, with input from these ministries will be presented. This meeting will provide a forum for dialogue on these critical issues, forming the basis for subsequent revision of the proposed action plan. In addition, a *Book of Best Practices* will be provided to meeting participants. This book, a compilation by health and mental health experts from developing and industrialized countries, will provide up-to-date knowledge and information on evidence-based practices within several different contexts.

Ensuring the field-level impact of this endeavor requires follow-up in dissemination and planned cooperation. After the December meeting, a team of experts from industrialized countries including Italy, the United States, and Japan, and mental health practitioners from postconflict and developing countries such as Peru, Uganda, Bosnia, Indonesia, and Rwanda, will be formed to provide on-site technical assistance for countries that foresee the need for such assistance in establishing mental health programs in the postconflict setting. This assistance will be provided in collaboration with MOH and local and international NGOs. In addition, the *Book of Best*

Practices will be widely disseminated and made available on the Internet, as World Bank operations managers, representatives of international agencies including WHO and the United Nations High Commissioner for Refugees, and interested NGOs will be invited to participate in all dissemination and consultation activities.

Project 1 Billion has received significant support from participating MOH from conflict-affected countries, international relief, development and charity organizations, scientific research and policy-based organizations, international policymakers, and scientific scholars. The resulting working partnership based on contextual realities and respect for evidence-based science will signify an international first effort to develop a mental health action plan where national health authorities play a key role in providing sustainable care to those suffering the psychological wounds of mass violence.

XI. CONCLUSION

In recent years, mass violence and acts of terrorism have taken a serious toll in loss of lives and livelihoods, resulting in the extreme traumatization of millions of individuals worldwide. The processes of globalization, the eradication of barriers both political and social, and the increasingly adopted view of health as an essential human right, have brought these issues of health to the fore of public concern and discussion. Medical practitioners, policymakers, and field-level researchers have grown increasingly aware of these outcomes through scientific and social research, and have widely acknowledged the inadequacy of existing international approaches to healing the psychological wounds of war in the postconflict context. Medical practitioners and policymakers within developing and industrialized countries are now urged to go one step further and take specific action to remedy existing flaws and to effect positive change. Project 1 Billion, a historic initiative based on cooperative partnership and scientifically valid treatments that promote healing, is now well poised to provide guidance in the development and provision of mental health services, and hope and the chance for recovery to those who deserve and so desperately need it.

For additional information on Project 1 Billion, see www.hprt-cambridge.org.

APPENDIX: PROJECT 1 BILLION MENTAL HEALTH ACTION PLAN

Project 1 Billion Scientific Committee

1. Mental Health Policy and Legislation

The MOH in postconflict countries are in an ideal situation to take over the responsibility for the design and implementation of a national mental health recovery plan that is culturally effective at the local level. Although the health and well-being of all citizens should be a national state goal, the MOH along with their allied ministries, such as education, labor, economic development, justice, and finance, are properly situated to assess and assure access to mental health care, provide science-based interventions, and provide mental health–related public health information to the general population.

The MOH should also be responsible for the coordination of all mental health activities by local and international NGOs, United Nations agencies, and international donors. MOH can also be responsible for developing and monitoring a simple, scientifically valid and reliable national mental health data system capable of informing national public health policy. This requires that the MOH, as the lead agency in mental health recovery, have a national mental health action plan that can be fully supported and financed by the national government through mental health policy and legislation.

1.1. MOH must work closely with national legislative and political authorities to assure that a mental health policy agenda exists, aimed at national and local postconflict recovery.

1.2. Establish a reasonable timetable (e.g., 5 years) and terms of reference at the onset of the mental health action plan for the legislative next step that will follow the completion of the initial action plan. A national mental health policy or action plan is the first step toward establishing mental health legislation through the country's parliamentary and legislative structures.

1.3. Conduct a national survey, at the beginning of the mental health recovery phase, of national and local resources, including institutions and practitioners capable of delivering a culturally effective mental health response.

1.4. Convene a series of meetings with key stakeholders and relevant experts to define the mental health needs of the general public and the training needs of national and local institutions and practitioners.

1.5. Establish a simple database and data-collection system for monitoring relevant mental health indices for adults and children to establish the mental health status of the general population at any given time and the changes in this status related to the relative effectiveness of mental health policy.

1.6. Guarantee national commitment of funding to assure a basic level of mental health care and prevention.

1.7. Impose requirements that all government health care projects have a mandatory mental health component and that all international programs (e.g., HIV/AIDS; landmines) have a mandatory mental health component.

2. Financing of Mental Health Recovery

Without adequate funding and financial support, no health or mental health action plan can be successful. To date, no major international donor, United Nations agency, or national government has established a clear set of guidelines for obtaining the financial resources for establishing and sustaining culturally effective mental health activities over time. It is the usual case that immediately after the close of a conflict, there is a large influx of international support for health, and sometimes mental health, activities. After this initial buildup of mental health resources, financial support is withdrawn, leading to the collapse of the promising, but embryonic, mental health initiative. Although initial donor support is short lived, mental health problems not only do not subside, but also usually grow in size and effect as the recovery phase encounters expected political and economic problems. At the outset of any international mental health intervention, MOH should decide who is going to pay for mental health services and prevention, and what is the relative percentage of financial support by international donors and the national government to sustain a mental health action plan over time.

2.1. Establish the unit costs for mental health services within the country's indigenous healing system in all relevant settings, such as community-based treatment facilities and hospitals. The indigenous healing system includes primary health care, the traditional healing system (i.e., religious and folk healers), family members, school-based counseling programs, local and international NGOs.

2.2. Define basic or minimum mental health services and determine costs. During the acute phase, international donors need to be asked to support the mental health aspect of the health reform, allocate resources to mental health programs, and develop a financing system to maintain continuing mental health care.

2.3. Decide the mechanisms for long-term financing, including contributions from international donors, the national social fund, patient fees, linkage to private business (e.g., using private enterprise to support mental health services) and voluntary/charitable contributions.

2.4. Establish a sustainable mental health financial plan that centralizes the financial resources of all contributors, including NGOs, that is a reasonable cost (i.e., provides decent minimum standards), and is cost efficient (primarily uses local labor and institutions whenever possible).

2.5. Establish a symbolic minimum payment by users (i.e., patients and clients). Mental health consumers are often the poorest segment of postconflict societies and rarely can make a substantial financial payment to support their mental health care. It is, however, essential that mental health patients/clients feel they are making at minimum a symbolic contribution to the mental health system. This must be done in a culturally appropriate way that does not place additional financial burden on the patient/client, but emphasizes the important value placed on their "support" of their mental health practitioners and institutions.

3. Science-Based Mental Health Services

Recent scientific studies have revealed the high prevalence of serious mental health disorders, such as depression and PTSD, in postconflict societies. Vulnerable groups such as sexually abused survivors, prisoners of war, and those families whose children and family members have disappeared or have been murdered are at particularly high risk for psychological and social problems. The mental health effects of conflict and other forms of extreme violence due to human aggression can be chronic and socially and economically disabling. Mental health problems, if untreated, can also develop into serious health problems, including hypertension, cardiovascular disease, diabetes, and cancer. Therefore, valid and reliable measures of emotional distress and psychosocial disabilities must be integrated into early screening identification and treatment.

Mental health training to build local capacities is necessary in many sectors of society, especially those that have direct contact with mental health problems on a daily basis. Local providers of mental health care in postconflict environments include primary care providers, nurses, schoolteachers and counselors, clergy, law enforcement agents, charity and voluntary agencies, local and international NGOs, traditional healers, and family members.

Emphasis should be on providing state-of-the-art scientifically proven interventions in local community settings with minimum use of stigmatizing institutions such as mental hospitals.

3.1. Support the development of a national set of science-based principles and best practices that are culturally relevant and feasible for all mental health interventions within the local postconflict environment.

3.2. Disseminate these principles and best practices widely at national and local levels. This dissemination should include the training of the *de facto* indigenous healing system: primary care practitioners, traditional healers, family members, school counselors, and local and international NGOs.

3.3. Monitor and evaluate all mental health services including those provided by international NGOs for their cultural competence, effectiveness, efficiency, and ethical standards. This can be achieved by establishing a simple set of evaluation criteria and can be used on a routine basis for monitoring and evaluation.

3.4. Link all specialized mental health services and practitioners to community-based services and the *de facto* mental health system. The few psychiatrists that exist can maximize their impact by providing consultation, liaisons, technical supervision, and training and evaluation support to the *de facto* mental health system. General hospital beds can replace the mental hospital for acute mental health care.

3.5. All international donors and United Nations agencies must allocate resources within their mental health activities for monitoring and evaluating the effectiveness of interventions; research dollars can also be allocated for mental health research in postconflict countries that identify new approaches to recovery.

3.6. Recruit local universities and scientists for mental health training evaluation and research. National universities and scientific centers are usually absent from the mental health action plans.

4. Continuing Mental Health Education

As a mental health capacity is being built in a postconflict society, an essential element of maintaining culturally valid, effective, and cost-efficient services and activities will be the development of a standardized program of continuing mental health education. Ongoing or continuing mental health education must be multidisciplinary and multisectoral to meet the training needs of all practitioners and institutions needed to achieve a successful mental health action plan. National training programs can guarantee recognition of local social and cultural norms and be based on available scientific evidence. National training standards can raise the educational bar for all providers, including national, local, and international agents.

4.1. Call together a national meeting of all key stakeholders from the indigenous healing communities (i.e., primary health care, traditional healing, religious institutions), community-based programs (i.e., schools, police), and international and local NGOs to establish continuing mental health educational goals, content and means of implementation.

4.2. Provide ongoing mental health training programs at three levels:

1. Lay persons including family members and survivors
2. Nondegree training for persons who already hold degrees (e.g., continuing medical education)
3. Specialized master's degree training in the care of survivors of mass violence, health, and mental health.

4.3. Provide opportunities for national and international fellowships (e.g., Fulbright Program) to those experts, scholars, and practitioners working in this area.

4.4. Develop new curricula to be introduced into health professional schools and schools of social work, public health administration, and economic development.

4.5. Provide incentives for ongoing continuing mental health education, including nationally recognized certificates of course completion, academic credit, and financial bonuses to those who have completed a program of continuing mental health education.

4.6. Control ongoing continuing mental health education at all levels for quality, efficacy and long-term impact. After administering testing, the MOH should offer a final certificate indicating that a high standard of knowledge and skills has been achieved.

4.7. Evaluate all training activities by international, national, and local agents for cultural competence, science-based practices, ethics, and cost-effectiveness.

5. Coordination of International Agencies

The coordination of health and mental health activities in postconflict countries is often characterized by anarchy. After an initial input of international agents and resources during the complex emergency phase, the recovery phase can lapse into an overall lack of governance of public health activities. MOH often do not have the human and economic resources or the mandate to develop, organize, and implement a national culturally effective system of mental health care. It is not uncommon for international and national efforts to be uncoordinated, leading to duplication and the development of parallel systems that can undermine the existing *de facto* indigenous healing system and prevent the building up of local capacity. Lack of the most efficient use of limited resources and the implementation of culturally incompetent services and programs is always a threat.

5.1. Identify and organize all international, national and local agencies, donors, and practitioners dealing with the recovery of citizens affected by mass violence into a working group.

5.2. Request international support to train managers capable of designing and implementing a mental health action plan.

5.3. Guarantee and implement fiscally transparent systems of governance for all aspects of the mental health action plan. This includes assuring donors of the proper use of human and financial resources.

5.4. Encourage and organize scientific cooperation at the international, regional, and local levels in all mental health–related areas. This includes international and national exchanges between national and international universities.

6. Mental Health Linkages to Economic Development

The mental health consequences of mass violence are no longer invisible. The Global Burden of Disease (GBD) study was the first major scientific overview to establish the economic and development costs of depression. The GBD of depression across nations was ranked fourth in 1990, preceded only by lower respiratory infection (ranked first), diarrheal diseases (ranked second), and prenatal diseases (ranked third). GBD data anticipate that by 2020 depression will move globally to rank second, and the disease burden caused by war will be ranked seventh.

Although the impact of depression on economic behavior in postconflict societies needs further clarification, high levels of hopelessness and despair, in some cases affecting more than 40% of citizens living in local towns and villages, is having a major negative effect on social and economic development.

In industrialized countries, the impact of mental illness on the labor market, measured in terms of job performance and productivity, has been well established. In the United States, depression is associated with the highest rate of work-related disability. For example, total annual cost in the United States due to depression in 1990 was estimated at USD 43.7 billion, owing to reduced productivity (55%), treatment costs (28%), and suicide-related mortality costs (17%). Those with depression have been found to be 27 times more likely to miss work, with 44% of those with depression reporting having missed at least 1 day of work in 3 months, compared with 2% of the general population. Research on PTSD has indicated that the average amount of days worked for people with PTSD is 3.6 days a month less than nontraumatized co-workers, resulting in an annual loss of USD 3 billion per year, measured in terms of productivity.

These data points to the significant economic costs of mental illness among highly traumatized civilian populations in the following areas:

- Days of work lost (per week)
- Quality of job performance
- Ability to plan for economic activities (e.g., farming)
- Increase in domestic violence
- Increase in high-risk behavior (e.g., HIV/AIDS)
- Increase in diabetes, cardiovascular disease, and stroke
- Premature death among the elderly
- Negative impact on social capital, neighborliness
- Higher suicide rates
- Poor school performance by children and adolescents

It is now urgent that governments in postconflict societies focus policies and programs on the linkages between mental health and economic development, while research is further clarifying this relationship.

6.1. Integrate governmental and nongovernmental activities between the mental health sector and the labor and social welfare sectors. This includes the coordination of all mental health activities with the Ministries of Labor, Education, and Social Welfare.

6.2. Promote, as a major aspect of the government's mental health activities, job production, job training, vocational training, and the development of economic productivity in the formal and informal work sector. Similarly, educational and vocational training must be made available to school-aged children and adolescents.

6.3. Design, implement, and link microenterprise activities to the country's indigenous healing system, including primary health care, traditional and spiritual healers, and international and local NGOs.

6.4. Design, implement, and link school-based programs to the country's indigenous healing system, including primary health care, traditional and spiritual healers, and international and local NGOs.

6.5. Establish indicators to monitor and evaluate the impact of economic and social development on the mental health status of the general population.

7. Mental Health Linkages to Human Rights

Linkage of a mental health framework to human rights is essential. Mental health services cannot function effectively in a society where human rights abuses are common and/or economic development remains poor with high rates of unemployment and poverty. The "chicken or egg" problem is clear in this context, because human rights abuses and poverty contribute to mental disability; similarly, enhanced mental health and well-being among citizens increases social capital, reduces disability, and argues strongly against the toxic social impact of ongoing violence. A mental health framework also contributes to the reduction of hatred and revenge and promotes ethnic reconciliation. Although the first job of a country's mental health system is to focus on the health and emotional well-being of its citizens, an effective system can be an important component of the country's development and promotion of human rights.

7.1. Recognize that poverty and violence are major risk factors producing negative mental health consequences in the general population. Although the health sector cannot "cure" poverty and violence, it can actively intervene at three levels:

1. *Patient/client level.* Provide social resources to aid patients/clients, including food, clothing, shelter, and work and educational opportunities.
2. *Family level.* Promote family resiliency by strengthening family resources and addressing family problems such as domestic violence.
3. *Community level.* Address at a public health level, through the media and other public health campaigns, the reduction of high-risk health behaviors (e.g., alcohol and drug abuse, unsafe promiscuous sex) by promoting family and community social capital and integrating marginal groups (e.g., child soldiers, orphans) into mainstream society.

7.2. Protect all health and mental health practitioners and their patients/clients from violence; guarantee that no health care practitioner or program engages in violence acts, including torture and other forms of human rights violations.

REFERENCES

1. Hurrell A, Woods N. Globalization and inequality. *Millennium J Int Stud* 1995;24:447–470.
2. Universal Declaration of Human Rights (1950). Adopted and proclaimed by General Assembly resolution 217 A (III) of 10 December 1948.
3. Annas GJ. Human rights and health: the Universal Declaration of Human Rights at 50. *N Engl J Med* 1998; 339:1778–1781.
4. World Health Organization. *World health report 2002: reducing risks, promoting healthy life.* Geneva: WHO, 2002.
5. Mabey D, Peelin RW, Ustianowsk A, et al. Tropical infectious diseases: diagnostics for the developing world. *Nat Rev Microbiol* 2004;2:231–240.
6. United Nations Development Programme. Human development report. New York: UNDP, 2003. Available at: http://hdr.undp.org/reports/global/2003. Accessed July 7, 2004.
7. United Nations Development Programme. Human development index reveals development crisis. New York: UNDP, 2003. Available at: http://www.undp.org/hdr2003/pdf/presskit/HDR03_PR4E.pdf. Accessed June 8, 2004.
8. Brogan P. *World conflicts.* 3rd ed. London: Bloomsbury, 1998.
9. World Bank. *Conflict, peace-building and development cooperation: the World Bank agenda.* Washington, DC: World Bank, 2002.
10. Sollenberg M, Wallensteen P. Patterns of major armed conflicts, 1990–2000. Appendix 1A to Seybolt TB. Major armed conflicts. In: Stockholm International Peace Research Institute. *SIPRI yearbook 2001: armaments, disarmament and international security.* Oxford: Oxford University Press, 2001. Available at: http://projects.sipri.se/conflictstudy/2001MACapp1a.pdf. Accessed July 7, 2004.
11. Carnegie Commission on Preventing Deadly Conflict. Preventing deadly conflict: final report with executive summary. Chapter 1: against complacency. Carnegie Corporation of New York. Available at: http://wwics.si.edu/subsites/ccpdc/pubs/rept97/text/1.htm. Accessed July 7, 2004.
12. US Committee for Refugees. *Country report: Sudan.* Washington, DC: USCR, 2002.
13. International Rescue Committee. Mortality in the Democratic Republic of the Congo: results from a nationwide survey [conducted September to November, 2003]. Available at: http://intranet.theirc.-org/docs/drc_mortality_iii_full.pdf. Accessed June 6, 2004.
14. US Committee for Refugees. World refugee survey. Washington, DC: USCR, 2000.
15. Human Rights Watch. Refugees. Available at: http://www.hrw.org/doc/?t=refugees&document_limit=0,2. Accessed June 14, 2003.
16. UNHCR in the UK: Public information: information and briefings: asylum issues. Available at: http://www.unhcr.org.uk/info/briefings/asylum_issues/. Accessed June 14, 2003.
17. Fox SH, Tang SS. The Sierra Leonean refugee experience: traumatic events and psychiatric sequelae. *J Nerv Ment Dis* 2000;188:490–495.
18. Weine SM, Becker DF, McGlashan TH, et al. Psychiatric consequences of "ethnic cleansing": clinical assessments and trauma testimonies of newly resettled Bosnian refugees. *Am J Psychiatry* 1995;152:536–542.
19. Mollica RF, Wyshak G, Lavelle J. The psychosocial impact of war trauma and torture on Southeast Asian refugees. *Am J Psychiatry* 1987;144:1567–1572.
20. Favaro A, Maiorani M, Colombo G, et al. Traumatic experiences, posttraumatic stress disorder, and dissociative symptoms in a group of refugees from former Yugoslavia. *J Nerv Ment Dis* 1999; 187:306–308.
21. Friedman MJ, Jaranson J. The applicability of the post-traumatic stress disorder concept to refugees. In: Marsella AJ, Bornemann T, Elkblad S, et al., eds. *Amidst peril and pain.* Washington, DC: American Psychological Association, 1994:207–228.
22. US Committee for Refugees. *World refugee survey 2004—warehousing issue.* Washington, DC: USCR, 2004.
23. Amowitz LL, Reis C, Lyons KH, et al. Prevalence of war-related sexual violence and other human rights abuses among internally displaced persons in Sierra Leone. *JAMA* 2002;287:513–521.

24. United Nations Children's Fund. State of the world's children: 1996. Available at: http://www.unicef.org/sowc96/. Accessed June 9, 2004.
25. Barlett S, Hart R, Satterthwaite D, et al. Cities for children: children's rights, poverty and urban management. London: Earthscan Publications, 1999:214.
26. Coalition to Stop the Use of Child Soldiers. *Child soldiers use 2003: a briefing on the 4th UN Security Council open debate on children and armed conflict.* London: Coalition to Stop the Use of Child Soldiers, 2004.
27. Derluyn I, Broekaert E, Schuyten G, et al. Post-traumatic stress in former Uganda child soldiers. *Lancet* 2004;363:861–863.
28. Human Rights Watch. Abducted and abused: renewed conflict in northern Uganda. *Human Rights Watch* 2003 July:15(12).
29. Deaths in World Trade Center terrorist attacks—New York City, 2001. *MMWR Morb Mortal Wkly Rep* 2002;51:16–18. Available at: http://www.cdc.gov/mmwr/preview/mmwrhtml/mm51SPa6.htm.
30. Massacre at Atocha: nearly 200 reported dead as toll mounts in Madrid bomb outrage. *Time* March 11, 2004. Available at: http://www.time.com/time/europe/eu/article/0,13716,599760,00.html. Accessed June 14, 2003.
31. Swahn MH, Mahendra RR, Paulozzi LJ, et al. Violent attacks on Middle Easterners in the United States during the month following the September 11, 2001 terrorist attacks. *Inj Prev* 2003;9: 187–189.
32. Centers for Disease Control and Prevention. Injuries and illnesses among New York City Fire Department rescue workers after responding to the World Trade Center attacks. *JAMA* 2002;288: 1581–1584.
33. Human Rights Watch. Human Rights Watch Afghanistan: new civilian deaths due to US bombing. October 29, 2001. New York: Human Rights Watch. Available at: http://www.hrw.org/press/2001/10/afghan1030.htm. Accessed June 14, 2003.
34. Human Rights Watch. Off target: the conduct of the war and civilian casualties in Iraq. New York: Human Rights Watch, 2003.
35. Mollica RF, Donelan K, Tor S, et al. The effect of trauma and confinement on functional health and mental health status of Cambodians living in Thai-Cambodia border camps. *JAMA* 1993;270: 581–586.
36. De Jong JP, Scholte WF, Koeter MWJ, et al. The prevalence of mental health problems in Rwandan and Burundese refugee camps. *Acta Psychiatr Scand* 2000;102:171–177.
37. Lopes Cardozo B, Talley L, Burton A, et al. Karenni refugees living in Thai-Burmese border camps: traumatic experiences, mental health outcomes and social functioning. *Soc Sci Med* 2004; 58:2637–2644.
38. Lopes Cardozo B, Vergara A, Agani F, et al. Mental health, social functioning, and attitudes of Kosovar Albanians following the war in Kosovo. *JAMA* 2000;284:569–577.
39. De Jong JTVM, Komproe IH, Van Ommeren M, et al. Lifetime events and posttraumatic stress disorder in 4 post conflict settings. *JAMA* 2001;286:555–562.
40. Bramsen I, van der Ploeg HM. Fifty years later: the long-term psychological adjustment of ageing World War II survivors. *Acta Psychiatr Scand* 1999;100:350–358.
41. Yehuda R, Schmeidler J, Wainberg M, et al. Vulnerability to posttraumatic stress disorder in adult offspring of Holocaust survivors. *Am J Psychiatry* 1998;155:1163–1171.
42. Mollica RF, Lopes Cardozo B, Osofsky HJ, et al. Scientific overview of the role of mental health in complex emergencies. *Lancet* 2004 *(in press).*
43. Rosner R, Powell S, Butollo W. Posttraumatic stress disorder three years after the siege of Sarajevo. *J Clin Psychol* 2003;59:41–55.
44. Yehuda R, Schmeidler J, Giller EL, et al. Relationship between posttraumatic stress disorder characteristics of Holocaust survivors and their adult offspring. *Am J Psychiatry* 1998;155:841–843
45. Mollica RF, McInnes K, Sarajlić N, et al. Disability associated with psychiatric comorbidity and health status in Bosnian refugees living in Croatia. *JAMA* 1999;282:433–439.
46. Mollica RF, Sarajlic N, Chernoff M, et al. Longitudinal study of psychiatric symptoms, disability, mortality and emigration among Bosnian refugees. *JAMA* 2001;286:546–554.
47. Paardekooper B, de Jong JTVM, Hermanns JMA. The psychological impact of war and the refugee situation on South Sudanese children in refugee camps in northern Uganda: an exploratory study. *J Child Psychol Psychiatry* 1999;40:529–536.
48. Hjern A, Angel B, Hofer B. Persecution and behavior: a report of refugee children from Chile. *Child Abuse Neglect* 1991;15:239–248.

49. Aziz A, Thabet M, Vostanis P. Post-traumatic stress reactions in children of war. *J Child Psychol Psychiatry* 1999;40:385–391.
50. Thabet AA, Abed Y, Vostanis P. Comorbidity of PTSD and depression among refugee children during war conflict. *J Child Psychol Psychiatry* 2004;45:533–542.
51. Nader K, Pynoos R, Fairbanks L, et al. A preliminary study of PTSD and grief among the children of Kuwait following the Gulf crisis. *Br J Clin Psychol* 1993;32:407–416.
52. Galea S, Ahern J, Resnick H, et al. Psychological sequelae of the September 11 terrorist attacks in New York City. *N Engl J Med* 2002;346:982–987.
53. Schuster MA, Stein BD, Jaycox L, et al. A national survey of stress reactions after the September 11, 2001, terrorist attacks. *N Engl J Med* 2001;345:1507–1512.
54. Ahern J, Galea S, Resnick H, et al. Television images and psychological symptoms after the September 11 terrorist attacks. *Psychiatry* 2002;65:289–300.
55. Bleich A, Gelkopf M, Solomon Z. Exposure to terrorism, stress-related mental health symptoms, and coping behaviors among a nationally representative sample in Israel. *JAMA* 2003;290:612–620.
56. Pfefferbaum B, North CS, Flynn BW, et al. The emotional impact of injury following an international terrorist incident. *Public Health Rev* 2001;29:271–280.
57. Pfefferbaum B, Pfefferbaum RL, Gurwitch RH, et al. Children's response to terrorism: a critical review of the literature. *Curr Psychiatry Rep* 2003;5:95–100.
58. Kawana N, Ishimatsu S, Kanda K. Psycho-physiological effects of the terrorist sarin attack on the Tokyo subway system. *Mil Med* 2001;166(12 Suppl):23–26.
59. World Health Organization. Mental health: responding to the call for action. Report by the Secretariat. Fifty-fifth World Health Assembly, provision agenda item 13.13, A55/18, April 11, 2002. Geneva: WHO. Available at: http://www.who.int/gb/ebwha/pdf_files/WHA55/ea5518.pdf. Accessed June 14, 2003.
60. Murray CJL, Lopez AD, eds. *The global burden of disease: a comprehensive assessment of mortality and disability from diseases, injuries, and risk factors in 1990 and projected to 2020.* Cambridge, MA: Harvard University Press, 1996.
61. Mollica RF. Invisible wounds: waging a new kind of war. *Sci Am* 2000;282:54–57.
62. Baingana, F. The World Bank. Mental health and conflict. Social development notes. conflict prevention and reconstruction. No. 13. October 2003. Available at: http://lnweb18.worldbank.org/ESSD/sdvext.nsf/67ByDocName/MentalHealthandConflictCPRNote13/$FILE/CPR13legal.pdf. Accessed June 16, 2004.
63. Gelder G, Lopez-Ibor JJ, Andreasen N. *New Oxford textbook of psychiatry.* Oxford: Oxford University Press, 2001.
64. World Health Organization/United Nations High Commissioner for Refugees. *Mental health of refugees.* Geneva: WHO, 1996.
65. Jones L. On a front line. *BMJ* 1995;310:1052.
66. Loga S, Ceric I, Stojak R, et al. Psychosocial research during the war in Sarajevo. *Med Arch* 1999; 53:139–144.
67. Rost K, Nutting P, Smith JL, et al. Managing depression as a chronic disease: a randomised trial of ongoing treatment in primary care. *BMJ* 2002;325:934.
68. Geddes J, Butler R. *Clinical evidence: mental health. Depressive disorders.* London: BMJ Publishing Group, 2002:74–89.
69. Mollica RF, Tor S, Lavelle J. *Pathway to healing.* Cambridge: Harvard Program in Refugee Trauma, 1998.
70. Hiegel JP. Use of indigenous concepts and healers in the care of refugees: some experiences from the Thai border camps. In: Marcella AJ, ed. *Amidst peril and pain: the mental health and well-being of the world's refugees.* Washington, DC: American Psychological Association, 1994.
71. Lavelle J, Tor S, Mollica RF, et al., eds. *Harvard guide to Khmer mental health.* Cambridge, MA: Harvard Program in Refugee Trauma, 1996.
72. Dybdahl R. Children and mothers in war: an outcome study of a psychosocial intervention program. *Child Dev* 2001;72:1214–1230.
73. Evaluation and Policy Analysis Unit and Health and Community Development Section, United Nations High Commissioner for Refugees. *Learning for a future: refugee education in developing countries.* Geneva: United Nations High Commissioner for Refugees, 2002.
74. UNESCO. Education in situations of emergency and crisis: challenges for the new century. Thematic studies. World Education Forum: Education for All 2000 Assessment. Dakar, Senegal April 26–28,

2000. France: UNESCO, 2001. Available at: http://unesdoc.unesco.org/images/0012/001234/123484e.pdf. Accessed July 8, 2003.
75. Agger I, Mimica J. *Psychosocial assistance to victims of war in Bosnia-Herzegovina and Croatia: an evaluation.* Brussels: ECHO, 1996.
76. Henderson DC, Mollica RF, Tor S, et al. Building primary care practitioners' confidence in mental health skills in a post-conflict society: a Cambodian example. *J Nerv Ment Dis* 2004 *(in press).*
77. World Health Organization. Mental health disorders in primary care. Geneva: WHO, 1998.
78. World Health Organization. *World health report 2001: mental health: new understanding, new hope.* Geneva: WHO, 2001.
79. Kleinman A. *Rethinking psychiatry: from cultural category to personal experience.* New York: The Free Press, 1988.
80. Bolton P, Ndogoni L. *Cross-cultural assessment of trauma-related mental illness (Phase II). A report of research conducted by World Vision Uganda and The Johns Hopkins University.* Baltimore: Johns Hopkins University, 2000.
81. Bisson J. *Clinical evidence: mental health. PTSD.* London: BMJ Publishing Group, 2002:120–126.
82. Bolton P, Bass J, Neugebauer R, et al. Group interpersonal psychotherapy for depression in rural Uganda: a randomized controlled trial. *JAMA* 2003;289:3117–3124.
83. Bryant RA, Harvey AG, Dang ST, et al. Treatment of acute stress disorder: a comparison of cognitive-behavioral therapy and supportive counselling. *J Consult Clin Psychol* 1998;66:862–866.
84. Bryant RA, Sackville T, Dang ST, et al. Treating acute stress disorder: an evaluation of cognitive-behaviour therapy and supportive counselling techniques. *Am J Psychiatry* 1999;156:1780–1786.
85. Weissman M, Markowitz J, Klerman G. *Comprehensive guide to interpersonal psychotherapy.* New York: Basic Books, 2000.
86. Rosen GM. Treatment fidelity and research on eye movement desensitization and reprocessing (EMDR). *J Anxiety Disord* 1999;13:173–184.
87. Acierno R, Hersen M, Van Hasselt VB, et al. Review of the validation and dissemination of eye-movement desensitization and reprocessing: a scientific and ethical dilemma. *Clin Psychol Rev* 1994;14:287–298.
88. Oswalt R, Anderson M, Hagstrom K, et al. Evaluation of the one-session eye-movement desensitization reprocessing procedure for eliminating traumatic memories. *Psychol Rep* 1993;73:99–104.
89. Welch KL, Beere DB. Eye movement desensitization and reprocessing: a treatment efficacy model. *Clin Psychol Psychother* 2002;9:165–176.
90. Oras R, Ezpeleta SC, Ahmad A. Treatment of traumatized refugee children with eye movement desensitization and reprocessing in a psychodynamic context. *Nord J Psychiatry* 2004;58:199–203.
91. Raphael B, Wilson JP, eds. *Psychological debriefing: theory, practice, and evidence.* New York: Cambridge University Press, 2000.
92. Foa E, Keane TM, Friedman MJ. Guidelines for treatment of PTSD. *J Traum Stress* 2000;13:4: 539–588.
93. Kessler RC, House JS, Turner JB. Unemployment and health in a community sample. *J Health Soc Behav* 1987;28:51–59.
94. Patel V. Poverty, inequality, and mental health in developing countries. In: Leon D, Walt G, eds. *Poverty, inequality and health: an international perspective.* Oxford, Oxford University Press, 2001: 247–261.
95. Saraceno B, Barbui C. Poverty and mental illness. *Can J Psychiatry* 1997;42:285–290.
96. Bloom D, Canning D, Jamison D. Good health increases wealth; more development aid needs to be directed towards health sectors. Washington, DC: Development Committee, World Bank and IMF, 2004.
97. Kapetanovic A. The prevalence of mental health disorders in primary health care. Unpublished data, 2002.
98. Geballe S. *The economic costs of mental illness and benefits of treatment.* New Haven: CT Voices for Children, 2001.
99. Kessler RC. Posttraumatic stress disorder: the burden to the individual and to society. *J Clin Psychiatry* 2000;61:4–12.
100. Walker EA, Katon W, Russo J, et al. Health care costs associated with posttraumatic stress disorder symptoms in women. *Arch Gen Psychiatry* 2003;60:369–374.
101. Mollica RF, Cui X, McInnes K, et al. Science-based policy for psychosocial interventions in refugee camps: a Cambodian example. *J Nerv Ment Dis* 2002;190:158–166.

102. World Bank. Social capital for development. Available at: http://www1.worldbank.org. Accessed September 13, 2004.
103. National Economic and Social Forum (NESF). The Policy Implications of Social Capital. Forum Report No. 28. Dublin, Ireland: National Economic and Social Forum, 2003.
104. Coletta NJ, Cullen ML. *Violent conflict and the transformation of social capital: lessons from Cambodia, Rwanda, Guatemala and Somalia.* Washington, DC: The World Bank, 2000.
105. Human Rights Watch. A dark and closed place: past & present human rights abuses in Foca. *Human Rights Watch* 1998 July;10(6). Available at: http://www.hrw.org/reports98/foca/. Accessed June 16, 2004.
106. Amnesty International. Report 2004. Bosnia and Herzegovina (summary). Available at: http://web.-amnesty.org/report2004/bih-summary-eng. Accessed June 16, 2004.
107. Boraine A, van Zyl P. Moving on requires looking back. Searching for the truth. Special English ed. Available at: http://www.dccam.org/Magazine/Special%20Issue%203/page_53.pdf. Accessed June 14, 2003 Phnom Penh: Documentation Center of Cambodia, 2003.
108. World Bank. *Annual report 1997.* Washington, DC: The World Bank, 1997.
109. Summerfield D. A critique of seven assumptions behind psychological trauma programmes in war-affected areas. *Soc Sci Med* 1999;48:1449–1462.
110. Mollica RF. Developing effective mental health policies and services for traumatized refugee patients. In: Koslow DR, Salett EP, eds. *Crossing cultures in mental health.* Washington, DC: Sietar International, 1989:101–115.
111. Gessler MC, Msuya DE, Nkunya MHH, et al. Traditional healers in Tanzania: sociocultural profile and three short portraits. *J Ethnopharmacol* 1995;48:145–160.
112. Mollica RF, McDonald L. Project 1 billion. Health Ministers of Post-conflict Nations Act on Mental Health Recovery. *UN Chronicle* 2003;4.
113. Fulbright New Century Scholars Program. Mental health 21: mental health policy and the recovery of conflict/post-conflict societies. September 23–24, 2002, Sarajevo, Bosnia-Herzegovina.
114. The Sphere Project. *Humanitarian charter and minimum standards in disaster response.* Oxford: Oxfam Publishing, 2000.

Subject Index